METHODS IN MOLECULAR BIOLOGY™

Series Editor
**John M. Walker
School of Life Sciences
University of Hertfordshire
Hatfield, Hertfordshire, AL10 9AB, UK**

For other titles published in this series, go to
www.springer.com/series/7651

Cancer Nanotechnology

Methods and Protocols

Edited by

Stephen R. Grobmyer and Brij M. Moudgil

University of Florida, Gainesville, FL, USA

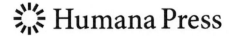

Editors
Stephen R. Grobmyer
Division of Surgical Oncology
Department of Surgery
University of Florida
PO Box 100286
Gainesville FL 32610
USA
stephen.grobmyer@surgery.ufl.edu

Brij M. Moudgil
Department of Materials
 Science and Engineering
Particle Engineering Research
 Center
University of Florida
P.O.Box 116005
Gainesville FL 32611
USA
bmoudgil@perc.ufl.edu

ISSN 1064-3745   e-ISSN 1940-6029
ISBN 978-1-60761-608-5   e-ISBN 978-1-60761-609-2
DOI 10.1007/978-1-60761-609-2
Springer New York Dordrecht Heidelberg London

Library of Congress Control Number: 2010920087

© Springer Science+Business Media, LLC 2010
All rights reserved. This work may not be translated or copied in whole or in part without the written permission of the publisher (Humana Press, c/o Springer Science+Business Media, LLC, 233 Spring Street, New York, NY 10013, USA), except for brief excerpts in connection with reviews or scholarly analysis. Use in connection with any form of information storage and retrieval, electronic adaptation, computer software, or by similar or dissimilar methodology now known or hereafter developed is forbidden.
The use in this publication of trade names, trademarks, service marks, and similar terms, even if they are not identified as such, is not to be taken as an expression of opinion as to whether or not they are subject to proprietary rights.
While the advice and information in this book are believed to be true and accurate at the date of going to press, neither the authors nor the editors nor the publisher can accept any legal responsibility for any errors or omissions that may be made. The publisher makes no warranty, express or implied, with respect to the material contained herein.

Cover illustration: Digitally modified transmission electron micrograph of ca. 50 nm multifunctional gold speckled silica (GSS) nanoparticle. Synthesized using microemulsions, GSS nanoparticles can be engineered and utilized as the mediators of cancer theranostics (Chapter 5).

Printed on acid-free paper

Humana Press is part of Springer Science+Business Media (www.springer.com)

Preface

Cancer nanotechnology is a rapidly emerging field which holds great promise for revolutionizing cancer detection, diagnosis, treatment, and cure. Furthermore, cancer nanotechnology holds the potential to ultimately improve access to cancer care worldwide.

Early detection of cancer at the cellular level, even before anatomic anomalies are visible, is critical to more efficacious and cost-effective diagnosis and therapeutic advances. Non-invasive techniques are required that are capable of reliably imaging at the molecular scale – 100–1,000 cells as opposed to the current techniques that require more than a million cells for accurate clinical diagnosis.

In developing clinically viable cancer therapeutic protocols, targeted and localized delivery of the drugs are the key challenges. In other words, the goal is to target the delivery of the anticancer drugs to selectively attack the cancer cells, with minimal toxicity of the healthy tissue and other undesirable side effects. Current protocols of systemic application of anticancer drugs greatly limit the maximal allowable dose of the drug in order to minimize severe side effects, yet the application of a higher dosage of anticancer drugs is necessary to overcome rapid elimination and non-specific distribution of the anticancer drugs into organs and tissues. This practice often leads to severe side effects including unintended damage to healthy tissue and organs.

Most cancer nanotechnology advances are primarily focused on developing Nano-engineered materials that can significantly impact non-invasive molecular scale imaging techniques and targeted delivery of drugs. Further, multifunctional nanostructures are being developed that can simultaneously serve as contrast agents for enhanced imaging and nano-vectors for targeted drug delivery or therapies. However, it is critical to identify/synthesize specific biomarkers, which, when conjugated to nanostructures, will target them only to specific tumor sites.

The achievement of the goals of nanotechnology-mediated early cancer detection and more efficacious therapies requires synergistic integration and convergence of a variety of disciplines. These include cancer biology, materials science and engineering, biomedical engineering, toxicology, computer science and engineering, chemistry, physics, and mathematics. The chapters in this book describe the most recent, cutting-edge, "how-to" approaches developed/employed by researchers in a variety of disciplines to identify cancer-specific biomarkers, construct suitable multifunctional targeted nanostructure platforms, and their enhanced imaging and therapeutic applications.

Our interest in and energy for completing this project is derived from the excitement generated by our interdisciplinary collaborations in cancer nanotechnology at the University of Florida. It is our hope that the information provided in this compendium will likewise excite and encourage others to engage in such similar interdisciplinary collaborative efforts that will yield new knowledge, for it is these types of collaborations that are essential for translating cancer nanotechnology into a clinical reality for those suffering from these devastating diseases.

We trust that both the established and those embarking on their maiden research voyage in the field of cancer nanotechnology will find this treatise valuable.

We are grateful to our distinguished group of international contributors who have made this project truly unique and relevant. Further, we thank the tireless efforts of outstanding colleagues including Drs. Sharma, Brown, and Iwakuma, who have helped make this work possible. We acknowledge the support of the Particle Engineering Research Center (PERC) and the Department of Surgery, University of Florida, and the following organizations: National Science Foundation, National Institute of Health, James Esther King Biomedical Research Program-Florida Department of Health, Bankhead Cooley Research Program-Florida Department of Health, and The Pat Adams Cancer Nanotechnology Research Fund. We thank our families for their patience and understanding of the time commitments necessary to conduct this and other important related work toward the cure of cancer. Finally, we thank the editing and production staff at Humana Press for their valued assistance.

Gainesville, FL *Stephen R. Grobmyer*
July 2009 *Brij M. Moudgil*

Contents

Preface . . . . *v*

Contributors . . . . *ix*

1. What Is Cancer Nanotechnology? 1
   Stephen R. Grobmyer, Nobutaka Iwakuma, Parvesh Sharma, and Brij M. Moudgil

2. Molecular-Targeted Therapy for Cancer and Nanotechnology 11
   Steven N. Hochwald

3. Enhanced Permeability and Retention (EPR) Effect for Anticancer Nanomedicine Drug Targeting 25
   Khaled Greish

4. Nanoparticle Characterization for Cancer Nanotechnology and Other Biological Applications 39
   Scott C. Brown, Maria Palazuelos, Parvesh Sharma, Kevin W. Powers, Stephen M. Roberts, Stephen R. Grobmyer, and Brij M. Moudgil

5. Multimodal Nanoparticulate Bioimaging Contrast Agents 67
   Parvesh Sharma, Amit Singh, Scott C. Brown, Niclas Bengtsson, Glenn A. Walter, Stephen R. Grobmyer, Nobutaka Iwakuma, Swadeshmukul Santra, Edward W. Scott, and Brij M. Moudgil

6. Gold Nanocages for Cancer Imaging and Therapy 83
   Leslie Au, Jingyi Chen, Lihong V. Wang, and Younan Xia

7. Nanoshells for Photothermal Cancer Therapy 101
   Jennifer G. Morton, Emily S. Day, Naomi J. Halas, and Jennifer L. West

8. Gold Nanorods: Multifunctional Agents for Cancer Imaging and Therapy 119
   Alexander Wei, Alexei P. Leonov, and Qingshan Wei

9. Polymeric Micelles: Polyethylene Glycol-Phosphatidylethanolamine (PEG-PE)-Based Micelles as an Example 131
   Rupa R. Sawant and Vladimir P. Torchilin

10. Fluorescent Silica Nanoparticles for Cancer Imaging 151
    Swadeshmukul Santra

11. Polymeric Nanoparticles for Drug Delivery 163
    Juliana M. Chan, Pedro M. Valencia, Liangfang Zhang, Robert Langer, and Omid C. Farokhzad

12. Synthesis, Characterization, and Functionalization of Gold Nanoparticles for Cancer Imaging 177
    Gary A. Craig, Peter J. Allen, and Michael D. Mason

13. Identification of Pancreatic Cancer-Specific Cell-Surface Markers for Development of Targeting Ligands 195
    David L. Morse, Galen Hostetter, Yoganand Balagurunathan, Robert J. Gillies, and Haiyong Han

14. Preparation and Characterization of Doxorubicin Liposomes 211
    Guoqin Niu, Brian Cogburn, and Jeffrey Hughes

15. PEGylated Nanocarriers for Systemic Delivery 221
    N.K. Jain and Manoj Nahar

16. Nanoparticle–Aptamer Conjugates for Cancer Cell Targeting and Detection . . . 235
    M. Carmen Estévez, Yu-Fen Huang, Huaizhi Kang, Meghan B. O'Donoghue, Suwussa Bamrungsap, Jilin Yan, Xiaolan Chen, and Weihong Tan

17. Targeting of Nanoparticles: Folate Receptor 249
    Sumith A. Kularatne and Philip S. Low

18. Magnetic Aerosol Targeting of Nanoparticles to Cancer: Nanomagnetosols 267
    Carsten Rudolph, Bernhard Gleich, and Andreas W. Flemmer

19. LHRH-Targeted Nanoparticles for Cancer Therapeutics 281
    Tamara Minko, Mahesh L. Patil, Min Zhang, Jayant J. Khandare, Maha Saad, Pooja Chandna, and Oleh Taratula

20. Antibody Targeting of Nanoparticles to Tumor-Specific Receptors: Immunoliposomes 295
    Miriam Rothdiener, Julia Beuttler, Sylvia K.E. Messerschmidt, and Roland E. Kontermann

21. Photoacoustic Tomography for Imaging Nanoparticles 309
    Zhen Yuan and Huabei Jiang

22. Current Applications of Nanotechnology for Magnetic Resonance Imaging of Apoptosis 325
    Gustav J. Strijkers, Geralda A.F. van Tilborg, Tessa Geelen, Chris P.M. Reutelingsperger, and Klaas Nicolay

23. Applications of Gold Nanorods for Cancer Imaging and Photothermal Therapy . . 343
    Xiaohua Huang, Ivan H. El-Sayed, and Mostafa A. El-Sayed

24. Use of Nanoparticles for Targeted, Noninvasive Thermal Destruction of Malignant Cells 359
    Paul Cherukuri and Steven A. Curley

25. Colloidal Gold: A Novel Nanoparticle for Targeted Cancer Therapeutics 375
    Anathea C. Powell, Giulio F. Paciotti, and Steven K. Libutti

26. Liposomal Doxorubicin and *nab*-Paclitaxel: Nanoparticle Cancer Chemotherapy in Current Clinical Use 385
    Alexander Gaitanis and Stephen Staal

Subject Index 393

Contributors

PETER J. ALLEN • *Department of Surgery, Memorial Sloan-Kettering Cancer Center, New York, USA*

LESLIE AU • *Department of Biomedical Engineering, Washington University, St. Louis, MO, USA*

YOGANAND BALAGURUNATHAN • *Computational Biology Division, Translational Genomics Research Institute, Phoenix, AZ, USA*

SUWUSSA BAMRUNGSAP • *Department of Chemistry and Department of Physiology and Functional Genomics, Shands Cancer Center and UF Genetics Institute, and McKnight Brain Institute, Center for Research at the Bio/Nano Interface, University of Florida, Gainesville, FL, USA*

NICLAS BENGTSSON • *Department of Molecular Genetics and microbiology, University of Florida, Gainesville, FL, USA*

JULIA BEUTTLER • *Institute of Cell Biology and Immunology, University of Stuttgart, Stuttgart, Germany*

SCOTT C. BROWN • *Department of Materials Science and Engineering, Particle Engineering Research Center, University of Florida, Gainesville, FL, USA*

JULIANA M. CHAN • *Department of Biology, Massachusetts Institute of Technology, Cambridge, MA, USA*

POOJA CHANDNA • *Department of Pharmaceutics, Rutgers, The State University of New Jersey, Piscataway, NJ, USA*

JINGYI CHEN • *Department of Biomedical Engineering, Washington University, St. Louis, MO, USA*

XIAOLAN CHEN • *Department of Chemistry and Department of Physiology and Functional Genomics, Shands Cancer Center and UF Genetics Institute, and McKnight Brain Institute, Center for Research at the Bio/Nano Interface, University of Florida, Gainesville, FL, USA*

PAUL CHERUKURI • *Department of Surgical Oncology and Experimental Therapeutics, University of Texas M. D. Anderson Cancer Center; Department of Chemistry, Smalley Institute for Nanoscale Science and Technology, Rice University, Houston, TX, USA*

BRIAN COGBURN • *Department of Pharmaceutics, University of Florida, Gainesville, FL, USA*

GARY A. CRAIG • *Department of Chemical and Biological Engineering, University of Maine, Orono, ME, USA*

STEVEN A. CURLEY • *Department of Surgical Oncology, University of Texas M. D. Anderson Cancer Center; Mechanical Engineering and Material Science, Rice University, Houston, TX, USA*

EMILY S. DAY • *Rice University, Houston, TX, USA*

IVAN H. EL-SAYED • *Department of Otolaryngology-Head and Neck Surgery, Comprehensive Cancer Center, University of California at San Francisco, San Francisco, CA, USA*

MOSTAFA A. EL-SAYED • *Laser Dynamics Laboratory, School of Chemistry and Biochemistry, Georgia Institute of Technology, Atlanta, GA, USA*

N. CARMEN ESTÉVEZ • *Department of Chemistry and Department of Physiology and Functional Genomics, Shands Cancer Center and UF Genetics Institute, and McKnight Brain Institute, Center for Research at the Bio/Nano Interface, University of Florida, Gainesville, FL, USA*

OMID C. FAROKHZAD • *Laboratory of Nanomedicine and Biomaterials, Department of Anesthesiology, Brigham Women's Hospital, Harvard Medical School, Boston, MA, USA*

ANDREAS W. FLEMMER • *Division of Neonatology, University Children's Hospital and Perinatal Center Grosshadern, Ludwig-Maximilian University, Munich, Germany*

ALEXANDER GAITANIS • *Division of Hematology and Oncology, Department of Medicine, University of Florida, Gainesville, FL, USA*

TESSA GEELEN • *Biomedical NMR, Department of Biomedical Engineering, Eindhoven University of Technology, Eindhoven, The Netherlands*

ROBERT J. GILLIES • *Department of Radiology, H. Lee Moffitt Cancer Center & Research Institute, Tampa, FL, USA*

BERNHARD GLEICH • *Zentralinstitut für Medizintechnik, Technische Universität München, Garching, Germany*

KHALED GREISH • *Department of Pharmaceuticals and Pharmaceutical Chemistry, and Utah Center for Nanomedicine, University of Utah, Salt Lake City, UT, USA*

STEPHEN R. GROBMYER • *Division of Surgical Oncology, Department of Surgery, University of Florida, Gainesville, FL, USA*

NAOMI J. HALAS • *Rice University, Houston, TX, USA*

HAIYONG HAN • *Clinical Cancer Research Division, Translational Genomics Research Institute, Phoenix, AZ, USA*

STEVEN N. HOCHWALD • *Department of Surgery, University of Florida, Gainesville, FL, USA*

GALEN HOSTETTER • *Translational Genomics Research Institute, Tissue Microarray Center, Phoenix, AZ, USA*

XIAOHUA HUANG • *Laser Dynamics Laboratory, School of Chemistry and Biochemistry, Georgia Institute of Technology, Atlanta, GA, USA*

YU-FEN HUANG • *Department of Chemistry and Department of Physiology and Functional Genomics, Shands Cancer Center and UF Genetics Institute, and McKnight Brain Institute, Center for Research at the Bio/Nano Interface, University of Florida, Gainesville, FL, USA*

JEFFREY HUGHES • *Department of Pharmaceutics, University of Florida, Gainesville, FL, USA*

NOBUTAKA IWAKUMA • *Division of Surgical Oncology, Department of Surgery, University of Florida, Gainesville, FL, USA*

N.K. JAIN • *Department of Pharmaceutical Sciences, Dr. H.S. Gour University, Sagar, India*

HUABEI JIANG • *Department of Biomedical Engineering, University of Florida, Gainesville, FL, USA*

HUAIZHI KANG • *Department of Chemistry and Department of Physiology and Functional Genomics, Shands Cancer Center and UF Genetics Institute, and McKnight Brain Institute, Center for Research at the Bio/Nano Interface, University of Florida, Gainesville, FL, USA*

JAYANT J. KHANDARE • *Department of Pharmaceutics, Rutgers, The State University of New Jersey, Piscataway, NJ, USA*

ROLAND E. KONTERMANN • *Institute of Cell Biology and Immunology, University of Stuttgart, Stuttgart, Germany*

SUMITH A. KULARATNE • *Department of Chemistry and Purdue Cancer Center, Purdue University, West Lafayette, IN, USA*

ROBERT LANGER • *Department of Chemical Engineering and Division of Health Science and Technology, Massachusetts Institute of Technology, Cambridge, MA, USA*

ALEXEI P. LEONOV • *Department of Chemistry, Purdue University, West Lafayette, IN, USA*

STEVEN K. LIBUTTI • *Tumor Angiogenesis Section, Surgery Branch, National Cancer Institute, Bethesda, MD, USA*

PHILIP S. LOW • *Department of Chemistry and Purdue Cancer Center, Purdue University, West Lafayette, IN, USA*

MICHAEL D. MASON • *Department of Chemical and Biological Engineering, University of Maine, Orono, ME, USA*

SYLVIA K.E. MESSERSCHMIDT • *Institute of Cell Biology and Immunology, University of Stuttgart, Stuttgart, Germany*

TAMARA MINKO • *Department of Pharmaceutics, Rutgers, The State University of New Jersey, Piscataway, NJ, USA*

DAVID L. MORSE • *Molecular and Functional Imaging, H. Lee Moffitt Cancer Center & Research Institute, Tampa, FL, USA*

JENNIFER G. MORTON • *Rice University, Houston, TX, USA*

BRIJ M. MOUDGIL • *Department of Materials Science and Engineering, Particle Engineering Research Center, University of Florida, Gainesville, FL, USA*

MANOJ NAHAR • *Department of Pharmaceutical Sciences, Dr. H.S. Gour University, Sagar, India*

KLAAS NICOLAY • *Biomedical NMR, Department of Biomedical Engineering, Eindhoven University of Technology, Eindhoven, The Netherlands*

GUOQIN NIU • *Department of Pharmaceutics, University of Florida, Gainesville, FL, USA*

MEGHAN B. O'DONOGHUE • *Department of Chemistry and Department of Physiology and Functional Genomics, Shands Cancer Center and UF Genetics Institute, and McKnight Brain Institute, Center for Research at the Bio/Nano Interface, University of Florida, Gainesville, FL 32611, USA*

GIULIO F. PACIOTTI • *CytImmune Sciences, Inc., Rockville, MD, USA*

MARIA PALAZUELOS • *Particle Engineering Research Center, University of Florida, Gainesville, FL, USA*

MAHESH L. PATIL • *Department of Pharmaceutics, Rutgers, The State University of New Jersey, Piscataway, NJ, USA*

ANATHEA C. POWELL • *Tumor Angiogenesis Section, Surgery Branch, National Cancer Institute, Bethesda, MD, USA*

KEVIN W. POWERS • *Particle Engineering Research Center, University of Florida, Gainesville, FL, USA*

CHRIS P.M. REUTELINGSPERGER • *Department of Biochemistry, Cardiovascular Research Institute Maastricht, University of Maastricht, Maastricht, The Netherlands*

STEPHEN M. ROBERTS • *Center for Environmental and Human Toxicology, University of Florida, Gainesville, FL, USA*

MIRIAM ROTHDIENER • *Institute of Cell Biology and Immunology, University of Stuttgart, Stuttgart, Germany*

CARSTEN RUDOLPH • *Department of Pediatrics, Ludwig-Maximilians University, Munich, Germany; Department of Pharmacy, Free University of Berlin, Berlin, Germany*

MAHA SAAD • *Department of Pharmaceutics, Rutgers, The State University of New Jersey, Piscataway, NJ, USA*

SWADESHMUKUL SANTRA • *Department of Chemistry and Biomolecular Science Center, NanoScience Technology Center, University of Central Florida, Orlando, FL, USA*

RUPA R. SAWANT • *Department of Pharmaceutical Sciences and Center for Pharmaceutical Biotechnology and Nanomedicine, Northeastern University, Boston, MA, USA*

EDWARD W. SCOTT • *Department of Molecular Genetics and Microbiology, University of Florida, Gainesville, FL, USA*

PARVESH SHARMA • *Department of Materials Science and Engineering, Particle Engineering Research Center, University of Florida, Gainesville, FL, USA; St. Stephen's College, Delhi University, Delhi, India*

AMIT SINGH • *Department of Materials Science and Engineering, Particle Engineering Research Center, University of Florida, Gainesville, FL, USA*

STEPHEN STAAL • *Division of Hematology and Oncology, Department of Medicine, University of Florida, Gainesville, FL, USA*

GUSTAV J. STRIJKERS • *Biomedical NMR, Department of Biomedical Engineering, Eindhoven University of Technology, Eindhoven, The Netherlands*

WEIHONG TAN • *Department of Chemistry and Department of Physiology and Functional Genomics, Shands Cancer Center and UF Genetics Institute, and McKnight Brain Institute, Center for Research at the Bio/Nano Interface, University of Florida, Gainesville, FL, USA*

OLEH TARATULA • *Department of Pharmaceutics, Rutgers, The State University of New Jersey, Piscataway, NJ, USA*

GERALDA A.F. VAN TILBORG • *Biomedical NMR, Department of Biomedical Engineering, Eindhoven University of Technology, Eindhoven, The Netherlands*

VLADIMIR P. TORCHILIN • *Department of Pharmaceutical Sciences and Center for Pharmaceutical Biotechnology and Nanomedicine, Northeastern University, Boston, MA, USA*

PEDRO M. VALENCIA • *Department of Chemical Engineering and Division of Health Science and Technology, Massachusetts Institute of Technology, Cambridge, MA, USA*

GLENN A. WALTER • *Department of Physiology and Functional Genomics, University of Florida, Gainesville, FL, USA*

LIHONG V. WANG • *Department of Biomedical Engineering, Washington University, St. Louis, MO, USA*

ALEXANDER WEI • *Department of Chemistry, Purdue University, West Lafayette, IN, USA*

QINGSHAN WEI • *Department of Chemistry, Purdue University, West Lafayette, IN, USA*

JENNIFER L. WEST • *Department of Bioengineering, Rice University, Houston, TX, USA*

YOUNAN XIA • *Department of Biomedical Engineering, Washington University, St. Louis, MO, USA*

JILIN YAN • *Department of Chemistry and Department of Physiology and Functional Genomics, Shands Cancer Center and UF Genetics Institute, and McKnight Brain Institute, Center for Research at the Bio/Nano Interface, University of Florida, Gainesville, FL, USA*

ZHEN YUAN • *Department of Biomedical Engineering, University of Florida, Gainesville, FL, USA*
LIANGFANG ZHANG • *Department of NanoEngineering, University of California-San Diego, La Jolla, CA, USA*
MIN ZHANG • *Department of Pharmaceutics, Rutgers, The State University of New Jersey, Piscataway, NJ, USA*

Chapter 1

What Is Cancer Nanotechnology?

Stephen R. Grobmyer, Nobutaka Iwakuma, Parvesh Sharma, and Brij M. Moudgil

Abstract

Cancer nanotechnology has the potential to dramatically improve current approaches to cancer detection, diagnosis, imaging, and therapy while reducing toxicity associated with traditional cancer therapy (1, 2). In this overview, we will define cancer nanotechnology, consider issues related to application of nanotechnology for cancer imaging and therapy, and broadly consider implications for continued development in nanotechnology for the future of clinical cancer care. These considerations will place in perspective the methodological approaches in cancer nanotechnology and subject reviews outlined in this volume.

Key words: Photothermal therapy, cancer therapy, photoacoustic tomography, cancer, nanotechnology, nanoparticle, nanotoxicology, active targeting, passive targeting, theranostics.

1. Introduction

"Nano" refers to nanometer which is 1×10^{-9} m. Nanotechnology is the engineering, characterization, and application of man-made structures on the scale of 1–100 nm in at least one dimension (3). Materials engineered on this scale have unique properties that are not seen with materials on larger scales and materials at this scale have a favorable profile for interaction with cell surface and intercellular structures (2–4). Cancer nanotechnology is the application of nanotechnology toward the "monitoring, repair, and improvement of human biologic systems" related to cancer (5). The transfer of cancer nanotechnology into routine clinical practice requires a multidisciplinary approach and relies upon careful clinical, ethical, and societal consideration (5).

Cancer nanotechnology has tremendous potential to safely revolutionize current approaches to cancer imaging, early diagnosis, treatment, and prevention of cancer (1).

2. Nanoparticles in Use for Cancer Nanotechnology

A wide variety of nanomaterials are currently under investigation and development for application relative to cancer nanotechnology. These include polymers, dendrimers, lipids, organometallic, and carbon based materials [reviewed extensively in (2, 6)]. Considerations on the selection of specific nanomaterials for cancer nanotechnology applications necessarily include biocompatibility, toxicity, size, surface chemistry, and their properties in biologic systems.

As described by Heath and Davis (7), nanoparticles have 4 unique properties that distinguish them from other cancer therapeutics (1): the nanoparticle, which can itself have therapeutic or diagnostic properties, can be designed to carry a large therapeutic "payload" (2); nanoparticles can be attached to multivalent targeting ligands which yield high affinity and specificity for target cells (3); nanoparticles can be made to accommodate multiple drug molecules that simultaneously allow combinatorial cancer therapy (4); and nanoparticles can bypass traditional drug resistance mechanisms.

Nanoparticles and nanoparticulate formulations of established therapeutics have been integrated into cancer therapeutics and ongoing clinical trials (8). These formulations offer improved efficacy and reduced toxicity compared to conventional therapeutics.

3. Nanotoxicology

Consideration must be given to the toxicological impacts of nanomaterials intended for human administration (9). Material, structure, size, size dispersion, agglomeration, shape, surface charge, surface chemistry, and adsorbed species are important and need to be considered as each of these characteristics ultimately effects not only biodistribution but patterns of clearance and ultimately toxicologic effects on end organs (10). Consideration also needs to be given to the ability of nanomaterials administered in vivo to suppress or stimulate the immune system as these factors can have significant impact on the wellbeing of the host (11).

There are no harmonized standards for assessing toxicology of nanomaterials and this remains a major challenge in the development of nanomaterials for human use. There is a need for reliable predictive assays that are much needed to accelerate the safe transition of nanomaterials toward human cancer applications (12).

4. Delivery of Nanomaterials to Cancer Sites

In order to achieve many imaging and therapeutic applications in cancer nanotechnology in vivo, nanomaterials must be delivered to sites of cancer (13). For many imaging and therapeutic applications, selective or preferential delivery of nanomaterials to sites of cancer would be optimal. Two general approaches have been utilized to accomplish this: passive targeting and active targeting (6).

4.1. Passive Targeting

Passive targeting of nanoparticles relies on abnormal gap junctions (100–600 nm) in the endothelium of tumor blood vessels for accumulation of nanoparticles in tumors (14). In order to achieve passive targeting of nanoparticles, engineering of particles with long-circulation half-lives [such as coating particles with hydrophilic polymer such as polyethylene glycol (PEG)] is most desirable and this type of construct favors passive accumulation of particles inside tumors (6, 13). Altered lymph drainage is a characteristic of tumors which favors retention of nanoparticles inside tumors. In general, small particle size is thought to favor intratumoral extravasation (15, 16). Particle composition and shape are also determinants of particle uptake, although these relationships have not been well characterized (4).

4.2. Active Targeting

Active targeting of nanoparticles relies on conjugation of a tumor-specific ligand(s) to nanoparticles for their specific delivery to tumor sites (17, 18). Targeting moieties that have been investigated include antibodies, peptides, cell surface ligands, and aptamers (13, 19). Targets in tumors have included tumor antigens, cell surface receptors that are internalized [e.g., folate receptors (20) and transferrin receptors (21)], and tumor vasculature (22). Active targeting has been extensively studied in preclinical models but has not been effectively translated into current clinical applications (13). In preclinical models, targeting has inconsistently led to increased accumulation in tumors (23, 24). In many instances, cancer cell uptake has been increased with targeting without increase in overall tumor accumulation of nanoparticles (23, 24). Development of novel, specific targeting strategies for nanoparticles to cancer remains an important area of active investigation.

4.3. Particle Characteristics and Biologic Interactions

The precise relationship between physicochemical properties of nanoparticles and their biodistribution continues to be poorly understood (10, 25). This is largely due to the complexity and variety of biological interactions between nanoparticles and the host as well as the widely varying properties of nanoparticles themselves (26) and the dynamic status of the biologic host. Particle characteristics change in different environments and should be measured in conditions as close to the point of application (e.g., in serum or in cell culture medium) as possible (10). As the relationship of the material properties of nanoparticles to intratumoral accumulation is poorly understood, studies that do not thoroughly characterize material properties likely will not reproduce consistent results (10). This remains an important area of ongoing investigation. An understanding of these principles will be essential to safe and reproducible utilization of nanomaterials for human cancer applications.

5. Nanoparticles as Imaging Contrast Agents

Nanoparticles have tremendous potential for traditional and emerging cancer imaging modalities. The ability to specifically engineer nanomaterials has the potential to improve contrast agent specificity, sensitivity, and functionality, leading to new paradigms in early cancer detection and image-guided cancer therapy (27). In addition, new nanoscale contrast agents are expected to exhibit reduced toxicity compared to traditional imaging contrast agents. Examples of nanoparticles applied as imaging contrast agents are described.

5.1. Magnetic Resonance Imaging Contrast Agents

A variety of nanoscale magnetic resonance imaging (MR) contrast agents have been developed (28). These particles have received significant attention, given the widespread use of MR in clinical practice currently (29). These contrast agents have been designed to improve detection sensitivity and may be biologically targeted to sites of cancer to offer imaging specificity (30). Further, nanoscale MR contrast agents have also been used to mediate noninvasive cancer therapy (e.g., Neutron capture therapy and radiofrequency ablation) and for targeted drug delivery (31).

5.2. Photoacoustic Imaging Contrast Agents

Photoacoustic tomography (PAT) is an emerging nonionizing imaging modality which combines high optical contrast and high ultrasound resolution (32). It uses pulsed laser light to generate light-induced acoustic signals which are measured (33). PAT with finite element reconstruction has been used to image nanoparticle containing millimeter-sized objects in vitro with high resolution (34). PAT images can also importantly be quantitatively reconstructed (34). Nanocages (35), carbon nanotubes (36), and gold-speckled silica particles (37) are among the particles which have been characterized as contrast agents for photoacoustic tomography.

5.3. Multimodal Imaging Contrast Agents

Advances in engineering at the nanoscale have permitted the development and characterization of new multimodal imaging contrast agents (27, 38). Multimodal contrast agents allow combinatorial imaging which can exploit unique advantages of distinct imaging modalities. Our group has recently described novel multimodal imaging contrast agents, gold-speckled silica particles, which function simultaneously as contrast agents for fluorescence imaging, photoacoustic imaging, and magnetic resonance imaging (37). Others, for instance, have described multimodal imaging (MR and fluorescence) with magnetic nanocrystals (39).

6. Nanoparticles for Drug Delivery

The functionality of engineered nanomaterials may be exploited to enhance specificity of drug delivery to sites of cancer, reduce toxicity, enhance therapeutic efficacy, and permit novel combinatorial cancer therapy. Liposomes were some of the earliest nanoscale vehicles used to deliver chemotherapeutic drugs to tumors (40). The preparation of drugs in liposomes allows enhanced delivery of drugs while reducing toxicity. Further, liposomes are amenable to surface conjugation and biologic targeting of delivery vehicles to cancer sites (24, 38). Numerous other nanoscale drug delivery vehicles have been and are currently under development including smart polymers which are pH sensitive, temperature sensitive, dendrimers, viral nanoparticles, carbon-based nanostructures, and polymers [reviewed in (41) and (30)].

Nanotechnology has enabled the development of combinatorial drug delivery systems using biologically targeted nanocarriers. Greater efficacy (and less toxicity) is achievable with higher concentrations of synergistic therapeutics specifically to sites of cancer. Sengupta et al., for instance, have developed a targeted "nanocell" which is designed to achieve temporal release of an antiangiogenic agent and cytotoxic chemotherapy at tumor sites (42). In a mouse model of cancer, the authors have demonstrated significantly enhanced efficacy compared to conventional therapeutics.

7. Nanoparticle-Mediated Novel Cancer Therapy

Engineered properties of nanoparticles are opening the door to new, noninvasive strategies for cancer therapy, not previously possible. This would include photothermal therapy, nanoparticle-enhanced radiotherapy, targeted combinatorial cancer therapy, and nanoparticle-enhanced radiofrequency cancer therapy.

7.1. Photothermal Therapy

Photothermal therapy relies on unique properties of nanoparticles which have high absorption in the NIR region. Nanoshells have been most extensively characterized as nanoscale mediators of photothermal ablation (52) have demonstrated thermal ablation of tumors in a mouse model following systemic injection of particles and exposure of tumors to NIR light. Other nanostructures including nanorods and carbon nanotubes which also strongly absorb in the near-infrared region have also been utilized for photothermal ablation of tumors.

7.2. Nanoparticle-Enhanced Radiotherapy

Gold nanoparticles have been demonstrated to enhance the effect of radiotherapy on tumors in vitro and in animal models of cancer. Hainfeld et al. have demonstrated improved efficacy of radiation therapy on mammary carcinomas in mice following intravenous administration of gold nanoparticles (43). Chang et al. have demonstrated similar effects in a mouse model of melanoma (44). This phenomenon suggests that the specific delivery of nanoparticles to cancer has the potential to enhance the efficacy of radiation therapy on cancer allowing dose reduction with reduced toxicity to surrounding normal tissues.

7.3. Nanoparticle-Enhanced Radiofrequency Therapy of Cancer

Radiofrequency ablation is an established approach to destroy tumors that traditionally has involved insertion of probes into tumors. Nanotechnology is enabling the development of noninvasive radiofrequency ablation of tumors. Gold nanoparticles have been demonstrated in vitro and in vivo to enhance cancer cell destruction in a noninvasive radiofrequency field (45, 46). Gannon et al. have also demonstrated the efficacy of single-wall carbon nanotubes as mediators of noninvasive radiofrequency ablation (47).

7.4. Nanoparticles for Cancer Theranostics

Theranostics is the new field focused on simultaneous diagnosis and treatment of a pathologic condition (48). Biocompatible nanoparticles are currently under development as cancer theranostic agents which would allow noninvasive diagnosis and precise cancer therapy (49). Such nanoparticle-mediated combinatorial strategies offer promise for accelerating treatment, reducing side-effects of treatment, and improving cancer cure rates.

8. Nanoparticles for Cancer In Vitro Diagnostics

Nanomaterials have the potential to significantly enhance both sensitivity and specificity of current in vitro diagnostic tests for cancer (30). Nanotechnology has the capacity to enable high-throughput multiplexed analyses in vitro, not previously possible (7). Numerous label-free nanoscale systems are in development which potentially will have important implications for clinical cancer care including nanowires, cantilevers, surface Plasmon resonance, and nanotubes (7, 30). Semiconductor quantum dots have been employed for enhanced tissue analyses (50, 51).

Acknowledgments

This work was supported by a James and Esther King Biomedical Research Award (06NIR-05-8356), State of Florida-Department of Health and the University of Florida, Patricia Adams Cancer Nanotechnology Research Fund; the DiMarco American Cancer Society IRG.

References

1. Cuenca, A. G., Jiang, H., Hochwald, S. N., Delano, M., Cance, W. G., and Grobmyer, S. R. (2006) Emerging implications of nanotechnology on cancer diagnostics and therapeutics. *Cancer* **107**(3), 459–466.
2. Alexis, F., Rhee, J. W., Richie, J. P., Radovic-Moreno, A. F., Langer, R., and Farokhzad, O. C. (2008) New frontiers in nanotechnology for cancer treatment. *Urol Oncol* **26**(1), 74–85.
3. Hartman, K. B., Wilson, L. J., and Rosenblum, M. G. (2008) Detecting and treating cancer with nanotechnology. *Mol Diagn Ther* **12**(1), 1–14.
4. De Jong, W. H. and Borm, P. J. (2008) Drug delivery and nanoparticles: applications and hazards. *Int J Nanomedicine* **3**(2), 133–149.
5. Duncan, R., Kreyling, W. G., Biosseau, P., Cannistraro, S., Coatrieux, J., Conde, J. P., Hennick, W., Oberleithner, H., and Rivas, J. (2005) ESF scientific forward look on nanomedicine. In European Science Foundation Policy Briefing. 1–6.
6. Cho, K., Wang, X., Nie, S., Chen, Z. G., and Shin, D. M. (2008) Therapeutic nanoparticles for drug delivery in cancer. *Clin Cancer Res* **14**(5), 1310–1316.
7. Heath, J. R. and Davis, M. E. (2008) Nanotechnology and cancer. *Annu Rev Med* **59**, 251–265.
8. Peer, D., Karp, J. M., Hong, S., Farokhzad, O. C., Margalit, R., and Langer, R. (2007) Nanocarriers as an emerging platform for cancer therapy. *Nat Nanotechnol* **2**(12), 751–760.
9. Maurer-Jones, M. A., Bantz, K. C., Love, S. A., Marquis, B. J., and Haynes, C. L. (2009) Toxicity of therapeutic nanoparticles. *Nanomed* **4**(2), 219–241.
10. Powers, K. W., Brown, S. C., Krishna, V. B., Wasdo, S. C., Moudgil, B. M., and Roberts, S. M. (2006) Research strategies for safety evaluation of nanomaterials. Part VI. Characterization of nanoscale particles for toxicological evaluation. *Toxicol Sci* **90**(2), 296–303.
11. Dobrovolskaia, M. A. and McNeil, S. E. (2007) Immunological properties of engineered nanomaterials. *Nat Nanotechnol* **2**(8), 469–478.
12. Marquis, B. J., Love, S. A., Braun, K. L., and Haynes, C. L. (2009) Analytical methods to assess nanoparticle toxicity. *Analyst* **134**(3), 425–439.

13. Lammers, T., Hennink, W. E., and Storm, G. (2008) Tumour-targeted nanomedicines: principles and practice. *Br J Cancer* **99**(3), 392–397.
14. Maeda, H. and Matsumura, Y. (1989) Tumoritropic and lymphotropic principles of macromolecular drugs. *Crit Rev Ther Drug Carrier Syst* **6**(3), 193–210.
15. Yuan, F., Dellian, M., Fukumura, D., Leunig, M., Berk, D. A., Torchilin, V. P., and Jain, R. K. (1995) Vascular permeability in a human tumor xenograft: molecular size dependence and cutoff size. *Cancer Res* **55**(17), 3752–3756.
16. Kong, G., Braun, R. D., and Dewhirst, M. W. (2000) Hyperthermia enables tumor-specific nanoparticle delivery: effect of particle size. *Cancer Res* **60**(16), 4440–4445.
17. Allen, T. M. (2002) Ligand-targeted therapeutics in anticancer therapy. *Nat Rev Cancer* **2**(10), 750–763.
18. Black, K. C., Kirkpatrick, N. D., Troutman, T. S., Xu, L., Vagner, J., Gillies, R. J., Barton, J. K., Utzinger, U., and Romanowski, M. (2008) Gold nanorods targeted to delta opioid receptor: plasmon-resonant contrast and photothermal agents. *Mol Imaging* **7**(1), 50–57.
19. Cho, K., Wang, X., Nie, S., Chen, Z., and Shin, D. M. (2008) Therapeutic nanoparticles for drug delivery in cancer. *Clinical Cancer Research* **14**(5), 1310–1315.
20. Santra, S., Liesenfeld, B., Dutta, D., Chatel, D., Batich, C. D., Tan, W., Moudgil, B. M., and Mericle, R. A. (2005) Folate conjugated fluorescent silica nanoparticles for labeling neoplastic cells. *J Nanosci Nanotechnol* **5**(6), 899–904.
21. Sahoo, S. K., Ma, W., and Labhasetwar, V. (2004) Efficacy of transferrin-conjugated paclitaxel-loaded nanoparticles in a murine model of prostate cancer. *Int J Cancer* **112**(2), 335–340.
22. Smith, B. R., Cheng, Z., De, A., Koh, A. L., Sinclair, R., and Gambhir, S. S. (2008) Real-Time Intravital Imaging of RGD-Quantum Dot Binding to Luminal Endothelium in Mouse Tumor Neovasculature. *Nano Lett* **8**(9), 2599–2606.
23. Kirpotin, D. B., Drummond, D. C., Shao, Y., Shalaby, M. R., Hong, K., Nielsen, U. B., Marks, J. D., Benz, C. C., and Park, J. W. (2006) Antibody targeting of long-circulating lipidic nanoparticles does not increase tumor localization but does increase internalization in animal models. *Cancer Res* **66**(13), 6732–6740.
24. Park, J. W., Benz, C. C., and Martin, F. J. (2004) Future directions of liposome- and immunoliposome-based cancer therapeutics. *Semin Oncol* **31**(6 Suppl 13), 196–205.
25. Hood, E. (2004) Nanotechnology: looking as we leap. *Environ Health Perspect* **112**(13), A740–A749.
26. Jabr-Milane, L. S., van Vlerken, L. E., Yadav, S., and Amiji, M. M. (2008) Multi-functional nanocarriers to overcome tumor drug resistance. *Cancer Treat Rev* **34**(7), 592–602.
27. Sharma, P., Brown, S., Walter, G., Santra, S., and Moudgil, B. (2006) Nanoparticles for bioimaging. *Adv Colloid Interface Sci* **123–126**, 471–485.
28. Jun, Y. W., Jang, J. T., and Cheon, J. (2007) Magnetic nanoparticle assisted molecular MR imaging. *Adv Exp Med Biol* **620**, 85–106.
29. Will, O., Purkayastha, S., Chan, C., Athanasiou, T., Darzi, A. W., Gedroyc, W., and Tekkis, P. P. (2006) Diagnostic precision of nanoparticle-enhanced MRI for lymph-node metastases: a meta-analysis. *Lancet Oncol* **7**(1), 52–60.
30. Pope-Harman, A., Cheng, M. M., Robertson, F., Sakamoto, J., and Ferrari, M. (2007) Biomedical nanotechnology for cancer. *Med Clin North Am* **91**(5), 899–927.
31. Sun, C., Lee, J. S., and Zhang, M. (2008) Magnetic nanoparticles in MR imaging and drug delivery. *Adv Drug Deliv Rev* **60**(11), 1252–1265.
32. Hoelen, C. G. A., de Mul, F. F. M., Pongers, R., and Dekker, A. (1998) Three-dimensional photoacoustic imaging of blood vessels in optical tissue. *Opt Lett* **23**, 648–650.
33. Copland, J. A., Eghtedari, M., Popov, V. L., Kotov, N., Mamedova, N., Motamedi, M., and Oraevsky, A. A. (2004) Bioconjugated gold nanoparticles as a molecular based contrast agent: implications for imaging of deep tumors using optoacoustic tomography. *Mol Imaging Biol* **6**(5), 341–349.
34. Yuan, Z. and Jiang, H. (2006) Quantitative photoacoustic tomography: recovery of optical absorption coefficient maps of heterogeneous media. *Appl Phys Lett* **88**(231101), 231101–231103.
35. Yang, X., Skrabalak, S. E., Li, Z. Y., Xia, Y., and Wang, L. V. (2007) Photoacoustic tomography of a rat cerebral cortex in vivo with au nanocages as an optical contrast agent. *Nano Lett* **7**(12), 3798–3802.
36. De la Zerda, A., Zavaleta, C., Keren, S., Vaithilingam, S., Bodapati, S., Liu, Z., Levi, J., Smith, B. R., Ma, T. J., and Oralkan, O. et al. (2008) Carbon nanotubes as photoacoustic molecular imaging agents in living mice. *Nat Nanotechnol* **3**(9), 557–562.

37. Sharma, P., Brown, S. C., Bengtsson, N., Zhang, Q., Walter, G. A., Grobmyer, S. R., Santa, S., Jiang, H., Scott, E., and Moudgil, B. (2008) Gold-speckled multimodal nanoparticles for noninvasive bioimaging. *Chemistry of Materials* **20**(19), 6087–6094.

38. McCarthy, J. R., Kelly, K. A., Sun, E. Y., and Weissleder, R. (2007) Targeted delivery of multifunctional magnetic nanoparticles. *Nanomed* **2**(2), 153–167.

39. Jun, Y. W., Huh, Y. M., Choi, J. S., Lee, J. H., Song, H. T., Kim, S., Yoon, S., Kim, K. S., Shin, J. S., and Suh, J. S. et al. (2005) Nanoscale size effect of magnetic nanocrystals and their utilization for cancer diagnosis via magnetic resonance imaging. *J Am Chem Soc* **127**(16), 5732–5733.

40. Moghimi, S. M., Hunter, A. C., and Murray, J. C. (2005) Nanomedicine: current status and future prospects. *Faseb J* **19**(3), 311–330.

41. Portney, N. G. and Ozkan, M. (2006) Nano-oncology: drug delivery, imaging, and sensing. *Anal Bioanal Chem* **384**(3), 620–630.

42. Sengupta, S., Eavarone, D., Capila, I., Zhao, G., Watson, N., Kiziltepe, T., and Sasisekharan, R. (2005) Temporal targeting of tumour cells and neovasculature with a nanoscale delivery system. *Nature* **436**(7050), 568–572.

43. Hainfeld, J. F., Slatkin, D. N., and Smilowitz, H. M. (2004) The use of gold nanoparticles to enhance radiotherapy in mice. *Phys Med Biol* **49**(18), N309–N315.

44. Chang, M. Y., Shiau, A. L., Chen, Y. H., Chang, C. J., Chen, H. H., and Wu, C. L. (2008) Increased apoptotic potential and dose-enhancing effect of gold nanoparticles in combination with single-dose clinical electron beams on tumor-bearing mice. *Cancer Sci* **99**(7), 1479–1484.

45. Gannon, C. J., Patra, C. R., Bhattacharya, R., Mukherjee, P., and Curley, S. A. (2008) Intracellular gold nanoparticles enhance noninvasive radiofrequency thermal destruction of human gastrointestinal cancer cells. *J Nanobiotechnol* **6**, 2.

46. Cardinal, J., Klune, J. R., Chory, E., Jeyabalan, G., Kanzius, J. S., Nalesnik, M., and Geller, D. A. (2008) Noninvasive radiofrequency ablation of cancer targeted by gold nanoparticles. *Surgery* **144**(2), 125–132.

47. Gannon, C. J., Cherukuri, P., Yakobson, B. I., Cognet, L., Kanzius, J. S., Kittrell, C., Weisman, R. B., Pasquali, M., Schmidt, H. K., and Smalley, R. E. et al. (2007) Carbon nanotube-enhanced thermal destruction of cancer cells in a noninvasive radiofrequency field. *Cancer* **110**(12), 2654–2665.

48. Tassinari, O. W., Caiazzo, R. J., Jr., Ehrlich, J. R., and Liu, B. C. (2008) Identifying autoantigens as theranostic targets: antigen arrays and immunoproteomics approaches. *Curr Opin Mol Ther* **10**(2), 107–115.

49. Santra, S., Kaittanis, C., Grimm, J., and Perez, J. M. (2009) Drug/dye-loaded, multifunctional iron oxide nanoparticles for combined targeted cancer therapy and dual optical/magnetic resonance imaging. *Small* **5**(16), 1862–1868.

50. Bruchez, M., Jr., Moronne, M., Gin, P., Weiss, S., and Alivisatos, A. P. (1998) Semiconductor nanocrystals as fluorescent biological labels. *Science* **281**(5385), 2013–2016.

51. Chan, W. C., Maxwell, D. J., Gao, X., Bailey, R. E., Han, M., and Nie, S. (2002) Luminescent quantum dots for multiplexed biological detection and imaging. *Curr Opin Biotechnol* **13**(1), 40–46.

52. O'Neal, D. P., Hirsch, L. R., Halas, N. J., Payne, J. D., West, J. L. (2004) Photothermal tumor ablation in mice using near infrared-absorbing nanoparticles. *Cancer Lett* **209**, 171–176.

Chapter 2

Molecular-Targeted Therapy for Cancer and Nanotechnology

Steven N. Hochwald

Abstract

In order to stop malignant tumor growth, >90% of a critical biochemical pathway needs to be blocked. Due to extraordinary advances in molecular biology, there is an increased understanding of rationale and relevant molecular targets in cancer. However, due to the heterogeneity of the molecular abnormalities in multiple tumor types, strategies designed to interfere with multiple molecular abnormalities will be necessary to impact survival. Nanoparticles have the potential to provide therapies not possible with other drug modalities. Researchers and clinicians must take advantage of these opportunities in order for nanotechnology to make an impact in the diagnosis and treatment of malignancy. A discussion of relevant targets either on the cell surface or the cytoplasm and strategies to achieve optimal drug targeting are the focus of this chapter.

Key words: Molecular targets, cancer, tyrosine kinases, nanoparticles, focal adhesion kinase, transforming growth factor beta.

1. Introduction

Despite recent advances in surgery, chemotherapy, and radiation treatment, survival of patients with advanced malignancy remains suboptimal. Fortunately, our understanding of the origins of cancer has changed dramatically over the last 25 years, owing in large part to the revolution in molecular biology that has changed all biomedical research. Powerful experimental tools are available to cancer biologists and have made it possible to uncover and dissect the complex molecular machinery operating inside normal and malignant cells. In addition, these tools have allowed researchers to pinpoint the defects that cause cancer cells to signal and proliferate abnormally.

We have learned that malignant cells are similar to normal cells in the signaling pathways that they use. However, cancer cells acquire aberrations that favor their growth in the complex environments of living tissues. This includes their ability to recruit blood vessels into tumor masses – the process of angiogenesis, their ability to invade and metastasize, and their ability to grow and divide indefinitely. Malignant tumors have growth kinetics that have been studied and predicted. Tumor cure requires elimination of all malignant cells and growth inhibition is not sufficient.

In order to stop malignant tumor growth, >90% of a critical biochemical pathway needs to be blocked. Thanks to an increased understanding of the biologic basis of cancer, investigators are turning to molecular-targeted therapy to further improve patient outcome. Since the software of a cancer cell has gone badly and progressively wrong, cancer cells are more vulnerable to specific and selective drugs. In fact, most of the intracellular messengers are binary: they are either switched on or off by phosphorylation or dephosphorylation. At any one time a number of positive and negative signals travel from the cell membrane to the nucleus. These signals are irreversibly altered in cancer cells. Recent years have seen the advent of a new generation of agents that directly target alterations in the malignant cell itself or the cells supporting tumor growth. This specific-targeted therapy should avoid the nonspecific toxicities that limit dosages that can be given with standard chemotherapy. Unfortunately, there are few cancers where inhibition of a single molecular defect at the center of the pathogenesis of the disease has been successful. Most cancers are complex and contain multiple genetic aberrations. Strategies designed to interfere with multiple molecular abnormalities will be necessary to impact survival.

2. Drug Target Selection

It is clear that cancer is caused by the accumulation of mutations in a cell that is permissive for expression of the malignant phenotype. Rarely, these mutations are inherited in the germline where they contribute to a hereditary predisposition to cancer. More commonly, these mutations are acquired with an increased frequency with increasing age. Cancer causing mutations include gain of function mutations that convert proto-oncogenes into oncogenes and loss-of-function mutations that inactivate tumor suppressor genes. Malignant transformation can also be due to epigenetic changes, such as alterations in DNA methylation that change gene expression patterns. These genetic and epigenetic changes are responsible for the cancer phenotype (1).

In humans, at least 4–6 rate limiting and causal mutations are required to transform normal cells into cancer cells (2). In designing a strategy targeting a particular tumor type, it is important to distinguish between mutations that are involved with the initiation of the malignancy from those many other mutations in the cancer cell that might be considered epiphenomenal or bystander mutations. Examples of such bystander mutations include up-regulation of genes as a result of chromosomal gain or deletion of genes as a result of chromosomal loss. In addition, in designing targeted therapy, it is also useful to separate cancer causing mutations from those mutations that are required continually to support the malignant phenotype. An example of genes supporting but not necessarily causing malignant behavior include those associated with resistance to apoptosis.

It is well recognized that cancers are heterogeneous, demonstrating both intratumor and intertumor heterogeneity, making targeted therapy problematic. To combat such heterogeneity, focusing on the causal genetic abnormalities within the tumor while ignoring the epiphenomenal changes may prove useful. Another approach is to focus on molecular pathways rather than on individual genes, because mutations in cancer cells likely act on pathways rather than individual proteins. For example, p53 is a tumor suppressor that under normal conditions induces apoptosis in response to DNA damage and carcinogenic symbols (3). p53 is a sequence-specific nuclear transcription factor that binds to defined consensus sites within DNA as a tetramer and affects the transcription of its target genes (4). p53 regulates these genes either by transcriptional activation (5) or by modulating other protein activities by direct binding (6). The p53-induced activation of target genes may result in the induction of growth arrest either before DNA replication in the G1 phase of the cell cycle or before mitosis in the G2 phase. There are many ways in which the p53 function may be altered in human cancers. p53 can be inactivated indirectly through binding to viral proteins, as a result of alterations in the *mdm2* or *p19*^{ARF} genes or by localization of the p53 protein to the cytoplasm. Due to multiple and diverse effects that an abnormality in a single gene can have on transcription and translation, broad-scale investigations on pathway regulation and perturbances are relevant. In this regard, there are now assays that can evaluate genes (DNA microarray), mRNA (taqman low-density array), or proteins on a large-scale basis in order to group or cluster similar tumors based on shared molecular complexity even if many variations exist at the level of individual genes.

All of the anticancer drugs in use today affect targets that are shared between normal cells and cancer cells, including proteins involved with fundamental processes such as DNA repair. The observations that certain drugs, especially molecularly targeted ones, can induce striking remissions indicate that relative differences between normal cells and cancer cells can be exploited for therapeutic gain. There are now multiple examples of cancers that seem to be dependent on or "addicted" to certain activated oncogenes. Such oncogene addiction might underlie the success of the molecular-targeted agents now in the clinic (7).

2.1. Passive Drug Targeting

Cancer nanotherapeutics have tremendous promise to solve several limitations of conventional drug delivery systems such as nonspecific biodistribution and targeting, lack of water solubility, low therapeutic indices, and poor oral bioavailability. Nanoparticles have been designed for optimal size and surface characteristics to increase their circulation time. Conventional surface nonmodified nanoparticles are usually trapped by the reticuloendothelial system and, therefore, have limited circulation time. However, the distribution of injected nanoparticles can be controlled by adjusting their surface features and their size. Most tumor-targeted nanomedicines currently in the clinic utilize passive targeting. This refers to the extravasation of the delivered drug into the interstitial fluid at the tumor site, taking advantage of locally increased tumor vascular permeability. In addition, solid tumors have minimal lymphatics, and extravasated nanoparticles are retained within the tumor for prolonged periods of time. This enhanced permeability and retention effect is currently the most important method for delivery of low molecular weight agents to tumors (8).

2.2. Active Drug Targeting

Lack of specificity with passive targeting by nanoparticles is a major drawback with this approach. Recently, investigators have attempted to include a targeting ligand or antibody in the nanocarrier in a process termed active nanoparticle targeting (9, 10). The ideal cell surface antigen and receptor that should be utilized for active targeting with these nanoparticles has not been found. Likely, it will be tumor specific. However, ideally it should be expressed only on tumor cells and not expressed on normal cells. In addition, it should be expressed in a homogeneous fashion on all targeted tumor cells. Finally, the cell surface antigens and receptors should not be shed into the blood circulation. Some of the molecular targets that have been successfully approached with kinase inhibitors or antibodies are discussed below.

2.3. Targets for Nanotechnology in Cancer

A large number of growth factors including platelet-derived growth factor (PDGF), epidermal growth factor (EGF), insulin-like growth factor-1 (IGF-1), fibroblast growth factor (FGF), and nerve growth factor (NGF) signal by inducing dimerization and activation of receptors that are protein tyrosine kinases. Dimerization enhances receptor autophosphorylation which stimulates enzymatic activity further and creates numerous binding sites for signal transduction components that contain SH2 (Src homology 2) or PTB (Phospho Tyrosine-Binding) domains. Tyrosine kinase receptors have variable number of tyrosine residues that are phosphorylated after activation and can recruit and bind different SH2/PTB domain proteins. Ligand binding to the receptor activates the signaling molecule through a variety of mechanisms including allosteric change, tyrosine phosphorylation, or contact with binding partners at the cell membrane. Many of these receptor-bound molecules channel into common pathways and many signaling routes serve similar and somewhat redundant purposes. Activation of receptor tyrosine kinase pathways leads to multiple changes in protein phosphorylation and activation of gene transcription (11). The major contributors to downstream activation from receptor tyrosine kinase activation include Ras/ERK and PI3K pathways (**Fig. 2.1**).

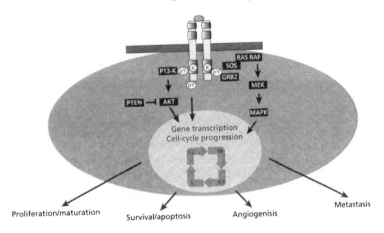

Fig. 2.1. Growth factor receptor.

3. Relevant Anti-neoplastic Targets for Nanotechnology on the Cell Surface

3.1. Epidermal Growth Factor Receptor (EGFR)

The human epidermal growth factor receptor (EGFR), HER, family of receptor proteins play an important role in tumorigenesis and progression of disease. HER1/EGFR and HER2 are the most widely studied HERs. In many cancers, HER1/EGFR expression is abnormal or up-regulated, indicative of a possible role in tumorigenesis (12–22). These proteins have formed the basis of extensive and growing drug development programs in both public and private research companies.

A range of potential therapeutic targets exist within the HER signaling system, both inside and outside the cell. Monoclonal antibodies and tyrosine kinase inhibitors, acting extracellularly and intracellularly, comprise two classes of agents most advanced in clinical development. Monoclonal antibodies were the earliest approach to targeting HERs, binding to the extracellular portion of the HER molecule, and preventing activation. Mouse monoclonal antibodies that inhibited these receptors were genetically engineered to contain human antibody motifs. Two examples are cetuximab (Erbitux), a HER1/EGFR-targeted mAb now in the late stages of clinical development in many cancers and approved for use in 2004 in metastatic colorectal carcinoma, in 2006 for head and neck cancer, and the HER2-specific trastuzumab (Herceptin), already established in the care of breast cancer patients.

Trastuzumab is the first HER-directed therapy to gain approval from the US Food and Drug Administration (FDA) for the treatment of patients with metastatic breast cancer. In preclinical studies, trastuzumab has been demonstrated to downregulate HER2, lead G_1 growth arrest and apoptosis, act as an angiogenic inhibitor, and have synergistic effect with doxorubicin, taxanes, vinorelbine, and flavopiridol in breast cancer cells (23–26). Response rates to trastuzumab given as a single agent ranged from 12 to 40%, in part depending on the method used to determine HER2 status and prior treatment received (24, 25, 27). Perhaps the most promising applications of trastuzumab mAb therapy will be in the adjuvant setting. Large randomized trials are being performed by the cancer cooperative groups in node-positive HER2 breast cancer patients. In these studies, trastuzumab is being added to the current chemotherapeutic regimen standard of care in an effort to improve response and survival.

On 12 February 2004, the FDA-approved cetuximab (Erbitux, Imclone Systems, Inc.) for use in combination with irinotecan, for the treatment of EGFR-expressing, metastatic colorectal carcinoma in patients who are refractory to irinotecan-based chemotherapy. This antibody was also approved for use as a single agent for the treatment of EGFR-expressing, recurrent metastatic colorectal carcinoma in patients who are intolerant to irinotecan-based chemotherapy. Cetuximab binds specifically to the EGFR on both normal and tumor cells, and competitively inhibits the binding of EGF and other ligands, such as transforming growth factor-alpha. Binding of cetuximab blocks phosphorylation and activation of receptor-associated kinases, resulting in inhibition of cell growth, induction of apoptosis, and decreased matrix metalloproteinase and vascular endothelial growth factor production.

Small molecule tyrosine kinase inhibitors (TKIs) are given orally and may be the most promising class of targeted agents currently in development. They block downstream signaling by inhibiting the intracellular portion of the target HER. Examples include gefitinib (Iressa) and erlotinib (Tarceva) which are both HER1/EGFR-targeted reversible TKIs. Other TKIs can be irreversible and can have single, dual, or pan HER specificity.

TKIs are in varying stages of development and several clinical trials, studying their toxicity and efficacy, are underway or have been completed.

3.2. c-Kit

Perhaps the most dramatic example demonstrating the potential of kinase-targeted therapy comes from gastrointestinal stromal tumor (GIST), the most common mesenchymal neoplasm of the intestinal tract. GISTs have a gain of function mutation in the kit proto-oncogene. Normally, kit protein is activated only when its ligand binds to it and induces receptor dimerization resulting in intracellular signaling and cell growth and survival. However, c-Kit is activated in GIST in the absence of its natural ligand resulting in unopposed neoplastic proliferation. STI571 was discovered at Novartis Pharmaceuticals during a search for inhibitors of platelet-derived growth factor receptor. STI571 selectively inhibits specific tyrosine kinases, including c-Kit, and has been shown to be an effective treatment for gastrointestinal stromal tumor (GIST) (28).

3.3. VEGF

Virtually, all existing anticancer drugs, and those in development, are designed to directly attack cancer cells by exploiting some property of the cancer cells that distinguishes them from normal cells. Antiangiogenic therapy is based on a fundamentally different approach: attacking a tumor's lifelines – its growing blood vessel supply – upon which tumor cells depend on oxygen and nutrients. Currently, there is a large and diverse group of drugs being developed and tested as angiogenesis inhibitors, e.g., monoclonal antibodies to VEGF, small molecule inhibitors of VEGF receptor-2 (which are expressed by activated endothelial cells of growing blood vessels, and convey pro-angiogenic signals into such cells after binding VEGF), or small peptide fragments of thrombospondin-1 (endogenous inhibitor of angiogenesis). In addition to specifically designed antiangiogenic drugs, evidence suggests that many other anticancer drugs which were not developed as angiogenesis inhibitors can actually express this activity. This group of antiangiogenic drugs include radiation, many chemotherapeutic agents, thalidomide, COX-2 inhibitors, and signal transduction inhibitors (Herceptin and STI571) (29).

Bevacizumab is a recombinant-humanized monoclonal antibody directed against vascular endothelial growth factor that has been recently studied in a variety of solid malignancies. When VEGF is targeted and bound to bevacizumab, it cannot stimulate the growth of blood vessels, thus denying tumors' blood, oxygen, and other nutrients needed for growth. Angiogenesis inhibitors such as bevacizumab have been studied, in the laboratory for three decades, with the hope they might prevent the growth of cancer. A recent Phase III randomized double blind study in 925 patients has demonstrated efficacy and safety when bevacizumab was added to irinotecan/5-fluorouracil/leucovorin chemotherapy as first-line therapy for metastatic colorectal cancer (30). In this study, the addition of bevacizumab, compared to placebo, resulted in an improved response rate, survival benefit, and time to progression. Median survival was increased by 4.5 months ($p = 0.00003$) and overall response increased by 10% ($p < 0.003$) in the bevacizumab arm. Relatively, few side-effects were demonstrated with the administration of bevacizumab, and most were related to mild increases in blood pressure that were easily controlled with oral anti-hypertensives. Of note, this is the first molecular-targeted antiangiogenic product that has been proven to delay tumor growth and more importantly, significantly extend the lives of patients. As a result, bevacizumab has been approved by the FDA as first-line treatment for metastatic colorectal cancer. However, other studies, including some in patients with breast cancer have not demonstrated a beneficial effect with the addition of bevacizumab. At present, the role of antiangiogenic-targeted therapy in other solid malignancies is not known.

3.4. IGF-1R

In normal and cancer cells, insulin-like growth factors (IGF-I and IGF-II) and their high-affinity binding proteins comprise a major superfamily of protein hormone that regulates cell growth, metabolism, and cell death. Several studies support the significance of the IGF-1 receptor-mediated mitogenic signal in cancer cells. Several members in the IGF family signaling pathway, including IGF-1, IGF-1R, IGF-2R, and IRS-1, are overexpressed in cancer (31–33). IGF-1 receptor antisense oligonucleotides constructs expressed as dominant negatives in adenovirus, anti-IGF-1R antibodies, and IGF-1R tyrosine kinase inhibitors have been shown to inhibit the proliferation of human cancer cells.

IGF-1 exerts its influence on protein, lipid, and carbohydrate metabolism through activation of IGF-1R. This tyrosine kinase cell surface receptor has selective binding affinity for IGF-1 but can bind both IGF-II and insulin with less affinity. Upon binding its ligand, IGF-1R undergoes conformational changes that trigger an intracellular signaling cascade through the insulin receptor substrates 1–4. These molecules activate the two main downstream signals of IGF-1R which are MAPK and PI3K.

Drug development aimed to inhibit the IGF-1R has recently expanded, and there are >25 molecules at different stages of development (34). The two most investigated strategies in preclinical models use monoclonal antibodies and tyrosine kinase inhibitors. Since IGF-1R shares 84% amino acid homology to the insulin receptor, IGF-1R presents a challenge for the development of specific small molecule inhibitors.

3.5. TGFβ

The TGFβ family of proteins includes cell surface receptors that respond to many ligands. Two types of receptor serine threonine kinases (Types I and II) are required to respond to TGFβ family ligands. Initial binding of ligand to the Type II receptor recruits Type I receptor which is subsequently phosphorylated. The Type I receptor then transmits signals to effector Smad proteins which provide transcription activation function. Although Smads are the major mediators of TGFβ signals, various MAPK pathways can be activated by TGFβ ligands. TGFβ proteins have many roles including acting as morphogens and promoting apoptosis. In cancer cells, TGFβ can exert an inhibitory effect on cell proliferation and are generally considered to act as tumor suppressors. The most prominent mechanisms by which TGFβ ligands can inhibit cell proliferation involve induction of CKI and repression of Myc (35). TGFβ pathway activity can be inhibited by elimination of Smad4 and selectively by loss of Type I or Type II receptors. The most frequent known mutation associated with human tumors is loss of Smad4 function (36). Mutations in the gene are seen in approximately 50% of pancreatic and colorectal adenocarcinomas.

4. Relevant Anti-neoplastic Targets for Nanotechnology in the Cytoplasm

4.1. FAK

Focal adhesion kinase (FAK) was discovered more than 15 years ago, as a protein that plays an important role in intracellular processes of cell spreading, adhesion, motility, survival, and cell cycle progression. FAK is one of the critical tyrosine kinases that is linked to the processes of tumor invasion and survival. The FAK gene encodes a nonreceptor tyrosine kinase that localizes at contact points of cells with extracellular matrix and is activated by integrin (cell surface receptor) signaling. FAK mRNA is up-regulated in invasive and metastatic human breast and colon cancer samples (37). At the same time, matched samples of normal colon and breast tissue from the same patients had almost no detectable FAK expression. This was the first evidence that FAK might be regulated at the level of gene transcription and other mechanisms (such as gene amplification). Subsequently, FAK has been demonstrated to be up-regulated at the protein level in numerous types of human tumors, including colon, breast, thyroid, ovarian, melanoma, and sarcoma (38–40). In addition, FAK has important binding partners, such as RIP (41), linking FAK with the death-receptor pathways; p53 (42), linking FAK with the apoptotic/survival nuclear pathways (43); VEGFR-3 (44), linking FAK with lymphogenesis and angiogenesis; and IGF-1R (45), linking FAK with the insulin growth factor receptor pathway, critical in pancreatic cancers. In addition, the regulatory promoter region of the FAK gene has been cloned and confirms transcriptional up-regulation in cancer cell lines. Recently, it was demonstrated that N-myc was able to bind the FAK promoter and up-regulate its expression in neuroblastoma cells (46).

4.2. FAK Inhibitors

Recently, Novartis Inc. developed novel FAK inhibitors down-regulating its kinase activity (47). The novel Novartis FAK inhibitor, TAE-226, recently was employed in brain cancer and effectively inhibited FAK signaling and caused apoptosis in these cells (48). TAE226 lacks specificity since it can also inhibit other signaling pathways in addition to FAK, such as IGFR-1. Another, ATP-targeting site inhibitor of FAK, Pfizer-PF-573,228 has been recently described (49). Another Pfizer inhibitor PF-562,271 with high specificity in inhibiting FAK activity has been shown to be effective in tumor xenograft models in vivo (50) and on bone tumors (51) and is now in clinical trials. In the future, detailed studies will be needed to address specificity of these drugs.

4.3. c-Src

The c-Src nonreceptor tyrosine kinase is overexpressed and activated in a large number of human malignancies and has been linked to the development of cancer and progression to distant metastases. These observations have led to the recent targeting of c-Src for the development of anticancer therapeutics, which show promise as a new avenue for cancer treatment. In addition to increasing cell proliferation, a key role of c-Src in cancer seems to promote invasion and motility, functions that might contribute to tumor progression. Another key role of c-Src is the regulation of specific angiogenic factors that promote tumor progression. Recent studies demonstrate that c-Src regulates constitutive VEGF and IL-8 expression (52).

c-Src also plays a crucial role in bone homeostasis, since inhibition or deletion of c-Src impairs the function of osteoclasts, the bone resorbing cells. Therefore, c-Src could be a target for the pharmacological treatment of cancers and their skeletal metastases. The pyrrolo-pyrimidines CGP77675 and CGP76030 (Novartis Pharma, Basel, Switzerland) have been shown to reduce the incidence of osteolytic lesions and visceral metastases and to decrease lethality in a bone metastasis mouse model. In addition, the purine-based c-Src inhibitor AP23451 and the dual c-Src/Abl inhibitors AP22408 and AP23236 proved efficacious in reducing bone metastases in preclinical studies (53).

5. Nanoparticle Therapeutics

Nanoparticles have the potential to provide therapies not possible with other drug modalities. The pharmacokinetics of nanoparticle administration can be fine-tuned by making them large enough to avoid single pass renal clearance and alterating surface properties to a significant extent to minimize nonspecific interactions with proteins and cells. However, in addition, targeted nanoparticles can be distinguished from other therapeutic entities by the following (1): Nanoparticles can be made to contain multiple-targeting ligands that can provide multivalent binding to cell surface receptors (2), can be made sufficiently large to accommodate multiple types of drug molecules (3), can bypass traditional means of drug-resistance mechanisms that involve cell surface protein pumps, because they enter the cell through endocytosis, and (4) can carry a large number of "effector" molecules that have no effect on pharmacokinetics or biodistribution (54).

References

1. Hanahan, D. and Weinberg, R. A. (2000) The hallmarks of cancer. *Cell* **100**, 57–70.
2. Hahn, W. C. and Weinberg, R. A. (2002) Modeling the molecular circuitry of cancer. *Nat Rev Cancer* **2**, 331–341.
3. Vogelstein, B., Lane, D., and Levine, A. J. (2000) Surfing the p53 network. *Nature* **408**, 307–310.
4. el-Deiry, W. S. (1998) Regulation of p53 downstream genes. *Semin Cancer Biol* **8**, 345–357.
5. Murphy, M., Ahn, J., Walker, K. K., Hoffman, W. H., Evans, R. M., Levine, A. J., et al. (1999) Transcriptional repression by wild-type p53 utilizes histone deacetylases, mediated by interaction with mSin3a. *Genes Dev* **13**, 2490–2501.
6. Guimaraes, D. P. and Hainaut, P. (2002) TP53: a key gene in human cancer. *Biochimie* **84**, 83–93.
7. Weinstein, I. B., Begemann, M., Zhou, P., Han, E. K., Sgambato, A., Doki, Y., et al. (1997) Disorders in cell circuitry associated with multistage carcinogenesis: exploitable targets for cancer prevention and therapy. *Clin Cancer Res* **3**, 2696–2702.
8. Lammers, T., Hennink, W. E., and Storm, G. (2008) Tumour-targeted nanomedicines: principles and practice. *Br J Cancer* **99**, 392–397.
9. Cho, K., Wang, X., Nie, S., Chen, Z. G., and Shin, D. M. (2008) Therapeutic nanoparticles for drug delivery in cancer. *Clin Cancer Res* **14**, 1310–1316.
10. Tolcher, A. W., Sugarman, S., Gelmon, K. A., Cohen, R., Saleh, M., Isaacs, C., et al. (1999) Randomized phase II study of BR96-doxorubicin conjugate in patients with metastatic breast cancer. *J Clin Oncol* **17**, 478–484.
11. Burgess, A. W. (2008) EGFR family: structure physiology signaling and therapeutic targets. *Growth Factors* **26**, 263–274.
12. Bartlett, J. M., Langdon, S. P., Simpson, B. J., Stewart, M., Katsaros, D., Sismondi, P., et al. (1996) The prognostic value of epidermal growth factor receptor mRNA expression in primary ovarian cancer. *Br J Cancer* **73**, 301–306.
13. Beckmann, M. W., Niederacher, D., Massenkeil, G., Tutschek, B., Beckmann, A., Schenko, G., et al. (1996) Expression analyses of epidermal growth factor receptor and HER-2/neu: no advantage of prediction of recurrence or survival in breast cancer patients. *Oncology* **53**, 441–447.
14. Bucci, B., D'Agnano, I., Botti, C., Mottolese, M., Carico, E., Zupi, G., et al. (1997) EGF-R expression in ductal breast cancer: proliferation and prognostic implications. *Anticancer Res* **17**, 769–774.
15. Fischer-Colbrie, J., Witt, A., Heinzl, H., Speiser, P., Czerwenka, K., Sevelda, P., et al. (1997) EGFR and steroid receptors in ovarian carcinoma: comparison with prognostic parameters and outcome of patients. *Anticancer Res* **17**, 613–619.
16. Fontanini, G., De Laurentiis, M., Vignati, S., Chine, S., Lucchi, M., Silvestri, V., et al. (1998) Evaluation of epidermal growth factor-related growth factors and receptors and of neoangiogenesis in completely resected stage I-IIIA non-small-cell lung cancer: amphiregulin and microvessel count are independent prognostic indicators of survival. *Clin Cancer Res* **4**, 241–249.
17. Fujino, S., Enokibori, T., Tezuka, N., Asada, Y., Inoue, S., Kato, H., et al. (1996) A comparison of epidermal growth factor receptor levels and other prognostic parameters

in non-small cell lung cancer. *Eur J Cancer* **32A**, 2070–2074.
18. Messa, C., Russo, F., Caruso, M. G., and Di, L. A. (1998) EGF, TGF-alpha, and EGF-R in human colorectal adenocarcinoma. *Acta Oncol* **37**, 285–289.
19. Rusch, V., Klimstra, D., Venkatraman, E., Pisters, P. W., Langenfeld, J., and Dmitrovsky, E. (1997) Overexpression of the epidermal growth factor receptor and its ligand transforming growth factor alpha is frequent in resectable non-small cell lung cancer but does not predict tumor progression. *Clin Cancer Res* **3**, 515–522.
20. Salomon, D. S., Brandt, R., Ciardiello, F., and Normanno, N. (1995) Epidermal growth factor-related peptides and their receptors in human malignancies. *Crit Rev Oncol Hematol* **19**, 183–232.
21. Uegaki, K., Nio, Y., Inoue, Y., Minari, Y., Sato, Y., Song, M. M., et al. (1997) Clinicopathological significance of epidermal growth factor and its receptor in human pancreatic cancer. *Anticancer Res* **17**, 3841–3847.
22. Walker, R. A. and Dearing, S. J. (1999) Expression of epidermal growth factor receptor mRNA and protein in primary breast carcinomas. *Breast Cancer Res Treat* **53**, 167–176.
23. Baselga, J., Tripathy, D., Mendelsohn, J., Baughman, S., Benz, C. C., Dantis, L., et al. (1996) Phase II study of weekly intravenous recombinant humanized anti-p185HER2 monoclonal antibody in patients with HER2/neu-overexpressing metastatic breast cancer. *J Clin Oncol* **14**, 737–744.
24. Cobleigh, M. A., Vogel, C. L., Tripathy, D., Robert, N. J., Scholl, S., Fehrenbacher, L., et al. (1999) Multinational study of the efficacy and safety of humanized anti-HER2 monoclonal antibody in women who have HER2-overexpressing metastatic breast cancer that has progressed after chemotherapy for metastatic disease. *J Clin Oncol* **17**, 2639–2648.
25. Nahta, R., Iglehart, J. D., Kempkes, B., and Schmidt, E. V. (2002) Rate-limiting effects of Cyclin D1 in transformation by ErbB2 predicts synergy between herceptin and flavopiridol. *Cancer Res* **62**, 2267–2271.
26. Xu, F., Lupu, R., Rodriguez, G. C., Whitaker, R. S., Boente, M. P., Berchuck, A., et al. (1993) Antibody-induced growth inhibition is mediated through immunochemically and functionally distinct epitopes on the extracellular domain of the c-erbB-2 (HER-2/neu) gene product p185. *Int J Cancer* **53**, 401–408.
27. Vogel, C. L., Cobleigh, M. A., Tripathy, D., Gutheil, J. C., Harris, L. N., Fehrenbacher, L., et al. (2002) Efficacy and safety of trastuzumab as a single agent in first-line treatment of HER2-overexpressing metastatic breast cancer. *J Clin Oncol* **20**, 719–726.
28. Braconi, C., Bracci, R., and Cellerino, R. (2008) Molecular targets in gastrointestinal stromal tumors (GIST) therapy. *Curr Cancer Drug Targets* **8**, 359–366.
29. Ellis, L. M. and Hicklin, D. J. (2008) VEGF-targeted therapy: mechanisms of anti-tumour activity. *Nat Rev Cancer* **8**, 579–591.
30. Hurwitz, H., Fehrenbacher, L., Novotny, W., Cartwright, T., Hainsworth, J., Heim, W., et al. (2004) Bevacizumab plus irinotecan, fluorouracil, and leucovorin for metastatic colorectal cancer. *N Engl J Med* **350**, 2335–2342.
31. Bergmann, U., Funatomi, H., Yokoyama, M., Beger, H. G., and Korc, M. (1995) Insulin-like growth factor I overexpression in human pancreatic cancer: evidence for autocrine and paracrine roles. *Cancer Res* **55**, 2007–2011.
32. Bergmann, U., Funatomi, H., Kornmann, M., Beger, H. G., and Korc, M. (1996) Increased expression of insulin receptor substrate-1 in human pancreatic cancer. *Biochem Biophys Res Commun* **220**, 886–890.
33. Ishiwata, T., Bergmann, U., Kornmann, M., Lopez, M., Beger, H. G., and Korc, M. (1997) Altered expression of insulin-like growth factor II receptor in human pancreatic cancer. *Pancreas* **15**, 367–373.
34. Rodon, J., DeSantos, V., Ferry, R. J., Jr., and Kurzrock, R. (2008) Early drug development of inhibitors of the insulin-like growth factor-I receptor pathway: lessons from the first clinical trials. *Mol Cancer Ther* **7**, 2575–2588.
35. Gomis, R. R., Alarcon, C., Nadal, C., Van, P. C., and Massague, J. (2006) C/EBPbeta at the core of the TGFbeta cytostatic response and its evasion in metastatic breast cancer cells. *Cancer Cell* **10**, 203–214.
36. Massague, J. and Gomis, R. R. (2006) The logic of TGFbeta signaling. *FEBS Lett* **580**, 2811–2820.
37. Weiner, T. M., Liu, E. T., Craven, R. J., and Cance, W. G. (1993) Expression of focal adhesion kinase gene and invasive cancer. *Lancet* **342**, 1024–1025.
38. Cance, W. G., Harris, J. E., Iacocca, M. V., Roche, E., Yang, X., Chang, J., et al. (2000) Immunohistochemical analyses of focal adhesion kinase expression in

benign and malignant human breast and colon tissues: correlation with preinvasive and invasive phenotypes. *Clin Cancer Res* **6**, 2417–2423.
39. Owens, L. V., Xu, L., Craven, R. J., Dent, G. A., Weiner, T. M., Kornberg, L., et al. (1995) Overexpression of the focal adhesion kinase (p125FAK) in invasive human tumors. *Cancer Res* **55**, 2752–2755.
40. Owens, L. V., Xu, L., Dent, G. A., Yang, X., Sturge, G. C., Craven, R. J., et al. (1996) Focal adhesion kinase as a marker of invasive potential in differentiated human thyroid cancer. *Ann Surg Oncol* **3**, 100–105.
41. Kurenova, E., Xu, L. H., Yang, X., Baldwin, A. S., Jr., Craven, R. J., Hanks, S. K., et al. (2004) Focal adhesion kinase suppresses apoptosis by binding to the death domain of receptor-interacting protein. *Mol Cell Biol* **24**, 4361–4371.
42. Golubovskaya, V. M., Finch, R., and Cance, W. G. (2005) Direct interaction of the N-terminal domain of focal adhesion kinase with the N-terminal transactivation domain of p53. *J Biol Chem* **280**, 25008–25021.
43. Golubovskaya, V. M. and Cance, W. G. (2007) Focal adhesion kinase and p53 signaling in cancer cells. *Int Rev Cytol* **263**, 103–153.
44. Garces, C. A., Kurenova, E. V., Golubovskaya, V. M., and Cance, W. G. (2006) Vascular endothelial growth factor receptor-3 and focal adhesion kinase bind and suppress apoptosis in breast cancer cells. *Cancer Res* **66**, 1446–1454.
45. Liu, W., Bloom, D. A., Cance, W. G., Kurenova, E. V., Golubovskaya, V. M., and Hochwald, S. N. (2008) FAK and IGF-IR interact to provide survival signals in human pancreatic adenocarcinoma cells. *Carcinogenesis* **29**, 1096–1107.
46. Beierle, E. A., Trujillo, A., Nagaram, A., Kurenova, E. V., Finch, R., Ma, X., et al. (2007) N-MYC regulates focal adhesion kinase expression in human neuroblastoma. *J Biol Chem* **282**, 12503–12516.
47. Choi, H. S., Wang, Z., Richmond, W., He, X., Yang, K., Jiang, T., et al. (2006) Design and synthesis of 7H-pyrrolo[2,3-d] pyrimidines as focal adhesion kinase inhibitors. Part 2. *Bioorg Med Chem Lett* **16**, 2689–2692.
48. Shi, Q., Hjelmeland, A. B., Keir, S. T., Song, L., Wickman, S., Jackson, D., et al. (2007) A novel low-molecular weight inhibitor of focal adhesion kinase, TAE226, inhibits glioma growth. *Mol Carcinog* **46**, 488–496.
49. Slack-Davis, J. K., Martin, K. H., Tilghman, R. W., Iwanicki, M., Ung, E. J., Autry, C., et al. (2007) Cellular characterization of a novel focal adhesion kinase inhibitor. *J Biol Chem* **282**, 14845–14852.
50. Roberts, W. G., Ung, E., Whalen, P., Cooper, B., Hulford, C., Autry, C., et al. (2008) Antitumor activity and pharmacology of a selective focal adhesion kinase inhibitor, PF-562,271. *Cancer Res* **68**, 1935–1944.
51. Bagi, C. M., Roberts, G. W., and Andresen, C. J. (2008) Dual focal adhesion kinase/Pyk2 inhibitor has positive effects on bone tumors: implications for bone metastases. *Cancer* **112**, 2313–2321.
52. Summy, J. M., Trevino, J. G., Lesslie, D. P., Baker, C. H., Shakespeare, W. C., Wang, Y., et al. (2005) AP23846, a novel and highly potent Src family kinase inhibitor, reduces vascular endothelial growth factor and interleukin-8 expression in human solid tumor cell lines and abrogates downstream angiogenic processes. *Mol Cancer Ther* **4**, 1900–1911.
53. Rucci, N., Susa, M., and Teti, A. (2008) Inhibition of protein kinase c-Src as a therapeutic approach for cancer and bone metastases. *Anticancer Agents Med Chem* **8**, 342–349.
54. Heath, J. R. and Davis, M. E. (2008) Nanotechnology and cancer. *Annu Rev Med* **59**, 251–265.

Chapter 3

Enhanced Permeability and Retention (EPR) Effect for Anticancer Nanomedicine Drug Targeting

Khaled Greish

Abstract

Effective cancer therapy remains one of the most challenging tasks to the scientific community, with little advancement on overall cancer survival landscape during the last two decades. A major limitation inherent to most conventional anticancer chemotherapeutic agents is their lack of tumor selectivity. One way to achieve selective drug targeting to solid tumors is to exploit abnormalities of tumor vasculature, namely hypervascularization, aberrant vascular architecture, extensive production of vascular permeability factors stimulating extravasation within tumor tissues, and lack of lymphatic drainage. Due to their large size, nano-sized macromolecular anticancer drugs administered intravenously (i.v.) escape renal clearance. Being unable to penetrate through tight endothelial junctions of normal blood vessels, their concentration builds up in the plasma rendering them long plasma half-life. More importantly, they can selectively extravasate in tumor tissues due to its abnormal vascular nature. Overtime the tumor concentration will build up reaching several folds higher than that of the plasma due to lack of efficient lymphatic drainage in solid tumor, an ideal application for EPR-based selective anticancer nanotherapy. Indeed, this selective high local concentration of nano-sized anticancer drugs in tumor tissues has proven superior in therapeutic effect with minimal side effects in both preclinical and clinical settings.

Key words: EPR effect, nanomedicines, half-life, targeted anticancer therapy, macromolecular drugs, tumor model, in vivo, biodistribution.

1. Introduction

Anticancer chemotherapy is one of the most notorious drugs known to human. The sole purpose of their use is cell killing, a task that usually achieved with high efficacy but little precision. Most anticancer chemotherapeutic agents used in clinic target dividing cells, regardless of its nature whether a dividing tumor cell or active intestinal epithelial cells, with same potency. The term of maximum tolerated dose thus is not based on the amount needed to cure the disease, conversely on the amount needed not to incapacitate the host. Alternatively, anticancer targeting proved to be a more effective approach with minimum toxicity. On the gross level, tumor vasculature proved to be a potential target for cancer treatment. Tumor vascular typically comprised of poorly aligned defective endothelial cells with wide fenestrations (up to 4 μm), lacking smooth muscle layer or innervations, with relatively wide lumen and impaired receptor function for vasoactive mediators especially angiotensin II; further they lack functional lymphatics (1–5). In addition, hyperproduction of vascular mediators, such as vascular endothelial growth factor, bradykinin, nitric oxide peroxynitrite, prostaglandins, and matrix metalloproteinases (6–10), contributes greatly to this hyperpermeability in tumor tissues. EPR effect involves two major components, first altered biodistribution, where the nano-size drug shows differential accumulation in the tumor tissues reaching higher concentration than that in the plasma or other organs (**Fig. 3.1A**), this effect is time dependent and can be reproduced in tumors of different size as shown in **Fig. 3.1B**. EPR effect is mainly the function of molecular weight with molecules ranging 40–800 kD can exhibit preferential tumor targeting (**Fig. 3.1C**).

The other aspect of EPR effect is increased plasma half-life of the nano-size drugs as their size exceeded the limit of renal excretion threshold, limiting their clearance (**Fig. 3.1D**). As pharmacological effect and plasma concentration are parallel, this phenomenon results in prolonged therapeutic effect in addition to targeting (11, 12). The gain expected from EPR effect is in the magnitude of 7- to 10-fold higher tumor concentration compared to equivalent doses of the same drug at low molecular weight form (13). EPR is a passive phenomenon that can be actively augmented by the following techniques related to the abnormalities of tumor vasculature.

1.1. Hypertension

In normal blood vessels, the smooth muscle layer responds to vascular mediators such as bradykinin, acetylcholine, NO, and calcium via the receptors on smooth muscle cells of blood vessels, and hence helps maintain constant blood flow volume (**Fig. 3.2 a B**). Raising the systolic blood pressure from 100 to 150 mm Hg for 15 min by infusing angiotensin II (AT II) into tumor-bearing rats caused 2- to 6-fold selective increase in tumor blood flow; blood flow in normal organs and tissues remained constant regardless of the induced blood pressure (14). When ^{51}Cr-labeled-SMANCS or ^{51}Cr-albumin was injected i.v. under AT-II-induced hypertension, 3-fold higher accumulation was achieved in tumor tissue compared to normotensive condition. Additionally, the amount of drug delivered to normal organs such as kidney and bone marrow was reduced because of the

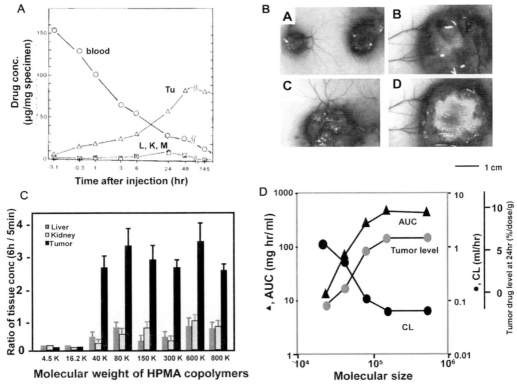

Fig. 3.1. Selective accumulation of Evans blue dye bound to albumin (70 kDa) in S 180 tumor in DdY mice. **a**, Blood concentration versus tumor, liver, kidney, and muscle. The graph represents the result of methods in **Section 3.2**. **b**, EBD accumulation in small tumor (A), large tumor (B), (C) shows the retention of the dye at 24 h and (D) is cross section of (B), the central region of the tumor is necrotic and avascular, and hence does not facilitate the uptake of nano-size EBD. **c**, The accumulation of ^{125}I-labeled *N*-(2-hydroxypropyl) methacrylamide (HPMA) copolymer in the solid tumor tissues. Note that large macromolecules, but not smaller ones, manifest progressive accumulation. **d**, The relation between molecular weight, AUC, tumor accumulation, and renal clearance. (Reproduced from 27 with permission from Imperial College Press.)

vasoconstriction occurring in normal organs under AT-II-induced hypertension. However, mitomycin C (334.3 Da) did not produce the same effect under the same experimental conditions (15). Better therapeutic effect could be demonstrated in the clinical setting, by using this method with SMANCS/Lipiodol for tumors such as cholangiocarcinoma, metastatic liver cancer, and renal cancer (16).

1.2. Bradykinin (BK)

BK-generating cascade is normally activated in tumor tissues and was found to be involved in accumulation of malignant ascitic and pleural fluids in cancer patients. Various human and rodent solid tumors express excessive levels of BK receptor B2 (7–9). BK is degraded by many peptidases, especially angiotensin-converting enzyme (ACE). Therefore, ACE inhibitors can cause local increase of BK levels at the tumor site. On the basis of these data, we used the ACE inhibitors enalapril and temocapril

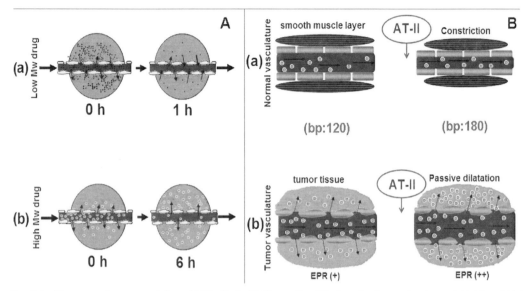

Fig. 3.2. Diagrammatic representation of EPR effect. (**A**) Shows the diffusion of a low molecular weight (*a*) and high molecular weight drug (*b*). Note progressive accumulation of macromolecular drug in the tumor tissues with time by the EPR effect. (**B**) Vascular leakage in relation to AT-II. Note that under AT-II-induced hypertensive state (**B**-*a*), vasoconstriction in the normal blood vessels occurs due to the presence of smooth muscle layer, while tumor vessels (**B**-*b*), passively dilate due to the absence of smooth muscle layer leading to enhanced extravasations of macromolecular drugs and hence augmentation of EPR effect. (Reproduced from 26 with permission from Elsevier.)

to inhibit BK degradation, this resulted in elevated BK level and further enhancement of the EPR effect (17). ACE inhibitors thus increase delivery of macromolecular drugs to tumors, even under normotensive conditions (**Fig. 3.3**).

1.3. Nitric Oxide (NO)

NO plays a key role in angiogenesis, cell proliferation, and EPR effect. NO is synthesized by NO synthase (NOS) from L-arginine. Consequently, inhibition of NO generation by NOS inhibitors as *N*-monomethyl-L-arginine was found to suppress tumor growth (7, 8, 10). NOS inhibitor irreversibly attenuated blood flow in R3230Ac rat mammary adenocarcinoma (18). In addition, we found that pro-matrix metalloproteinases (proMMPs) are activated by peroxynitrite (ONOO–), which is produced extensively in tumor and inflammatory tissues (19). Clinically, we have utilized the vasodilator effect of NO to increase the delivery of the nanomedicine drug SMANCS to tumor site in hepatocellular carcinoma by local injection of isosorbide dinitrate (ISDN) into the tumor-feeding artery (**Fig. 3.4**).

1.4. Photodynamic Therapy (PDT)

When a photosensitizer is administrated systemically or locally and subsequently activated by illumination with visible light, this leads to the generation of reactive oxygen species. This effect has active role in enhancing tumor vascular permeability (20, 21). The concentration of nano-size FITC-dextran was 5-fold higher

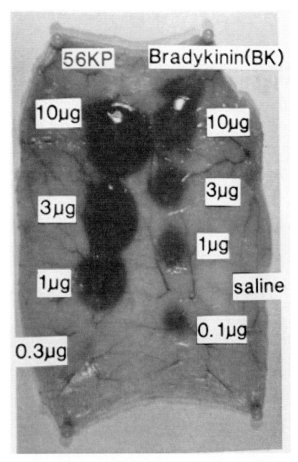

Fig. 3.3. Enhancement of permeability in the skin of guinea pig after SC injection of various doses of BK and the 56 kDa protease which induces kallikrein–kinin system. EBD was injected intravenously after 10 min of SC injection. The results show the enhancement of permeability at 6 h after injection of EBD.

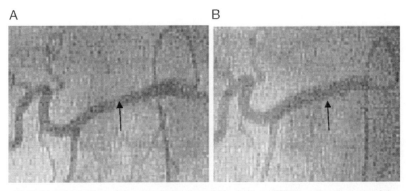

Fig. 3.4. The effect of local injection of the vasodilator isosorbide dinitrate (ISDN) on the diameter of the proper hepatic artery (*arrow*): (**a**) before ISDN and (**b**) after ISDN injection. Note the 187% increase in the vessel diameter (**b**), this technique was successfully used in the clinic to enhance SMANCS targeting into hepatic tumors.

in orthotropic MatLyLu rat prostate tumors treated with the photosensitizer verteporfin, at 15 min following light irradiation, compared to nonirradiated control group (21). Photosensitization causes endothelial cell microtubule depolymerization and induces the formation of actin stress fibers. Thus, endothelial cells were found to retract, leading to the formation of intercellular gaps, which result in enhanced vascular permeability. In addition, endothelial cell damage leads to the establishment of thrombogenic sites within the vessel lumen, and this initiates a physiological cascade of responses including platelet aggregation, the release of vasoactive molecules, leukocyte adhesion, and increases in vascular permeability (20). We have used the photosensitizer ZnPP to enhance tumor permeability and could achieve 3-fold higher accumulation of the Evans blue dye in tumor tissue after 5 min irradiation with ambient light (**Fig. 3.5**).

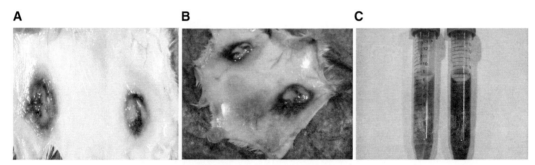

Fig. 3.5. Enhancement of the EPR effect by photodynamic therapy (PDT). (**a**), EBD concentration in S-180 murine sarcoma without PDT. (**b**) 15 min after injection of 5 mg/kg ZnPP photosensitizer, animals were injected with EBD 10 mg/kg. After another 30 min of ZnPP injection, animals were irradiated for 5 min at 50.000 Lux, 4 h after irradiation animals were scarified and EBD was quantified. (**c**), ZnPP-mediated photoactivity enhanced the EPR effect by 3-fold magnitude.

2. Materials

2.1. Establishment of In Vivo Tumor Model

1. Mouse sarcoma S-180 cells, ATCC Number TIB-66 (Manassas, VA).
2. Male DdY mice, 6 weeks old weighing 30–35 g (SLC, Inc., Shizuoka, Japan).
3. Isoflurane (MWI Veterinary Supply, MERIDIAN, ID).
4. Isoflurane vaporizer system (V3000PK, Parkland Scientific, Coral Springs, FL).

2.2. Demonstration of EPR Effect in Tumor Model

1. Evans blue dye (EBD) (Sigma Chemical Co., St. Louis, MO).
2. Formamide reagent grade, 98% (Sigma Chemical Co., St. Louis, MO).
3. Isoton II (Coulter Corporation, Miami, FL).

2.3. Styrene Maleic Acid (SMA) – Micelle Preparation

1. SMA (Kuraray Ltd., Kurashiki, Japan).
2. 1-Ethyl-3-(3-dimethylaminopropyl) carbodiimide (EDAC) (Dojindo, Kumamoto, Japan).
3. Doxorubicin (Sigma Chemical Co., St. Louis, MO).
4. Amicon ultrafiltration system (YM-10 membrane; cut-off molecular size of 10 kDa) (Millipore, Bedford, MA).

2.4. Pharmacokinetics of Nano-sized Micelle of Doxorubicin Versus Free Drug

1. ^{14}C Doxorubicin hydrochloride, 91.9% radio chemically pure with a specific radioactivity of 3.5 MBq/mg (Amersham, Buckinghamshire, UK).
2. Soluene-350 (Packard Instruments, Groningen, the Netherlands).
3. Hionic Fluor LSC cocktail (Packard Instruments, Meriden, CT).
4. Beta liquid scintillation counters (LSC-5100, Aloka, Tokyo, Japan).

3. Methods

3.1. Establishment of In Vivo Tumor Model

1. Inject 5×10^6 S-180 cells in 1 mL PBS into the right lower quadrant of the abdomen of DdY mice using 27-G needle.
2. Observe animals for 7–10 days, this is a proper time to aspirate the resulting ascetic fluid of tumor; longer time will result in bloody aspirate.
3. Euthanize animal using CO_2 for 2 min.
4. Place the animal on its side and insert G18 needle mounted 10 mL syringe into the most gravity-dependent point and aspirate cells.
5. Cells to be diluted with five times cold sterile PBS and centrifuged at 800 rpm at 4°C for 5 min to remove proteins and blood from cancer cells, repeat for two times or until the cell precipitates become clear.
6. Repeat Steps 1–5 for another extra passage before inducing SC tumor to insure high tumorgenic ability of cells.
7. Count a small sample of cell (5 µL) using trypan blue dye in hemocytometer.
8. Prepare 2×10^6 cells per 200 µL PBS and keep in ice.
9. Anesthetize animals using 3–4% isoflurane for 2–3 min in induction chamber of the vapor anesthesia system, then move animals to warm heated blanket, and use nose cone for anesthesia.

10. Shave two bilateral dorsal sites where tumor injection is intended.

11. Lay anesthetized animal ventrally, raise a dorsal skin fold with a tweezers, clean it with gauze soaked in 70% ethanol, and at near horizontal angel, insert the 27 G needle mounted on 1-mL syringe, inject cell slowly to prevent leakage from injection site. The development of SC bleb indicates successful injection.

12. Follow the animal daily for 7–10 days, at this time usually animal will develop tumors of 5–7 mm diameter which are optimal for EPR-related studies.

3.2. Demonstration of EPR Effect in Tumor Tissues

1. Dissolve Evans blue dye (EBD) in DW at final concentrations of 1 mg/mL, and then adjust the concentration to give final dose of 10 mg/kg of mice weight in 0.2 mL.

2. As the tumor reaches the diameter of 7 mm, immobilize the animal in immobilization chamber and inject 0.2 EBD in saline into the tail vein.

3. At each time point of evaluation, euthanize animals in CO_2 chamber for 2 min.

4. Place the animal ventrally and through midline incision, expose inferior vena cava, collect 0.2 mL of blood, and mix instantly with 2.8 mL of Isoton II, followed by centrifugation at 800 rpm for 5 min, then read by spectrophotometer at 620 nm.

5. After blood collection, cut the diaphragm and expose the heart, grasp the heart with tweezers, and using 20-mL syringe with 24-G needle, inject 20 mL of saline slowly into the left side of the heart to remove the dye from the blood component of any organ.

6. Expose the dorsal skin having the tumor, visually document the EBD color in the tumor tissue in contrast to surrounding skin using camera, remove the tumor from the base using surgical scissor, weigh, and add to 3 mL formamide.

7. Collect sample from other tissue similarly, weigh, and add to 3 mL formamide.

8. Incubate at 60°C water bath with shaking for 48 h to extract EBD.

9. Read by spectrophotometer at 620 nm and convert the reading into μg EBD/mg tissue using standard curve of EBD.

3.3. Preparing SMA-Micelles

1. Dissolve SMA powder in water at pH 5.0 at 10 mg/mL.

2. Dropwise add doxorubicin solution in DW at a concentration of 10 mg/mL.

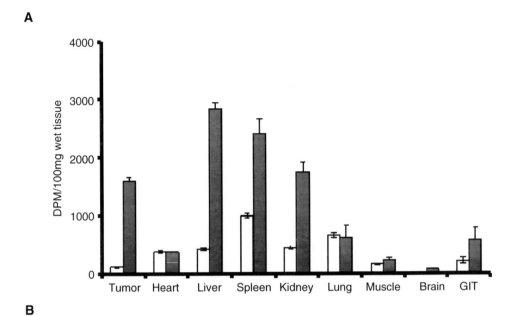
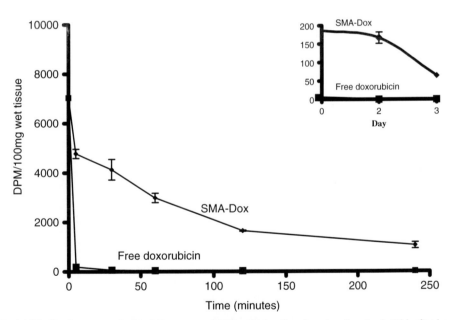

Fig. 3.6. (a) Micellar drug concentration in tumor was 13 times higher than free drug in animals 24 h after i.v. administration. (b) The $t^{1}/_{2}\,\alpha$ (half-life) of SMA-Dox micelles increased about 400-fold, while the area-under-concentration (AUC) time curve was 25 times greater than that of free drug when calculated for up to 3 days, the graph describes the result of method in **Section 3.4**. (Reproduced from 13 with permission from Elsevier.)

3. Add water soluble carbodiimide (EDAC) 10 mg/mL. The solution will precipitate.

4. Wash precipitates by centrifugation at 8,000 rpm for 5 min twice, and then reconstitute in pH 7, leave for 60 min to totally solubilize the micelles.

5. Wash and concentrate the micelle to one-tenth of the original volume by ultrafiltration with the Amicon ultrafiltration, repeat three times.

6. Measure concentration of the resulting micelle through UV, comparing it to standard curve of the absorbance of free doxorubicin.

3.4. Pharmacokinetics and Drug Distribution

1. Use animal model as described in **Section 3.1**.

2. Divide animals into two groups, control the group to receive radio-labeled free doxorubicin, and test the group to receive radio-labeled SMA-Dox micelles. Inject 5 mg/kg of doxorubicin equivalent through the tail vein in a 0.2-mL volume saline.

3. At scheduled time points, euthanize mice in CO_2 and collect blood samples from the inferior vena cava as in Step 4 of **Section 3.2**.

4. Inject 20 mL of saline to remove blood components from the blood vessels in the tissues as in Step 5 of **Section 3.2**, then collect and weigh tumor tissues, liver, kidney, gastrointestinal tract (GIT), heart, lung, brain, and muscles.

5. Mix each 100 mg sample of tissue with 1 mL of Soluene-350, solubilize the mixtures by incubation at 60°C for 4 h, after which add to 10 mL of Hionic Fluor LSC cocktail.

6. Measure the radioactivity of plasma and various tissues by using a beta liquid scintillation counter (**Fig. 3.6**).

4. Notes

1. Both xenogeneic and syngeneic animal models can be used; syngeneic model is preferred as it ensures natural tumor vessels development accounting for role of immunomodulators secreted by infiltrating neutrophils and macrophages on the tumor vasculature (22, 23).

2. Cancer cells should be passaged in animals twice before starting the final experiment.

3. Cell number needed to establish tumor in animals can vary from one tumor cell line to the other, usually ranges from 1 to 5 million cell per injection site.

4. Number of animal per experiment is chosen according to the time points, many points needed to be selected to reflect both the pharmacokinetics of free drug and the nano-sized drug (5, 30,120, 480, 720 min, and 1–2 days) are example of the time points that can be used.

5. Tumor size of 5–7 mm in diameter (7–10) must be used; larger tumor size tends to have poor vascularization as tumor necrosis develops centrally with collapse of the fragile tumor vasculature (**Fig. 3.1B, D**). Animals having under- or over-grown tumors should be removed.

6. Metastatic models can be used, however, metastatic tumor tends to show poor EPR effect due to its more deranged vessel development (24).

7. When injecting the tumor cells subcutaneously, avoid the hind limb of the animal as rapid growth of the tumor can affect animal mobility.

8. The use of SMA-micelles is experimental example; it can be substituted with any nano-sized drug of molecular weight above 40 kDa (**Fig. 3.1C**).

9. The injected dose calculation should be based on the active ingredient (cargo) dose, not on the total gram value of injected material including the polymer carrier.

10. Many macromolecular drug combine with plasma protein changing their in vivo molecular weight and biological properties, this phenomenon is species specific (25).

11. In the previous experimental examples, UV and radioactivity detection methods were used, in addition fluorescence properties could also be used. However, radioactivity detection is the most accurate and time efficient.

12. Ideal experiment should delineate the concentration of the carrier polymer from the drug cargo, double labeling of both the carrier polymer and the drug carrier can address this issue.

13. Expected gain of EPR effect is ∼7- to 10-fold higher tumor concentration compared to free low molecular weight drug, combining passive EPR targeting with hypertension, ISDN, PDT, or ACE inhibitor can result in up to 30-fold higher tumor accumulation (26).

14. EPR effect is not limited to pharmacokinetics and biodistribution, the main benefit is more effective anticancer therapy with fewer side effects. In vivo anticancer assay and toxicity study complement the study of EPR effect.

15. EPR effect can also similarly be demonstrated in inflammatory tissue, however, less retention time is always observed compared to tumor tissues (11).

Acknowledgments

The author gratefully acknowledges the support of Prof. Hiroshi Maeda. The EPR effect was first described and extensively studied by Prof. Maeda's group. Techniques related to EPR effect, described in this chapter, were developed by Maeda's group in the Department of Microbiology, Kumamoto University, Japan.

References

1. Folkman, J. (1971) Tumor angiogenesis: therapeutic implications. *N Engl J Med* **285**, 1182–1186.
2. Skinner, S. A., Tutton, P. J., and O'Brien, P. E. (1990) Microvascular architecture of experimental colon tumors in the rat. *Cancer Res* **50**, 2411–2417.
3. Yuan, F., Salehi, H. A., Boucher, Y., Vasthare, U. S., Tuma, R. F., and Jain, R. K. (1994) Vascular permeability and microcirculation of gliomas and mammary carcinomas transplanted in rat and mouse cranial windows. *Cancer Res* **54**, 4564–4568.
4. Folkman, J. (1995) Angiogenesis in cancer, vascular, rheumatoid and other disease. *Nat Med* **1**, 27–31.
5. Hashizume, H., Baluk, P., Morikawa, S., McLean, J. W., Thurston, G., Roberge, S., Jain, R. K., and McDonald, D. M. (2000) Openings between defective endothelial cells explain tumor vessel leakiness. *Am J Pathol* **156**, 1363–1380.
6. Noguchi, Y., Wu, J., Duncan, R., Strohalm, J., Ulbrich, K., Akaike, T., and Maeda, H. (1998) Early phase tumor accumulation of macromolecules: a great difference in clearance rate between tumor and normal tissues. *Jpn J Cancer Res* **89**, 307–314.
7. Wu, J., Akaike, T., and Maeda, H. (1998) Modulation of enhanced vascular permeability in tumors by a bradykinin antagonist, a cyclooxygenase inhibitor, and a nitric oxide scavenger. *Cancer Res* **58**, 159–165.
8. Maeda, H., Akaike, T., Wu, J., Noguchi, Y., and Sakata, Y. (1996) Bradykinin and nitric oxide in infectious disease and cancer. *Immunopharmacology* **33**, 222–230.
9. Maeda, H., Matsumura, Y., and Kato, H. (1988) Purification and identification of [hydroxyprolyl3]bradykinin in ascitic fluid from a patient with gastric cancer. *J Biol Chem* **263**, 16051–16054.
10. Doi, K., Akaike, T., Horie, H., Noguchi, Y., Fujii, S., Beppu, T., Ogawa, M., and Maeda, H. (1996) Excessive production of nitric oxide in rat solid tumor and its implication in rapid tumor growth. *Cancer* **77**, 1598–1604.
11. Matsumura, Y. and Maeda, H. (1986) A new concept for macromolecular therapeutics in cancer chemotherapy: mechanism of tumoritropic accumulation of proteins and the antitumor agent smancs. *Cancer Res* **46**, 6387–6392.
12. Seymour, L. W., Miyamoto, Y., Maeda, H., Brereton, M., Strohalm, J., Ulbrich, K., and Duncan, R. (1995) Influence of molecular weight on passive tumour accumulation of a soluble macromolecular drug carrier. *Eur J Cancer* **31A**, 766–770.
13. Greish, K., Sawa, T., Fang, J., Akaike, T., and Maeda, H. (2004) SMA-doxorubicin, a new polymeric micellar drug for effective targeting to solid tumours. *J Control Release* **97**, 219–230.
14. Suzuki, M., Hori, K., Abe, I., Saito, S., and Sato, H. (1981) A new approach to cancer chemotherapy: selective enhancement of tumor blood flow with angiotensin II. *J Natl Cancer Inst* **67**, 663–669.
15. Li, C. J., Miyamoto, Y., Kojima, Y., and Maeda, H. (1993) Augmentation of tumour delivery of macromolecular drugs with reduced bone marrow delivery by elevating blood pressure. *Br J Cancer* **67**, 975–980.
16. Greish, K., Fang, J., Inutsuka, T., Nagamitsu, A., and Maeda, H. (2003) Macromolecular therapeutics: advantages and prospects with special emphasis on solid tumour targeting. *Clin Pharmacokinet* **42**, 1089–1105.
17. Tanaka, S., Akaike, T., Wu, J., Fang, J., Sawa, T., Ogawa, M., Beppu, T., and Maeda, H. (2003) Modulation of tumor-selective vascular blood flow and extravasation by the stable prostaglandin 12 analogue beraprost sodium. *J Drug Target* **11**, 45–52.
18. Meyer, R. E., Shan, S., DeAngelo, J., Dodge, R. K., Bonaventura, J., Ong, E. T., and Dewhirst, M. W. (1995) Nitric oxide synthase inhibition irreversibly decreases

perfusion in the R3230Ac rat mammary adenocarcinoma. *Br J Cancer* **71**, 1169–1174.
19. Okamoto, T., Akaike, T., Sawa, T., Miyamoto, Y., van der Vliet, A., and Maeda, H. (2001) Activation of matrix metalloproteinases by peroxynitrite-induced protein S-glutathiolation via disulfide S-oxide formation. *J Biol Chem* **276**, 29596–29602.
20. Dougherty, T. J., Gomer, C. J., Henderson, B. W., Jori, G., Kessel, D., Korbelik, M., Moan, J., and Peng, Q. (1998) Photodynamic therapy. *J Natl Cancer Inst* **90**, 889–905.
21. Chen, B., Pogue, B. W., Luna, J. M., Hardman, R. L., Hoopes, P. J., and Hasan, T. (2006) Tumor vascular permeabilization by vascular-targeting photosensitization: effects, mechanism, and therapeutic implications. *Clin Cancer Res* **12**, 917–923.
22. Nozawa, H., Chiu, C., and Hanahan, D. (2008) Infiltrating neutrophils mediate the initial angiogenic switch in a mouse model of multistage carcinogenesis. *Proc Natl Acad Sci USA* **33**, 12493–12498.
23. Furuya, M. and Yonemitsu, Y. (2008) Cancer neovascularization and proinflammatory microenvironments. *Curr Cancer Drug Targets* **4**, 253–265.
24. Nagamitsu, A., Inuzuka, T., Greish, K., and Maeda, H. (2007) SMANCS Dynamic therapy for various advanced solid tumors and promising clinical effects enhanced drug delivery by hydrodynamic modulation with vascular mediators, particularly angiotensin II, during arterial infusion. *DDS* **22**, 510–522.
25. Pahlman, I. and Gozzi, P. (1999) Serum protein binding of tolterodine and its major metabolites in humans and several animal species. *Biopharm Drug Dispos* **2**, 91–99.
26. Iyer, A. K., Khaled, G., Fang, J., and Maeda, H. (2006) Exploiting the enhanced permeability and retention effect for tumor targeting. *Drug Discov Today* **11**, 812–818.
27. Greish, K., Arun, I., Fang, J., and Maeda, H. (2006) Enhanced permeability and retention (EPR) effect and tumor-selective delivery of anticancer drugs. In *Delivery of Protein and Peptide Drugs in Cancer.* V. P. Torchilin(Ed.), Imperial College Press, London, 37–52.

Chapter 4

Nanoparticle Characterization for Cancer Nanotechnology and Other Biological Applications

Scott C. Brown, Maria Palazuelos, Parvesh Sharma, Kevin W. Powers, Stephen M. Roberts, Stephen R. Grobmyer, and Brij M. Moudgil

Abstract

Nanotechnology is actively being used to develop promising diagnostics and therapeutics tools for the treatment of cancer and many other diseases. The unique properties of nanomaterials offer an exciting frontier of possibilities for biomedical researchers and scientists. Because existing knowledge of macroscopic materials does not always allow for adequate prediction of the characteristics and behaviors of nanoscale materials in controlled environments, much less in biological systems, careful nanoparticle characterization should accompany biomedical applications of these materials. Informed correlations between adequately characterized nanomaterial properties and reliable biological endpoints are essential for guiding present and future researchers toward clinical nanotechnology-based solutions for cancer. Biological environments are notoriously dynamic; hence, nanoparticulate interactions within these environments will likely be comparatively diverse. For this reason, we recommend that an interactive and systematic approach to material characterization be taken when attempting to elucidate or measure biological interactions with nanoscale materials. We intend for this chapter to be a practical guide that could be used by researchers to identify key nanomaterial characteristics that require measurement for their systems and the appropriate techniques to perform those measurements. Each section includes a basic overview of each measurement and notes on how to address some of the common difficulties associated with nanomaterial characterization.

Key words: Nanomaterial characterization, nanotoxicology, particulates, characterization techniques, cancer nanotechnology, nanoparticles.

1. Introduction

Nanotechnology holds significant promise for catalyzing the development of new, paradigm changing tools and treatments for the diagnosis, treatment, and potential eradication of cancer. The impact of cancer nanotechnology is anticipated to be large and far-reaching as evidenced by the dramatic increase in scientific literature relating to this topic. Engineered nanoparticulate systems, are attractive for a wide range of biomedical applications due to their unique properties. Differences between the physiochemical behavior of bulk materials and nanoparticulates can be large, and sometimes unexpected. These differences are often attributed to their high surface area to mass ratio, quantum or physical confinement effects, or other lesser known phenomena that become prevalent when materials become ultrasmall.

It is becoming increasingly evident that nanoscale features and particulate matter can have a dramatic affect on physiological systems. Protein adsorption (1–3) and cellular function (e.g., adhesion, differentiation, growth, motility, and morbidity) (4–9) have been shown to be significantly altered by the presence of nanoscale asperities and chemical domains. In recent years, the potential risks associated with nano-sized materials have been recognized by both government agencies and academic research groups alike (10, 11). However, few systematic investigations into the specific properties of nanoscale particulate materials that result in altered biological response have been conducted. The majority of the researches attempting to assess the risks or benefits associated with nanoparticulates fail to provide adequate characterization of the administered materials. This lack of detail hinders the delineation of fundamental nanoparticulate attributes that result in biological responses and may invalidate comparisons between different studies.

For instance, in the field of particle toxicology, several authors have demonstrated that for some materials a better fit of the dose–response relationship is achieved by using surface area – rather than mass – as the dosimetric unit for particles of the "same material" but of different size (12–16). Although these examples appear convincing, the lack of adequate nanoparticle characterization in these studies draws questions as to the fundamental mechanisms involved. Are the results a direct manifestation of enhanced exposure to the inherent particle surface properties, or do they merely illustrate that contamination probability increases with increasing surface area? It can be argued that smaller particles simply serve as more efficient carriers of environmental toxins to the biological environment, based on surface area and energetic considerations. Because of the lack of materials characterization, carbon nanotube materials were originally believed to be highly cytotoxic; however, it is now suggested that much of the perceived toxicity was due to residual catalyst used in making the materials rather than the nanostructures themselves (11, 17). These examples illustrate just a couple of the many "loose ends" that can be used to contest results when adequate particle characterization is not present. It is not uncommon for the surface properties, shape, crystal structure, dissolution profiles, and surface reactivity of particles with identical chemical composition to change with respect to their size and/or method of synthesis, not to mention the type and extent of trace chemical contaminants that might be present. Proper biological assessment of nanomaterials needs to include detailed characterization in order to address these and other related issues.

The administration of nanomaterials to biological systems results in a complex dynamic cascade of biotic/abiotic physicochemical interactions that ultimately define the materials behavior, disposition, and fate in physiological environments. To make strides in cancer nanotechnology, it is important that both biological and nanomaterial systems are well understood, both when separate and when together. A thorough materials analysis is imperative for drawing fundamental insights into the behavior of nanomaterials in vivo, in vitro, and to facilitate comparisons with other researchers. Informed correlations between adequately characterized nanomaterial properties and reliable biological end points are essential for guiding present and future researchers toward clinical nanotechnology-based solutions for cancer.

To date, few nanotoxicology studies and even fewer cancer nanotechnology research studies have characterized the administered nanoparticulate materials with enough thoroughness to contribute to a mechanistic understanding of the structure–property relationships regarding the implication of nanomaterials in normal and/or diseased hosts. In biological fluids, nanoparticle characteristics such as particle-size distribution and surface chemistry often change due to fluid–particle interactions (e.g., biomolecule/ion adsorption, dissolution, and oxidation). Therefore, particle characterization should be conducted both (i) on the material prior to administration (as received from manufacturer or in the original preparation) and (ii) under physiologically relevant conditions (e.g., in media, plasma and other biological fluids) (18, 19). Further, the influence of possible mechanical interactions such as fluid shear or tissue movement-induced interactions should not be neglected (20, 21).

The development of nanotechnologies for biomedical applications and nanotoxicology research involve complex problems that require multidisciplinary expertise from diverse fields such as medicine, chemistry, toxicology, chemical engineering and materials science to arrive at adequate solutions. Since the key parameters affecting the biological activity of nanomaterials may vary widely and are largely unknown, it is recommended that the characterization of test materials be as broad and comprehensive as possible (18, 19). A series of guidelines and/or recommended practices for characterization of nanomaterials for toxicity assessment have been developed with the aid of several national and international working groups (10, 11, 18, 19, 22–24). It is further recommended that an interactive and systematic approach to material characterization be taken when attempting to elucidate or measure biological interactions with nanoscale materials. Biological environments are notoriously dynamic; hence, nanoparticulate interactions within these environments will likely be comparatively diverse. Extrapolation or generalization of these interactions to that of different nanomaterials and/or organisms is cautioned until a fundamental understanding of the mechanisms governing these phenomena is acquired.

The research community is currently working to develop reference protocols for nanomaterial characterization. Most of these are still under development and are expected to vary significantly with technique and the materials to be tested. The National Cancer Institute (NCI) is leading this effort through a collaboration with the National Institute of Standards and Technology (NIST) (25). Various protocols developed for the testing of preclinical toxicology, pharmacology, and efficacy of nanoparticles and devices are available on the Nanotechnology Characterization Laboratory (NCL) web site (22). The full list of recommended physiochemical characterization protocols is still under development and as of the time this chapter, only one protocol has been made publicly available, despite the recognized need for thorough and systematic nanoparticle characterization. The available protocol describes nanoparticle-size measurement in aqueous media using dynamic light scattering and is openly available (26). Other protocols and best practices are expected in the near future.

The following sections provide an overview of important characterization parameters, methods, and general recommendations that can be applied to describe materials used for cancer nanotechnology.

2. Methods

2.1. Sampling and Storage

Meaningful characterization of any material starts with the proper collection and storage of representative samples for analysis. Nanomaterials can be very homogenous and monodispersed in nature or quite the opposite. It is important to collect as much information as possible from the manufacturer. This will greatly facilitate the characterization of the as-received materials. The amount of material acquired should be enough for both the biological assessment and the material characterization experiments and ideally should come from the same lot or batch. Nanomaterials can greatly vary in their properties depending on the manufacturing method, age, and storage conditions, thus consistency between the characterization results and the biological observations will only be guaranteed if the same batch of material is used for all experiments. All nanomaterials to be tested should be stored in a manner that inhibits sample degradation (e.g., under inert atmospheres). In many instances, nanomaterials may be functionalized by a biomolecule and received in a lyophilized state or as a frozen suspension. Storage at reduced temperatures to prevent the degradation of the attached biomolecules is recommended; however, the implication of these storage conditions on the nanomaterials should not go unchecked. Some best practices when sampling powders recommended by the National Institute of Standards and Technology (27) include

- When possible sample from a "flowing" powder by using standard apparatus like the spinning riffler. Small samples and/or light materials with tendency to suspend in air may need to be sampled by scooping. If that is the case powder should be properly mixed and subsamples should be taken from different areas of the bulk.

- If possible, take the sample from a liquid suspension to avoid exposure to airborne nanoparticles and to facilitate dispersion. Dispersant aids may be used to measure the "primary" particle size but should not be used for toxicity assessment unless they are biocompatible and biorelevant (e.g., lung surfactant on inhalation exposures).

- Avoid contamination by using clean utensils and storing materials in properly sealed containers. Stability of properties should be checked overtime to account for potential aging of the particles and other potential instabilities of the samples.

Although sampling from well-dispersed nanoparticulate suspensions is usually not a major issue, special care should be exercised with samples that aggregate and rapidly settle. These suspensions should be agitated as need (e.g., mild vortexing) prior to aliquoting.

2.2. Size Distribution and Shape Information

Particle-size distribution. Particle size is the most frequently reported nanoparticle attribute in nanoparticle research studies; however, it is routinely insufficiently characterized. This is a critical oversight since emerging evidence illustrates that biological interactions with nanoparticulate materials can be size dependent. The deposition profile of inhaled particulate matter, the ability of particles to translocate within the body, cellular uptake, and adsorbed biomolecule activity are just a few of the biotic/abiotic interactions that are dependent on particle size (11). For diagnostic and therapeutic applications, nanoparticle pharmacokinetics and tumor targeting capacity can be dramatically influenced by particle size (28). Particulate systems are seldom perfectly monodispersed (particularly in biological environments) and normally consist of population of particles or aggregates that fall within different size classes. For broad or aggregated distributions, the common practice of reporting a single mean particle size, or values obtained from the manufacturer without verification, is inadequate and often misleading. Mean values are also highly dependent on the weighting factor (e.g., number weighted or volume weighted distributions) used to report or depict the particle size. Particle-size distributions (PSDs) depicted in both number and volume percent distributions, as indicated in **Fig. 4.1**, are helpful in assessing the nature of particulate systems and are recommended to be reported in this manner. Corresponding tabular statistical data are also encouraged. By reporting more than one particle mean, a more complete depiction of the PSD is achieved. Differences in the mean values are indicative of polydispersity in size and/or extent of agglomeration. The breadth and shape of the size distribution is often not reflected in the mean values reported by the manufacturers as calculated from the BET surface area measurements. It is always recommended that manufacturer reported values are confirmed by independent methods to ensure accuracy.

Important issues to consider when measuring particle-size distributions include

– Experiments should be planned to ensure that a sufficient amount of particles (and/or agglomerates) are available for statistically reliable determination of size distribution of the

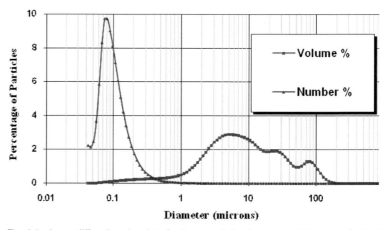

Fig. 4.1. Laser diffraction size data for "nanoscale" polymeric particles manufactured for animal trials. Note the apparent difference in size when depicted as a number distribution versus a volume distribution. This is due to the fact that volume scales as the cube of the particle diameter. Each curve, if presented by itself, would give an incomplete picture of the particle-size distribution of the sample. (Data courtesy of the Particle Engineering Research Center and Disc Dynamics Inc.)

sample in the to-be-administered state and after exposure to physiological fluids.

- As the polydispersity of a sample increases, it becomes necessary to measure a larger number of particles to accurately portray the size distribution (29). Fractionation and microscopy techniques are recommended for polydisperse samples.

- Nanoscale particulates may be difficult to maintain in a dispersed state. Potential sample segregation when sampling and/or while measuring PSD should be taken into account. The presence large agglomerates might not be detected within the size range suitable for the measurement technique used. If instability and/or large agglomerates are suspected, sample size segregation (e.g., centrifugation, filtration) and a combination of sizing techniques (e.g., dynamic light scattering and laser diffraction) may be needed for a representative PSD depiction.

- Particle diameters obtained from most available techniques are often calculated on the basis of an equivalent sphere (e.g., the diameter of a sphere having equal mass, surface area or settling velocity). These "equivalent sphere" models enable one to conveniently plot size distributions of irregularly shaped systems using a single value (diameter) along a single axis. However, if particle shape deviates significantly from spherical, the size calculated from these techniques becomes increasingly unreliable. For this reason, it is recommended that some form of microscopy is used to identify the shape characteristics of the nanoparticulate materials for verification of results measured by other means.

- Microscopy can provide valuable information regarding size, shape, morphology, etc. Electron microscopy (EM) offers the resolution needed to analyze nanomaterials. However, in order to provide a statistically valid representation of the full-size distribution, one must ensure that enough particles are examined.

- Multiple techniques should be used wherever possible to develop a more complete understanding of the system. It is preferred that at least one size fractionation or ensemble technique and a suitable microscopic technique are used where feasible.

Table 4.1 shows a number of techniques used to measure nanoparticles in and outside of physiological fluids along with advantages and disadvantages of the methods.

Particle shape. Most nanoparticulate materials contain populations of particles with different characteristic three-dimensional geometries and surface morphologies. A number of properties, such as dissolution rate, aggregation behavior, surface energy,

Table 4.1
Particle population sizing techniques applicable to nanoparticle systems

Technique	Size range	Advantages	Limitations
Ensemble sizing techniques			
Dynamic light scattering (DLS) (42, 27)	0.6 nm–6 μm (density dependent)	Minimal sample preparation and loss during measurement, small sample volume, can be integrate for electrophoresis (zeta potential) measurements	Poor technique for polydisperse/broad systems, not applicable for fast-settling particle systems
Small angle X-ray (SAX)/neutron scattering (43), X-ray diffraction (XRD) (47)	1 nm–1 μm	Good for solid-state-embedded systems	Requires high-concentrations of particles, cumbersome
Acoustic and electroacoustic techniques (45)	5 nm–100 μm	Good for concentrated systems, can be used for electrophoresis measurement	High concentration of particles required (~1 wt%), poor resolution
Static light scattering (SLS) (27)	>10 nm	Radius of gyration determination for polymeric nanomaterials, can be used to interpret particle/molecular interactions via second viral coefficient measurements	Larger particle sizes/molecular weights require multiple measurements
Laser diffraction	20–3 mm	Broad dynamic range – wet or dry measurements	Assumes spherical particles – shape effects unknown
Size fractionation techniques			
Centrifugal sedimentation (42, 27)/disc centrifuge/analytical ultracentrifuge	> 5 nm, density dependent	Good for broad-size distributions, can be used with whole blood and other physiological fluids	May require cumbersome sample preparation
Electrospray ionization time of flight mass spectroscopy (27)	1 nm–3 μm (100 to > 100 MDa)	Can be used with laser ablation for particle chemical composition analysis	Expensive, representative sampling difficult, multiple detectors required for full range, Rayleigh breakup could skew results

(continued)

Table 4.1 (continued)

Technique	Size range	Advantages	Limitations
Field flow fractionation (FFF) (27)	2 nm–200 μm	Good resolution of size distributions	Must be used in conjunction with other techniques (e.g., light scattering)
Size exclusion chromatography (SEC) (43, 44)	1 nm–2 μm	Good resolution, small sample volume	Slow, requires good calibration
Microscopy techniques			
Atomic force microscopy (AFM) (27)	~1 nm–microns	Good resolution and three-dimensional imaging (wet or dry), can be used to characterize surface material properties simultaneously with imaging	Prone to tip-induced artifacts, tedious
Scanning electron microscopy (SEM) (42, 46)	0.4 nm–several microns	Good resolution and imaging, sample topography information, can be combined with elemental analysis	Artifacts from sample preparation and required vacuum
High resolution-/scanning-/transmission electron microscopy (HR-/S-/TEM) (42, 46)	0.08 nm–microns	Atomic resolution, crystallographic, and detailed elemental analysis possible	Low sample throughput, expensive and time-consuming, biological samples can be complex to prepare
Optical dark field – Brownian motion	~70 nm–5 μm	Good for distributions, inexpensive optical technique, measured in liquids	Limited lower size limit, requires homogeneous fluid

surface area, exposure and availability of active/catalytic/reactive sites – among others – are intricately linked to shape at the nanoscale. It is quite possible that differences in geometrical and morphological profiles will have substantially different biological consequences. Inhaled fiber toxicity provides a classical example – a number of studies have illustrated that the aspect ratio and length of inhaled fibers is directly related to their clearance rate and observed toxicity (11). However, particle shape can have greater ramifications than simply modulating phagocytic ability and in vivo retention. For instance, if one compares the properties of a single nano-sized crystallite of the same material in platelet and spheroid form, the spatial distribution of surface atoms (exposed crystalline planes, steps, etc.) on the two particles will be significantly different. This can result in strikingly different surface energies, surface reactivities, and stereochemical biomolecular proclivities that have the potential to alter their inherent biological action. Further, particle shape can also have ramification when it comes to mechanical interactions. For instance, it has been recently shown that as the diameter of rod-shaped nanomaterials decreases, the amount of force necessary to puncture cell membranes is dramatically reduced to values comparable to the normal forces exerted by native undulations of living cell plasma membranes (20).

Currently, the combination of microscopic techniques and image analysis appears to be best suited for identifying particles of various shapes. For nanomaterials (<100 nm), some form of electron or atomic force microscopy is normally required to capture images with the necessary resolution. However, explicit care must be taken during sample preparation and analysis to prevent artifacts from contaminants and aggregates and avoid bias due to orientation effects – particularly when the method only provides two-dimensional images (e.g., TEM). Since the majority of these techniques require measurement in liquid-free states, additional care must be placed to avoid drying artifacts from the suspending media (e.g., salt crystals, aggregation). Shape distribution quantification for regularly shaped particles (e.g., fibers, platelets) is possible; however, irregularly shaped systems pose complications associated with choosing appropriate shape parameters (e.g., aspect ratio, sphericity, convexity) that make quantification a formidable challenge.

It should be noted that a few ensemble and size fractionation particle-sizing methods are capable of providing some information regarding the shape of particle systems; however, these methods typically have limited resolution and may not provide representative data for irregularly shaped systems. Particle shape is very difficult to quantify at the nanoscale. Representative micrographs should be taken to provide an indication of particle shape distributions but quantification may not be practical, with the exception of consistently shaped particulates or known consequences of shape variation.

2.3. State of Dispersion

The state of dispersion of nanoparticulate systems refers to the relative number of agglomerates (clusters of multiple particulates) in comparison to primary (single) particles in a suspending medium. Particle agglomeration and agglomerate size have been shown to play a role in the ability of macrophages to phagocytize particles and in the tendency for particle uptake and translocation through tissues, lymph, or circulatory system (30, 31). The agglomeration of aerosol particulates is also known to modulate lung deposition profiles. Furthermore, the state of aggregation of nanomaterials has recently been shown to affect the dose–response relationship of nanomaterials further complicating comparative analysis (21). Despite these finding, the state of dispersion of nanoparticles prior to, during, and after administration is rarely measured. The absence of this information could lead to widely skewed interpretations of experimental findings since it is evident that agglomeration state may lead to significant variations in the effective nanomaterial dose and largely modulate their fate and transport in vivo.

In liquids, the dispersion of nanoparticulate systems is controlled by an intricate balance of surface and intermolecular forces involving particle–particle interactions and those between particles and surrounded solvated and adsorbed molecular species. Slight perturbations in the properties of the surrounding environment (e.g., pH, ionic strength, concentrations of molecular constituents) can significantly modify the dispersion of nanoparticulate systems. Whether a particle remains a single-dispersed particle or forms an agglomerate is primarily dependent on three main factors: (1) the combined distant-dependent contribution from attractive (e.g., van der Waals, electrostatic, hydrophobic) and repulsive (e.g., steric, electrostatic, and hydration) forces between the two interacting surfaces (2), the probability for nanoparticle–nanoparticle collisions or close particle–particle approaches at the nanometer scale, and (3) the relative mechanical or thermal energy possessed by the particles when the interaction occurs. The latter can be extremely important in biological systems where surface adsorbates are typically heterogeneous with conformation-dependent surface properties. In such systems, there may exist complex interactions where repulsion is favored at low collision forces and attraction is favored at higher collision forces. The direct measurement of nanoparticle–nanoparticle interaction forces in biological fluids is tedious, but possible through the use of advanced nanoparticle-terminated probe technologies and the use of atomic force microscopy (32). Both particle size and shape can further modulate these interactions. These parameters dictate the effective surface area participating in the surface force engagement as the nanomaterials approach. Because this area is typically proportional to the overall force exerted, it has significant ramifications for the propensity of agglomeration particularly when only weak attractive forces are present. For instance, the interaction force experienced by two cross-cylinders is approximately twice that experienced by two spheres of the same diameter. Furthermore, if the cylinders are aligned, the interaction force would be dependent on the cylinder length and could be greater than 1,000 times the force experienced by spherical particles (21, 33). Hence, a material may have a low probability to agglomerate in the spherical state but may form significant agglomerates when prepared as rod-like materials.

In biological environments, the state of nanoparticulate dispersion is likely to be a transient process linked to the dynamic and competitive adsorption/desorption of biomolecules at their surface and presiding mechanical interactions mediated by fluid flow and/or tissue movement. Often researchers attempt to prevent or delay aggregation by adding highly hydrated molecules such as polyethylene glycol (PEG) or polysaccharides (e.g., dextran) to particle surfaces. These adsorbed or preferably chemically attached species inhibit the osponization of particles by inhibiting the adsorption of biomolecules on their surface and also inhibit agglomeration by inducing repulsive steric forces.

The state of dispersion is typically assessed by comparison of particle-size distributions measured under different conditions. By monitoring time-dependent changes in particle-size distribution when an initially dispersed suspension is subjected to a test environment, a qualitative assessment of agglomeration potential can be made. In most cases, a before and after depiction of PSD data is presented at carefully monitored time points and under controlled system parameters. When assessing state of dispersion of nanoparticle for biological applications the following should be noted:

- The balance of forces that define the state of agglomeration can be rapidly altered by small changes on the suspension properties (e.g., temperature, lack of/presence of mechanical interactions) therefore measurements should be performed under environments/conditions as close to the biological system of interest as possible.

- When measuring PSD and state of agglomeration, the characteristics of the surrounding biological fluid should be considered. This is of special importance when using physiological media that could contain molecules in the same size range as the particles to be measured or any exhibit other properties that could interfere with the technique (e.g., absorbance).

- Agglomeration rate and floc strength studies should be pursued when agglomerate-induced effects appear evident (34).

2.4. Surface Area and Porosity

The unique interactions between nanoparticulate materials and biological systems are believed by many to predominantly result from their surface properties. Indeed, several investigations have shown that the biological consequences of insoluble nanoparticulate exposures scale with surface area rather than mass (11). Specific surface area (e.g., m^2/g) of the dosed particles should always be reported when feasible. The surface area of nanoparticulate materials is preferably measured through the physical adsorption of an inert gas (typically nitrogen) using the method of Brunauer, Emmett, and Teller (BET). However, surface area measurements by this method can only be performed on dry powders, a major limitation in many cases.

The BET surface area includes both the external geometrical surface and the surface area of any open internal pores. Information on the population distribution of micropores (< 2 nm) and mesopores (2–50 nm) within the particles can be measured via multilayer isotherm analysis and adsorption and desorption isotherm hysteresis. Knowledge of both the internal and the external surface area of nanoparticulate materials can be useful when trying to mechanistically understand fundamental surface-borne nano–bio interactions.

There are a number of nanoparticle systems, whose porosity and surface area cannot be sufficiently probed by gas sorption due artifacts that arise from either sample drying or difficult sample recovery. Hydrated polymeric nanoparticle systems, micro- and nanoemulsion systems, nanolyposomes, dendrimers, fullerenes, and atmospheric particulates are just a few. The surface area of these systems can be estimated through particle sizing (e.g., DLS, cryo-TEM/AFM/SEM for wet systems and dynamic mobility analysis for dry systems). For aqueous suspensions, potentiometric titrations can sometimes be used assuming a uniform distribution of surface ionization groups. Under ideal situations, the adsorption and desorption isotherms (alternatively, uptake and leaching) of probe molecules from solution may also be used to approximate both surface area and porosity; however, it should be noted that the extent of surface area available to molecules in solution may change with environment-induced particle surface properties (e.g., solvent-induced swelling, salting-out phenomena).

2.5. Surface Properties

As mentioned earlier, the surface properties of nanoparticulate materials contribute greatly to the extent and mechanism of their biological interactions. Surface composition, energy, charge, reactivity, and opsonization – among others – are expected to modulate nanoparticle interactions with biomolecules and biological systems. Characterizing the full spectrum of surface properties for each nanoparticle system would be timely and costly and not essential in most cases. Because of this, it is especially recommended that an interactive approach to surface characterization be under taken. It is further suggested that a sample of the particulates (as-prepared and as-administered) be stored under inert conditions (e.g., under argon gas for dry powders, and cryogenic preservation of particle suspensions) to enable future analysis if necessary. At the very minimum, the surface composition and structure of nanomaterials should be measured on the particles in their original pre-administered state and post-exposure to biological environments when feasible (18).

Surface composition/atomic arrangement. The molecular composition and structure of the surface of nanoparticles will ultimately define their energy, charge, and reactivity; however, the prediction of these properties – especially for nanomaterials in biological systems – is difficult with current scientific approaches. A list of techniques applicable for identifying the surface composition and atomic arrangement of nanoparticles is given in **Table 4.2**. The following should be kept in mind when analyzing surface composition of nanoparticulate systems:

- It is recommended to directly measure the elemental composition of nanomaterials, pre- and post-administration, since many of these systems are subject to trace surface contaminants that are often not detectable via bulk composition analysis.

- Many of the methods used for surface characterization require ultrahigh vacuum environments ($<10^{-7}$ Pa). In some cases, the surface properties and bonding structure of some materials have been shown to change under such conditions. Because of this, care should be taken when interpreting and extrapolating results to the biological setting. ESCA, XPS, and SIMS, in particular, have been extensively used for characterizing nanoparticles and correlating biomaterial surface properties to physiological end points (35).

- Where feasible post-exposure examination of changes in surface composition and structure should be performed. Care must be taken to prevent/identify artifacts from the washing and removal of biomolecules from the surface of the particles either as a required step or as a collateral consequence of the analysis.

Surface energy/wettability. The role of surface energy in biocompatibility of materials has been identified in applications such as medical implants, catheters, and stents (35). Nanoparticle aggregation, dissolution, opsonization, and bioaccumulation behavior are just some of the properties linked to surface energy and wettability. The surface energy of nanoparticle systems can

Table 4.2
Surface analysis techniques applicable to nanoparticulate systems

Technique	Penetration depth[1]	Sample required	Applications	Limitations
Extended X-ray absorption fine structure spectroscopy (EXAFS) (50)	Few Å	Few mg	Surface atom packing, Surface–substrate interactions, colloid samples can be used	Crystalline materials only
Low-/high-energy electron diffraction (LEED/HEED) (48)	Few Å	< μg	Surface crystal structure and phase identification	Applicable only for single crystals, high-to-ultrahigh vacuum required
Secondary ion mass spectroscopy (SIMS) (53)	Few Å	μg–mg	Surface elemental analysis with depth profiling	Not quantitative, surface damage, low mass resolution, high-to-ultrahigh vacuum required
X-ray absorption near edge spectroscopy (XANES) (50)	Few Å	Few mg	Ionicity/atomic charge, surface–substrate interactions, colloid samples can be used	Needs further advances in theory to interpret the data
X-ray emission spectroscopy (XES) (54)	Few Å	Few mg	Surface composition	High-to-ultrahigh vacuum required
Auger electron spectroscopy (AES) (48)	1–5 nm	μg–mg	Surface composition	Insulators cannot be used without flood gun due to significant charging, surface damage, high-to-ultrahigh vacuum required
X-ray photoelectron spectroscopy (XPS)/electron spectroscopy for chemical analysis (ESCA) (55)	1–5 nm	μg–mg	Surface chemical analysis	Poor spatial resolution, not suitable for trace analysis, high-to-ultrahigh vacuum required

(continued)

Table 4.2 (continued)

Technique	Penetration depth[1]	Sample required	Applications	Limitations
High resolution-/scanning-/transmission electron microscopy (HR-/S-/TEM) (49, 53)	1–5 nm	< μg	Local structure and morphology	Sample preparation difficult, e-beam can damage organic materials, high-to-ultrahigh vacuum required
Energy loss spectroscopy (ELS), high resolution-/electron energy loss spectroscopy (HR-/EELS) (49)	Few nm	< μg	Surface composition and elemental mapping	Performed with TEM and thus requires thin sections, high-to-ultrahigh vacuum required
Scanning electron microscopy (SEM) (52)	Microns	mg–g	Surface morphology	Sample charging, high-to-ultrahigh vacuum required
Atomic force microscopy (AFM), scanning probe microscopy (SPM)	None or varies with mode	< μg	Surface morphology, material composition, surface interactions analysis, nanomechanical analysis, multiple advanced modes available for specialized applications (e.g., electrostatic force microscopy, magnetic force microscopy, scanning tunneling microscopy)	Typically low throughput, artifact prone, tends to be tedious

[1] Penetration depth of radiation source.

be measured through heat of immersion microcalorimetry studies or through contact angle measurements with various liquids. It should be noted that the surface energy values derived from different methods are not necessarily interchangeable. Multiple theories for deriving surface energy can potentially be used, such as those devised by Zismann, Van Oss, and Folkes (36). In some cases, contact angle measurements can also be used to estimate the acid–base character of nanoparticle surfaces – which is useful in understanding phenomena such as hydrogen bonding. Gas sorption studies with various volatized liquids or thermogravometric analysis of the evaporation of solvents may alternatively be used to gain some qualitative insights into the wettability of nanoparticulate systems (36).

Dynamic and static contact angle measurements can be performed to directly determine apparent particle wettabilility within biological fluids. Phospholipids, proteins, and other biomolecules are known to adsorb to surfaces in physiological fluids thus changing their wettability and other surface properties. Phase-partitioning experiments can also be designed to determine relative surface wettability in biologically relevant fluids (36).

Surface charge. The surface charge of nanoparticulate systems will influence their state of agglomeration, and the adsorption of ions and biomolecules at their interface, cellular uptake potential, and intracellular distribution. The average surface charge of a particulate system is usually approximated through zeta potential measurements (37). These measurements involve quantifying the velocity of particle movement in an applied electric field. The particle mobility depends on the charge experienced at the interface between the stagnant fluid layer that travels with the particle and the bulk liquid. This interface is known as the shear plane. The term zeta potential technically refers to the sign and magnitude of charge at the shear plane and depends on the adsorbed species at the surface and the ionic strength of the surrounding solution. Changes in zeta potential are indicative of the adsorption, exchange, and ionization of molecules within the shear plane and at the particle surface. Zeta potentials of nanoparticles are typically measured by electrophoresis or electroacoustophoresis methods. Potentiometric titrations can also be used to acquire particle charge information.

The zeta potential value derived from particulate materials is typically highly dependent on pH, electrolyte, and the presence of any potential adsorbates. Hence, single zeta potential values alone do not provide much information. The magnitudes of zeta potentials can also largely vary by measurement technique and mathematical interpretation. It is recommended that both a relevant zeta potential value a simple electrolyte system (e.g., at a set in pH 1 mM KCl) is provided along with the isoelectric point (IEP), or pH when the zeta potential is zero, under identical electrolyte conditions. The IEP is determined by pH titration. It should be noted that this pH also corresponds to the point of zero charge at the apparent surface. Both the zeta potential and the IEP of the particle in controlled monovalent electrolyte and zeta potential values in relevant biological fluids should be reported. It should be noted, however, that a particle system can consist of populations of particles that have different surface charges. Although zeta potentials should be characterized as distributions – much like particle sizes – currently few instruments are available that are capable of providing zeta potential distributions for nanomaterials.

- For each material, zeta potential measurements should be performed in pure water with a small amount (1–10 mM) of monovalent background electrolyte (e.g., KCl). It is recommended that the IEP is also determined in the same system and this pH value should be reported with zeta potential values (sign and magnitude) to provide an indication of surface charge.
- The type theory used for zeta potential calculation should also be disclosed (e.g., Smoluchowski, Huckel, Henry, and others) and the limitations of these theories should be recognized.
- Zeta potential measurements can be performed on nanoparticles in biological fluids; however, care must be taken to ensure that appropriate measures are taken to avoid artifacts from the high ionic strength and biomolecules encountered in these fluids.
- In whole biological fluids, the zeta potential measured is often of an adsorbed biomolecular layer and is often indicative of a Donnan layer potential rather than the underlying surface potential.
- Particle-size-independent theories (e.g., Smoluchowski, Huckel) are recommended when reporting values for agglomerating systems, soft particles (e.g., dendrimers), non-spherical particles, particles with a soft adsorbate layer, and porous materials due to the limitations of current theories.

Surface reactivity. Due to their large surface area, surface reactive nanomaterials can have untold consequences on interacting cells and biological species. Moreover, nanoparticulates that are able to actively participate in oxidation/reduction reactions can largely skew many biological assays. The surface reactivity of nanoparticles can be measured through comparative microcalorimetry or through a number of electrochemical methods. Usual practice includes the use of molecular probes that are monitored for degradation or changes in oxidative state when exposed to the nanomaterial of interest. When monitoring particle reactivity in biological fluids, losses in sensitivity and artifacts are likely and should be evaluated. The choice of method will depend on the types of molecular transformations that occur at the particle surface (18).

Surface adsorption of biomolecules (opsonization). Ultimately, cellular and tissue interactions between nanoparticles in biological fluids will be mediated by the molecules adsorbed at their surface. The biospecies adsorbed to the nanoparticle surface and their relative activity can dramatically impact nanoparticle uptake by cells. As well, there is some indication that they may regulate and direct translocation. The adsorption of biomolecules to foreign surfaces has been shown to be peculiarly selective, in many cases, the adsorption process leads to the preferential enrichment of a select subset of proteins at the surface (38). It is interesting to note that some of the adsorbed molecules only become responsive to cellular interactions upon adsorption to a surface. For instance, free fibronectin does not bind to platelets, whereas bound fibronectin causes cell adhesion (35). With emerging evidence illustrating that smaller sized nanoparticles may interact with some biomolecules without causing denaturalization (3), questions arise as to the fate of these particles and consequent cellular interactions in vivo, and attention should be paid to the route of exposure.

Protein/biomolecule adsorption has traditionally been measured through the use of radio-labeled molecules; however, this approach significantly restricts the measurable biomolecule population (35). In recent years, matrix-assisted laser desorption ionization tandem mass spectroscopy (MALDI MS/MS) and electrospray ionization tandem mass spectroscopy (ESI MS/MS) have become widely used for these types of studies. Additional, complementary techniques that are useful in further diagnosing biomolecule adsorbed state are found in **Table 4.3**.

2.6. Bulk and Chemical Properties

Bulk and chemical properties refer to whole particle material descriptors rather than those that are surface specific. There are a wide variety of physical and chemical properties that can potentially be measured for nanoparticulate systems (e.g., heat capacitance, thermal/electrical conductivity, dielectric constant, modulus, density, magnetic properties). However, particle composition, dissolution/solubility, and crystallinity have been most frequently correlated with unique biological end points, and therefore will be focused upon here for initial nanoparticle screenings.

Atomic/molecular composition. By having an indication of total nanoparticle constituents, decisions can be made as to design subsequent tests to evaluate the availability of potential constituent toxins from nanoscale materials to biological systems in which they are exposed. A number of techniques are available for analyzing bulk nanoparticle composition. Selections of these techniques are presented in **Table 4.4**.

Table 4.3
Adsorbate analysis techniques applicable nanoparticle systems

Technique	Sample required	Advantages	Disadvantages
Circular dichroism spectroscopy (CDS) (56)	µg–mg	Structural changes of adsorbed optically active biomolecules, applicable to liquid phase	Arbitrary reference protein, incompatibility with certain buffers
Electron paramagnetic resonance spectroscopy (EPR)/electron spin resonance (ESR) (57)	µg–g	Surface chemical structure and bonding, applicable to liquid phase	Applicable to systems with unpaired e^-, difficult to quantify, further computer analysis needed
Fourier transform infrared spectroscopy (FTIR), attenuated total reflection (ATR), diffuse reflectance infrared Fourier transform (DRIFT) (58)	pg–g	Intermolecular bonding information, identification of binding sites, applicable to aqueous phase	Not applicable to all inorganic materials, presence of water, voids, and defects may obscure the spectrum
Photoacoustic spectroscopy (PAS) (59)	µg–g	Surface composition of adsorbed species	Gas atmosphere needed for measurement
Surface-enhanced Raman spectroscopy (SERS) (60)	µg–mg	Detection of adsorbates, study of adsorbate–metal interactions	Applicable only to rough metal surfaces
Sum frequency generation (SFG) (48)	pg–g	Surface chemical composition, orientation of adsorbed proteins, applicable to liquid interface	Can be applied only to interfaces
Thermal desorption spectroscopy (TDS), temperature-programmed desorption spectroscopy (TPD), flash desorption spectroscopy (FDS) (48)	µg–mg	Identification and quantification of adsorbate and adsorbate–surface bond strength, used in conjunction with other techniques such as mass analyzer	Can cause sample damage, fragments with similar charge/mass ratio can cause interferences in detection
Ultraviolet photoelectron spectroscopy (UPS) (61)	µg–mg	Electronic nature of adsorbate–substrate interaction	High-to-ultrahigh vacuum required

Table 4.4
Bulk composition analysis techniques applicable to nanoparticulate systems

Technique	Sample required	Applications	Limitations
FTIR, ATR, DRIFT (58, 62)	pg–g	Molecular structure and composition, intermolecular bonding information, applicable to aqueous phase	Not applicable to all inorganic materials, presence of water, voids, and defects may obscure the spectrum
Raman (58)	μg–g	Molecular structure and composition, applicable to aqueous phase	Fluorescence can obscure spectrum, sample damage due to heating
EDS, EPMA, WDS (62)	μg–g	Elemental composition and distribution	Low sensitivity, high-to-ultrahigh vacuum required
UV/Vis (58)	ng–mg	Quantitative analysis, applicable to aqueous phase	Cannot determine molecular structure, spectrum consists of broad bands
ICP (63, 64)/ICP-MS	ng–μg levels (analyte dependent)	Quantitative analysis, trace element analysis, applicable to aqueous phase	Spectral overlap, high concentration of other element can reduce the trace element intensity
XRF, WDXF, EDXF (64)	mg–g	Qualitative and quantitative elemental composition	Cannot be used for elements below Al, standards required for quantitative analysis, high-to-ultrahigh vacuum required
HAADF-STEM (58, 64)	<40 nm thickness	Quantitative elemental mapping	Low resolution, poorer signal-to-noise ratio, high-to-ultrahigh vacuum required
Mossbauer, γ-ray spectroscopy (65)	Few mg	Chemical shifts of nuclei, intra-molecular bonding information of magnetic atom	Limited to magnetic ions such as Fe
NMR (solution (66)/solid state (67))	0.5–3 mL, μg–mg	Chemical structure determination, detailed conformational and configurational information, diffusion of molecular species	Limited to nuclei with magnetic moments, spectral overlap for amorphous solids in solid-state NMR

(continued)

Table 4.4 (continued)

Technique	Sample required	Applications	Limitations
NAA	pg–mg	Trace analysis of elements, applicable to all states of materials with minimal preparation	Neutron source required
MS (68)	ng–μg	Detection and quantitative analysis	Limited resolution
LIF (69)	μg–mg	Quantitative analysis of chemicals	Fluorescence interference from other species (hydrocarbons), low signal-to-noise ratio

FTIR – Fourier transform infrared spectroscopy; ATR – attenuated total reflection; DRIFT – diffuse reflectance infrared Fourier transform spectroscopy; EDS – energy dispersive X-ray spectrometry; EPMA – electron probe microanalysis; WDS – wavelength dispersive spectrometry; UV/vis – ultraviolet-visible light spectroscopy; ICP – inductively coupled plasma; XRF – X-ray fluorescence spectroscopy; WDXF – wavelength dispersive X-ray fluorescence spectrometry; EDXF – energy dispersive X-ray fluorescence spectrometry; HAADF-STEM – high angle annular dark field-scanning tunneling electron microscopy; NMR – nuclear magnetic resonance; NAA – neutron activation analysis; MS – mass spectroscopy; LIF – laser-induced fluorescence; HV – high vacuum; UHV – ultrahigh vacuum.

- Careful attention should be paid to statistical sampling and the detection limits of the methods used to identify elemental constituents.

Solubility. Dissolution of materials, even those with low solubilities, can have a dramatic effect on their behavior and/or toxicity in vivo. Nanoparticles are likely to exhibit greater solubility and more rapid dissolution than larger sized particles of the same materials. Depending on the solubility, a nanoparticle's dosimetrics and potential biological mechanisms can be very different from what might be expected for larger particles or bulk materials. Since the adsorption of biomolecules and other factors can modulate the dissolution process, the propensity for nanoparticulate materials to dissolve in biological fluids should be directly measured where applicable. Although changes in particle size can provide some indication of dissolution, the use of a technique that monitors the concentration of dissolved nanoparticle content in solution such as various forms of mass spectroscopy (e.g., ICP-MS) is preferred.

Crystallinity. Crystal structures of particulate systems have been shown to dramatically impact the toxicity of materials. Perhaps the most recognized example is the clear distinction between the toxicological profiles of amorphous and crystalline silica – amorphous silica is apparently benign, whereas crystalline silica (quartz) is cytotoxic and carcinogenic (39, 40). For this reason, the crystal structure of nanoparticulate systems should always be evaluated. The crystal structure of nanoparticle systems can be

Table 4.5
Crystal structure analysis techniques applicable to nanoparticulate systems

Technique	Sample required	Comments
Transmission electron microscopy – selected area diffraction (TEM-SAD) (71)	Single particle	Can be performed while imaging, high-to-ultrahigh vacuum required
Scanning tunneling microscopy (STM)	Single particle	Performed while imaging, surface crystallinity and atom mapping, requires conductive samples, tedious
X-ray diffraction (XRD) (70)	mg–g	Chemical composition information, time consuming, large volume of sample required, not good for particle size <7 nm
Low-energy electron diffraction (LEED), high-energy electron diffraction (HEED) (48)	mg–g	Surface structure information, probe area must be single crystalline, high-to-ultrahigh vacuum required
X-ray absorption spectroscopy (XAS), X-ray absorption near edge spectroscopy (XANES) (71)	mg–g	Oxidation state and coordination environment, colloid samples can be used, needs further advances in theory to interpret the data

analyzed with the use of methods described in **Table 4.5**. It should be noted that some nanomaterials have been shown to change their crystal structure depending on the suspending solution environment (41); therefore, it may be of interest to monitor the crystal structure of nanoparticulate materials in the biofluids to which they are exposed. Methods such as XAS and XRD (with some modification) are applicable to liquid suspensions. When possible, attention should be placed on the surface crystal structure (e.g., as measured via STM or interpreted through TEM-SAD) and the presence of microstructure defects such as dislocations and staking faults – since these two variables are likely to mediate nanoparticle reactivity.

3. Concluding Remarks

The successful development of new nanomaterials as diagnostic and therapeutic tools will depend on the proper evaluation and understanding of their interactions with biological entities and their potential for inadvertent toxicities. These correlations can only be established with a thorough understanding of nanoparticle properties obtained through reliable characterization of those nanomaterials. This chapter addresses several nanoparticle attributes that may lead to significant biological interactions and identifies techniques and recommended practices that can be used for their evaluation in and outside biological media. Regardless of the technique applied, detailed scrutiny of sample preparation procedures, equipment limitations, and measurement protocols is necessary to ensure reliable data are obtained. When possible, relevant national- and international-standardized practices should be consulted as guides for performing measurements. Additionally, national and academic centers like the Nanotechnology Characterization Laboratory (NCL) can be called upon for assistance in characterization.

Nanoparticulate systems provide new challenges to cancer researchers, toxicologist, engineers, and scientists alike, requiring new protocols and more advanced techniques for characterizing nanoparticulate systems in biological contexts. The active and promising research in this field should catalyze novel methods and the development of additional tools that will ultimately allow the translation of these technologies into products and solutions in the near future.

Acknowledgments

The authors acknowledge the financial support of the State of Florida Center of Excellence for Nano-Bio Sensors (CNBS), the Florida Biomedical Research Program, the National Science Foundation (CBET-0853707; NIRT 0506560), and the Particle Engineering Research Center (PERC) at the University of Florida. Any opinions, findings, and conclusions or recommendations expressed in this material are those of the authors and do not necessarily reflect those of the National Science Foundation.

References

1. Mueller, W. G., et al. (2001) Large-scale chromatin decondensation and recondensation regulated by transcription from a natural promoter. *Mol Biol Cell* **12**, 357A–357A.
2. Jiang, X., et al. (2005) Effect of colloidal gold size on the conformational changes of adsorbed cytochrome c: probing by circular dichroism, UV-visible, and infrared spectroscopy. *Biomacromolecules* **6**(1), 46–53.
3. Vertegel, A. A., Siegel, R. W., and Dordick, J. S. (2004) Silica nanoparticle size influences the structure and enzymatic activity of adsorbed lysozyme. *Langmuir* **20**(16), 6800–6807.
4. Hartgerink, J. D., Beniash, E., and Stupp, S. I. (2001) Self-assembly and mineralization of peptide-amphiphile nanofibers. *Science* **294**(5547), 1684–1688.
5. Ito, A., et al. (2004) Tissue engineering using magnetite nanoparticles and magnetic force: heterotypic layers of cocultured hepatocytes and endothelial cells. *Tiss Eng* **10**(5–6), 833–840.
6. Teixeira, A. I., Nealey, P. F., and Murphy, C. J. (2004) Responses of human keratocytes to micro- and nanostructured substrates. *J Biomed Mater Res A* **71A**(3), 369–376.
7. Catledge, S. A., et al. (2004) Mesenchymal stem cell adhesion and spreading on nanostructured biomaterials. *J Nanosci Nanotechnol* **4**(8), 986–989.
8. Berry, C. C., et al. (2005) The fibroblast response to tubes exhibiting internal nanotopography. *Biomaterials* **26**(24), 4985–4992.
9. Yim, E. K. F., et al. (2005) Nanopattern-induced changes in morphology and motility of smooth muscle cells. *Biomaterials* **26**(26), 5405–5413.
10. Thomas, K. and Sayre, P. (2005) Research strategies for safety evaluation of nanomaterials, part I: evaluating the human health implications of exposure to nanoscale materials. *Toxicol Sci* **87**(2), 316–321.
11. Oberdorster, G., Oberdorster, E., and Oberdorster, J. (2005) Nanotoxicology: an emerging discipline evolving from studies of ultrafine particles. *Environ Health Perspect* **113**(7), 823–839.
12. Brown, D. M., et al. (2001) Size-dependent proinflammatory effects of ultrafine polystyrene particles: a role for surface area and oxidative stress in the enhanced activity of ultrafines. *Toxicol Appl Pharmacol* **175**(3), 191–199.
13. Donaldson, K., et al. (2002) The pulmonary toxicology of ultrafine particles. *J Aerosol Med Deposition Clear Effect Lung* **15**(2), 213–220.
14. Donaldson, K., Li, X. Y., and Macnee, W. (1998) Ultrafine (nanometre) particle mediated lung injury. *J Aerosol Sci* **29**(5–6), 553–560.
15. Oberdorster, G., et al. (1992) Role of the alveolar macrophage in lung injury – studies with ultrafine particles. *Environ Health Perspect* **97**, 193–199.
16. Tran, C. L., et al. (2000) Inhalation of poorly soluble particles. II. Influence of particle surface area on inflammation and clearance. *Inhalat Toxicol* **12**(12), 1113–1126.
17. Kagan, V. E., et al. (2006) Direct and indirect effects of single walled carbon nanotubes on RAW 264.7 macrophages: role of iron. *Toxicol Lett* **165**(1), 88–100.
18. Powers, K. W., et al. (2006) Research strategies for safety evaluation of nanomaterials. Part VI. characterization of nanoscale particles for toxicological evaluation. *Toxicol Sci* **90**(2), 296–303.
19. Tervonen, T., et al. (2009) Risk-based classification system of nanomaterials. *J Nanoparticle Res* **11**(4), 757–766.

20. Vakarelski, I. U., et al. (2007) Penetration of living cell membranes with fortified carbon nanotube tips. *Langmuir* **23**(22), 10893–10896.
21. Brown, S. C., et al. (2007) Influence of shape, adhesion and simulated lung mechanics on amorphous silica nanoparticle toxicity. *Adv Powder Technol* **18**(1), 69–79.
22. NCL_NIST 2007 <http://ncl.cancer.gov/working_assay-cascade.asp>.
23. OECD, List of Manufactured Nanomaterials and List of Endpoints for Phase One of the OECD Testing Programme. 2008.
24. Warheit, D. B., et al. (2008) Health effects related to nanoparticle exposures: environmental, health and safety considerations for assessing hazards and risks. *Pharmacol Ther* **120**(1), 35–42.
25. http://ncl.cancer.gov/.
26. http://ncl.cancer.gov/NCL_Method_NIST-NCL_PCC-1.pdf.
27. Jillavenkatesa, A. and Kelly, J. F. (2002) Nanopowder characterization: challenges and future directions. *J Nanoparticle Res* **4**(5), 463–468.
28. Perrault, S. D., et al. (2009) Mediating tumor targeting efficiency of nanoparticles through design. *Nano Lett* **9**(5), 1909–1915.
29. Masuda, H. and Iinoya, K. (1971) Theoretical study of the scatter of experimental data due to particle-size-distribution. *J Chem Eng Jpn* **4**(1), 60–66.
30. Renwick, L. C., Donaldson, K., and Clouter, A. (2001) Impairment of alveolar macrophage phagocytosis by ultrafine particles. *Toxicol Appl Pharmacol* **172**(2), 119–127.
31. Nemmar, A., et al. (2001) Passage of intratracheally instilled ultrafine particles from the lung into the systemic circulation in hamster. *Am J Respir Crit Care Med* **164**(9), 1665–1668.
32. Vakarelski, I. U., et al. (2007) Nanoparticle-terminated scanning probe microscopy tips and surface samples. *Adv Powder Technol* **18**(6), 605–614.
33. Israelachvili, J. N. (1985) *Intermolecular and Surface Forces: With Applications to Colloidal and Biological Systems.* Academic Press, London; Orlando, FL, xv, 296p.
34. Jarvis, P., et al. (2005) A review of floc strength and breakage. *Water Res* **39**(14), 3121–3137.
35. Ratner, B. D. (2004) *Biomaterials Science: An Introduction to Materials in Medicine,* 2nd ed. Elsevier Academic Press, Amsterdam; Boston, xii, 851p.
36. Neumann, A. W. and Spelt, J. K. (1996) *Applied Surface Thermodynamics. Surfactant Science Series,* v. 63. M. Dekker, New York, xii, 646p.
37. Adamson, A. W. and Gast, A. P. (1997) *Physical Chemistry of Surfaces,* 6th ed. Wiley, New York, xxi, 784p.
38. Wasdo, S. C., et al. (2008) Differential binding of serum proteins to nanoparticles. *Int J Nanotechnol* **5**(1), 92–115.
39. Borm, P. J. A., et al. (2001) The quartz hazard revisited: the role of matrix and surface. *Gefahrstoffe Reinhaltung Der Luft* **61**(9), 359–363.
40. Tsuji, J. S., et al. (2006) Research strategies for safety evaluation of nanomaterials, part IV: risk assessment of nanoparticles. *Toxicol Sci* **89**(1), 42–50.
41. Zhang, H. Z., et al. (2003) Water-driven structure transformation in nanoparticles at room temperature. *Nature* **424**(6952), 1025–1029.
42. Bootz, A., et al. (2004) Comparison of scanning electron microscopy, dynamic light scattering and analytical ultracentrifugation for the sizing of poly(butyl cyanoacrylate) nanoparticles. *Eur J Pharm Biopharm* **57**(2), 369–375.
43. Fritz, H., Maier, M., and Bayer, E. (1997) Cationic polystyrene nanoparticles: preparation and characterization of a model drug carrier system for antisense oligonucleotides. *J Colloid Interface Sci* **195**(2), 272–288.
44. Bootz, A., et al. (2005) Molecular weights of poly(butyl cyanoacrylate) nanoparticles determined by mass spectrometry and size exclusion chromatography. *Eur J Pharm Biopharm* **60**(3), 391–399.
45. Dukhin, A. S., et al. (1999) Electroacoustic phenomena in concentrated dispersions: new theory and CVI experiment. *Langmuir* **15**(20), 6692–6706.
46. Sjostrom, B., et al. (1995) Structures of nanoparticles prepared from oil-in-water emulsions. *Pharm Res* **12**(1), 39–48.
47. Borchert, H., et al. (2005) Determination of nanocrystal sizes: a comparison of TEM, SAXS, and XRD studies of highly monodisperse COPt3 particles. *Langmuir* **21**(5), 1931–1936.
48. Unterhalt, H., Rupprechter, G., and Freund, H. J. (2002) Vibrational sum frequency spectroscopy on Pd(111) and supported Pd nanoparticles: CO adsorption from ultrahigh vacuum to atmospheric pressure. *J Phys Chem B* **106**(2), 356–367.
49. Park, S. H., et al. (2005) Effects of silver nanoparticles on the fluidity of bilayer

50. Gilbert, B., et al. (2004) Analysis and simulation of the structure of nanoparticles that undergo a surface-driven structural transformation. *J Chem Phys* **120**(24), 11785–11795.
51. Nakamura, R. and Sato, S. (2002) Oxygen species active for photooxidation of n-decane over TiO2 surfaces. *J Phys Chem B* **106**(23), 5893–5896.
52. Duffin, R., et al. (2001) Aluminium lactate treatment of DQ12 quartz inhibits its ability to cause inflammation, chemokine expression, and nuclear factor-kappa B activation. *Toxicol Appl Pharmacol* **176**(1), 10–17.
53. Chakraborty, B. R., et al. (2005) TOF-SIMS and laser-SNMS investigations of dopant distribution in nanophosphors. *Nanotechnology* **16**(8), 1006–1015.
54. Guo, J. H. (2003) Synchrotron radiation, soft-X-ray spectroscopy and nanomaterials. *Int J Nanotechnol* **1**(1–2), 193–225.
55. Kim, S. H., et al. (2005) Target-specific cellular uptake of PLGA nanoparticles coated with poly(L-lysine)-poly(ethylene glycol)-folate conjugate. *Langmuir* **21**(19), 8852–8857.
56. Li, T. H., et al. (2004) Circular dichroism study of chiral biomolecules conjugated nanoparticles. *Nanotechnology* **15**(10), S660–S663.
57. Wanner, M., et al. (2005) Treatment of citrate-capped Au colloids with NaCl, NaBr and Na2SO4: a TEM, EAS and EPR study of the accompanying changes. *Colloid Polymer Sci* **283**(7), 783–792.
58. Burt, J. L., et al. (2004) Noble-metal nanoparticles directly conjugated to globular proteins. *Langmuir* **20**(26), 11778–11783.
59. Santos, J. G., et al. (2005) Use of the photoacoustic spectroscopy in the investigation of biocompatible magnetic fluids. *J De Physique Iv* **125**, 27–30.
60. Kneipp, K., et al. (1999) Ultrasensitive chemical analysis by Raman spectroscopy. *Chem Rev* **99**(10), 2957–2976.
61. Gunhold, A., et al. (2003) Nanostructures on La-doped SrTiO3 surfaces. *Anal Bioanal Chem* **375**(7), 924–928.
62. Lang, H. G., et al. (2004) Synthesis and characterization of dendrimer templated supported bimetallic Pt-Au nanoparticles. *J Am Chem Soc* **126**(40), 12949–12956.
63. Dai, L. J., et al. (1999) Insulin stimulates Mg2+ uptake in mouse distal convoluted tubule cells. *Am J Physiol Renal Physiol* **277**(6), F907–F913.
64. Utsunomiya, S., et al. (2004) Direct identification of trace metals in fine and ultrafine particles in the Detroit urban atmosphere. *Environ Sci Technol* **38**(8), 2289–2297.
65. Marchetti, S. G. and Mercader, R. C. (2003) Magnetism of nanosized oxide systems investigated by Mossbauer spectroscopy. *Hyperfine Interact* **148**(1–4), 275–284.
66. Hung, C. H. and Whang, W. T. (2005) Effect of surface stabilization of nanoparticles on luminescent characteristics in ZnO/poly(hydroxyethyl methacrylate) nanohybrid films. *J Mater Chem* **15**(2), 267–274.
67. Ladizhansky, V., Hodes, G., and Vega, S. (2000) Solid state NMR study of water binding on the surface of CdS nanoparticles. *J Phys Chem B* **104**(9), 1939–1943.
68. Ostblom, M., et al. (2005) On the structure and desorption dynamics of DNA bases adsorbed on gold: a temperature-programmed study. *J Phys Chem B* **109**(31), 15150–15160.
69. Huang, Y. F., Huang, C. C., and Chang, H. T. (2003) Exploring the activity and specificity of gold nanoparticle-bound trypsin by capillary electrophoresis with laser-induced fluorescence detection. *Langmuir* **19**(18), 7498–7502.
70. Choi, H. C., et al. (2004) Characterization of the structures of size-selected TiO2 nanoparticles using X-ray absorption spectroscopy. *Appl Spectr* **58**(5), 598–602.
71. Cheng, G. and Guo, T. (2002) Surface segregation in Ni/Co bimetallic nanoparticles produced in single-walled carbon nanotube synthesis. *J Phys Chem B* **106**(23), 5833–5839.

Chapter 5

Multimodal Nanoparticulate Bioimaging Contrast Agents

Parvesh Sharma, Amit Singh, Scott C. Brown, Niclas Bengtsson, Glenn A. Walter, Stephen R. Grobmyer, Nobutaka Iwakuma, Swadeshmukul Santra, Edward W. Scott, and Brij M. Moudgil

Abstract

A wide variety of bioimaging techniques (e.g., ultrasound, computed X-ray tomography, magnetic resonance imaging (MRI), and positron emission tomography) are commonly employed for clinical diagnostics and scientific research. While all of these methods use a characteristic "energy–matter" interaction to provide specific details about biological processes, each modality differs from another in terms of spatial and temporal resolution, anatomical and molecular details, imaging depth, as well as the desirable material properties of contrast agents needed for augmented imaging. On many occasions, it is advantageous to apply multiple complimentary imaging modalities for faster and more accurate prognosis. Since most imaging modalities employ exogenous contrast agents to improve the signal-to-noise ratio, the development and use of multimodal contrast agents is considered to be highly advantageous for obtaining improved imagery from sought-after imaging modalities. Multimodal contrast agents offer improvements in patient care, and at the same time can reduce costs and enhance safety by limiting the number of contrast agent administrations required for imaging purposes. Herein, we describe the synthesis and characterization of nanoparticulate-based multimodal contrast agent for noninvasive bioimaging using MRI, optical, and photoacoustic tomography (PAT)-imaging modalities. The synthesis of these agents is described using microemulsions, which enable facile integration of the desired diversity of contrast agents and material components into a single entity.

Key words: Multimodal nanoparticles, water-in-oil microemulsions, magnetic resonance imaging, optical imaging, photoacoustic tomography, gold-speckled silica.

1. Introduction

Advances in nanoscience and nanotechnology are expected to have significant impact in the biomedical arena leading to vast improvements in diagnostics and therapy. The fabrication of nanoconstructs with engineered features and surface characteristics has provided researchers with invaluable tools to investigate the complex biological environments. One such area in the biomedical field has been the development of multimodal contrast agents (i.e., those which can be imaged simultaneously or in succession by more than one imaging modality). Because different imaging methods vary in terms of spatial and temporal resolution, sensitivity, penetration depth, etc., imaging with complimentary imaging tools is highly attractive (1–4). This approach offers the potential to integrate the advantages of different techniques while at the same time surmounting the limitations of one another (5, 6). For example, MRI (one of the most commonly used clinical imaging modalities) can provide soft-tissue contrast, nearly unlimited tissue penetration and high levels of safety (since it employs nonionizing radio waves); however, compared to other methods, it has low sensitivity. Optical imaging (OI) e.g., fluorescence-based imaging (7, 8), on the other hand, suffers from poor-tissue penetration limiting its use for deep-tissue imaging; however, it can provide high material sensitivity. The combination of MRI and OI capabilities enables one to gather information from a sample that would be nearly impossible to obtain from either independently, by enabling high sensitivity with cellular resolution in vivo. Such multimodal contrast agents are expected to be useful as diagnostics and assist in real-time guidance in intraoperative surgical resections of sensitive pathologies such as brain tumors (9).

Additionally, multimodal contrast agents can help in the technical advancement of emerging imaging techniques (10–12). For instance, PAT (also known as optoacoustic imaging) is an emerging noninvasive imaging modality that employs nonionizing radiation (visible to near-infrared light) to produce contrast with high sensitivity and temporal/spatial resolution (13–16). In this method, the absorption of pulsed incident light by the biological tissue induces a series of thermoelastic expansion events that produce an acoustic signal which is collected and reconstructed into an image of the object. Blood vessels (14), tumors (13, 17), tumor angiogenesis (18), and hemoglobin oxygenation (19) have been imaged by PAT. The development of multimodal contrast agents for PAT and MRI offers advantages such as development of PAT as an independent imaging tool to provide high-resolution 3D imagery noninvasively and with relatively low cost. In the future, PAT imaging may permit high-resolution in vivo imaging for patients who cannot be imaged by MRI because of metallic implants or debris.

In this chapter, the synthesis, characterization, and functional evaluation of multimodal nanoparticulate contrast agents using water-in-oil microemulsions (reverse/inverse micelles) are described. In contrast to macroemulsion systems, microemulsions have ultralow interfacial tensions, are thermodynamically stable and optically clear. In reverse microemulsions, the water molecules form surfactant-stabilized nanodroplets in a bulk organic phase (20, 21). The size of these water droplets or nanoreactors can be carefully changed by manipulation of the water to surfactant molar ratio, known as W_0. The selection of surfactant/co-surfactant, oil, water, temperature can have profound effects on the size and shape of the synthesized material, thus providing versatility in this approach. The fundamentals and scope of microemulsion-mediated nanoparticle synthesis have been covered exhaustively (22–26). The applications of microemulsions for synthesis of fluorescent, magnetically doped, and gold-speckled silica nanoparticles as contrast agents for bioimaging applications are discussed in the following sections.

2. Materials

All reagents employed for the synthesis of multimodal nanoparticles were reagent grade and used without further purification. Tetraethylorthosilicate (TEOS), 3-(aminopropyl)triethoxysilane (APTS), tris(2,2′-bipyridyl)dichlororuthenium(II) hexahydrate (RuBpy), $Cd(CH_3COO)_2 \cdot 2H_2O$, $Mn(CH_3COO)_2$, Na_2S, and $Zn(CH_3COO)_2 \cdot 2H_2O$, dioctyl sulfosuccinate (Aerosol OT or AOT), Triton X-100 (TX-100), n-hexanol, 3-(trihydroxysilyl) propyl methylphosphonate, monosodium salt solution (42 wt% in water), O-[2-(3-mercaptopropionylamino)ethyl]-O′-methylpolyethylene glycol, gold chloride, heptane, and cyclohexane were purchased from Aldrich Chemical Co. Inc. N-(Trimethoxysilylpropyl) ethyldiaminetriacetic acid trisodium salt (TSPET) (45 wt% solution in water) was purchased from Gelest Co. Gadolinium acetate, and hydrazine hydrate were obtained from Acros Organics and ammonium hydroxide (NH_4OH, 28–30 wt%) was obtained from the Fisher Scientific Co. Deionized (DI) water (NANOpure, Barnstead) was used for the preparation of all solutions.

3. Methods

Multimodal contrast agents for MR-Optical and MR-PAT imaging have been synthesized using the water-in-oil microemulsions. The reverse micellar approach offers many advantages over other bottom-up synthesis methods such as sol–gel and layer-by-layer deposition. Because particle synthesis is nucleated and carried out within the "water pools" (nano-vessels), particles resulting from this method are typically of nanodimensions. Further, manipulation of W_0 allows flexibility in the tuning of the water core thus permitting an easy control over the particle size. However, it must be noted that the overall reaction and particle formation process within the microemulsions are influenced by collision rates and inter-droplet reactant exchange as well as reaction kinetics and resulting surface chemistries (27, 28). One of the main highlights of using reverse micelles approach is that it enables the production of nanoparticles with a narrow particle size distribution. Because of this feature, it has been used exhaustively for the synthesis of highly regular nanoparticles, such as dye-doped silica, gold, and quantum dots (Qdots). Another advantage of using the reverse micelles is the ability to fabricate particles that are readily water dispersible, which is an important requirement for the majority of biological applications. Reverse micelles also help fabricate core-multiple shell particles in a one-pot reaction, thus enabling integration of multiple functional features uniformly in individual particles.

3.1. Design of Multimodal Particles

Herein, we describe the synthesis of Gadolinium (Gd) chelated fluorescent core (dye-doped silica/quantum dots) and Gd-chelated gold-speckled silica nanoparticles as contrast agents for MR-Optical and MR-PAT. The multimodal nanoparticles construct comprises the following components:

1. Core: Both MR-Optical and MR-PAT particles consist of a fluorescent core, onto which the rest of the architecture is built. The ability to image these particles optically through fluorescence is built in either synthesizing Qdots as core or by the incorporation of fluorescent dye molecules into the silica core.

2. MRI active shell: The MR property is integrated into the constructs by modification of the surface of the silica core with metal complexing ligands which help in chelation of paramagnetic Gd ions.

3. PAT active surface: The PAT contrast generating ability is generated by the deposition of irregular, gold-speckled nanoparticles on the Gd-doped silica matrix.

4. Particle dispersion and surface conjugation: Over and above the optical/MR/PAT active particles, further surface modification may be required to improve the dispersion of the particles in biological media and for introducing functional groups which would enable bioconjugation to targeting molecules such as antibodies, peptides, and receptor-specific ligands.

3.2. Synthesis of MR-Optical Multimodal Contrast Agents

The overall one-pot synthesis of fluorescent dye-doped and Gd-chelated silica nanoparticles in nonionic microemulsions is described below:

3.2.1. Synthesis of Fluorescent Core

The water-in-oil (w/o) microemulsion was prepared by mixing 1.77 g Tx-100, 7.7 mL cyclohexane, 1.6 mL n-hexanol, and 340 μL water (*see* **Note 1**). n-Hexanol acts as a co-surfactant to the nonionic surfactant. The contents of the mixture were stirred for 10 min to obtain an optically transparent solution. A volume of 40 μL of 0.10 M RuBpy solution was added to the above microemulsion and stirred for 10 min. Next, 50 μL of TEOS was added to the microemulsion and allowed to equilibrate throughout the microemulsion. After 30 min of stirring 100 μL of NH$_4$OH was injected into the microemulsion to initiate TEOS hydrolysis and polymerization. The size of the silica nanoparticles, prepared in w/o microemulsions can be changed by varying the W_0 and/or reactant concentrations (29–31). In general, the decrease in W_0 in Tx-100/cyclohexane/water microemulsions has been shown to increase the size of the silica nanoparticles (29, 30).

3.2.2. MRI Active Shell

The incorporation of the paramagnetic Gd in the nanoparticle is achieved by its binding to the chelating groups introduced on the silica nanoparticle. These groups are incorporated on the silica core by the addition of 50 μL TEOS to the above microemulsion, stirring for 30 min, followed by the addition of 25 μL TSPET (*see* **Note 2**). The microemulsion is stirred vigorously during the addition of silane chelating agent and continued to stir for additional 24 h. During this period, TSPET co-condenses with TEOS and introduces chelating groups on the surface of the silica nanoparticle. A volume of 100 μL of 0.10 M Gd acetate solution was added next, followed by further stirring for 24 h. TSPET binds to Gd ions through its five coordination sites, though binding of some Gd ions to the silanol groups on the silica surface cannot be completely ruled out. **Figure 5.1** shows the

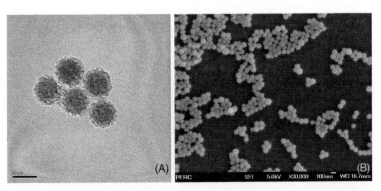

Fig. 5.1. Representative (**a**) TEM of 50 nm and (**b**) SEM of 100 nm multimodal silica nanoparticles synthesized using Tx-100 w/o microemulsion.

representative electron microscopy pictures for 50 and 100 nm multimodal silica nanoparticles.

3.2.3. Surface Modification

In order to be able to perform bioconjugation of the resultant particles with targeting ligands such as proteins, peptides, and antibodies, the particle surface is modified to introduce NH_2 functional groups on the particle surface. However the introduction of the amine groups leads to a decrease in the zeta potential of the particle, thus negatively affecting its dispersability in aqueous-buffered medium. To improve the dispersion of the particles subsequent to chelation of Gd, and to introduce primary amine groups on nanoparticles surface, Schroedter's protocol (32) with slight modifications has been adopted (33, 34). The surface of the particles is postcoated by the addition of 50 μL TEOS, 40 μL THPMP (with vigorous stirring for 5 min) and 10 μL of APTS to the above microemulsion and stirring for another 24 h. The co-condensation of THPMP ($pK_a = 2.0$) together with APTS ($pK_a = 9.0$) and TEOS produces a resultant zeta potential of ∼−35 mV, thus aiding the dispersion of the nanoparticles. Similar modifications have also been carried out on the surface of silica-coated multimodal CdS:Mn/ZnS (35) and CdS:Mn/ZnS-Gd Qdots (34) to improve their aqueous dispersion. The synthesis of the multimodal Qdots is described in a separate section.

3.2.4. Extraction and Washing of Nanoparticles

The nanoparticles were extracted from the microemulsion by addition of ∼4–5 mL of 200 proof ethanol with continuous stirring. The stirring was stopped after a couple of minutes and the resulting mixture was allowed to stand for 10 min. Additions of ethanol lead to complete crashing of the reverse micelles and resulted in the formation of two immiscible layers of ethanol and oil (cyclohexane). The nanoparticles accumulated in bottom ethanol layer and were separated by centrifugation after which they aggregated in pellet form. The top layer of surfactants, ethanol, and oil was carefully removed and replenished with 200 proof ethanol. The solution was vortexed and sonicated to redisperse the particles followed by another round of centrifugation. For complete removal of the surfactant (see **Note 3**) the particles were washed four times with ethanol and five times with water. After final water washing the nanoparticles were redispersed in nanopure water. The optical and MR contrast generating ability of the particles is demonstrated by labeling the J774 mouse macrophage cells with the multimodal nanoparticles and imaging by optical and MRI as shown in **Fig. 5.2**.

3.3. Synthesis of MR-Optical Multimodal Quantum Dots

The synthesis of Gd-doped CdS:Mn/ZnS/Silica Qdots as multimodal Qdots is described below. In this construct RuBpy-doped silica core (**Section 3.2.1**) is replaced by Mn-doped CdS core, ZnS shell Qdots as the highly fluorescent part of the multimodal

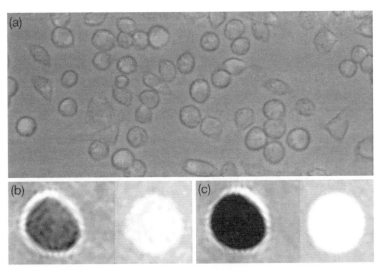

Fig. 5.2. (a) In vitro image of cultured J774 mouse macrophage cells labeled overnight with RuBpy–Gd particles. Merged image, 20× brightfield/Texas red. (b) T1w spin-echo sequence, TR/TE = 1500/7 ms, of live J774 cells at 4.7T magnetic field strength. *Left:* RuBPy–Gd-labeled cells, *Right:* Unlabeled control cells. Due to the extremely short transverse relaxation time of the labeled cells, positive contrast is not obtained. Longitudinal relaxation times (T1) for labeled versus unlabeled cells were determined to be 0.24 versus 2.13 s. (c) T2w spin-echo image, TR/TE = 1500/32 ms, of the same cells depict the rapid transverse relaxation as a complete loss of signal from the labeled cells. Transverse relaxation times (T2) for labeled versus unlabeled cells were determined to be 14.5 versus 239.4 ms (all MRI data were analyzed using Paravision 3.0.2 software).

particles, and the Gd is chelated to the silica shell on Qdots to integrate the MR activity. **Figure 5.3** shows the TEM image of the multimodal Qdots and the schematic representation of the design of the construct. Qdots have many advantages over the dye-doped silica core in terms of increased photostability, broad

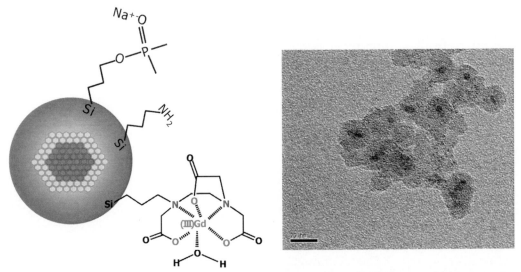

Fig. 5.3. Schematic representation of a silica-coated CdS:Mn/ZnS core/shell quantum dot functionalized by APTS, THPMP, and TSPETE, and a transmission electron microscopic image of Gd-Qdots (the scale bar in TEM image is 20 nm).

absorption and sharp emission spectra, and large Stokes shift (36) which are useful for many cell-labeling and cell-tracking experiments. However, the long-term toxicity of Qdots due to leaching of Cd ions, particularly in acidic biological environments, limits their applications, especially for clinical implementation. CdS:Mn/ZnS Qdots used in this study have fluorescence emission at ~590 nm with 400 nm excitation.

3.3.1. Synthesis of CdS:Mn/ZnS Core

The overall synthesis of the multimodal Qdots was carried out in AOT/heptane/water w/o microemulsion. Initially, 0.2 M AOT solution in heptane was prepared. The microemulsions were prepared by adding 3.6 mL of Cd:Mn acetate solution [$Cd(CH_3COO)_2 \cdot 2H_2O$ (0.096 g), $Mn(CH_3COO)_2$ (0.0012 g)] in 100 mL 0.2M AOT in small aliquots while stirring continuously. Similarly, Na_2S (0.5624 g in 10.8 mL H_2O) and $Zn(CH_3COO)_2 \cdot 2H_2O$ (0.61 g in 10.8 mL H_2O) microemulsions were formed separately by slow addition to 300 mL 0.2M AOT. All the solutions were allowed to stir till optically clear microemulsions were obtained (*see* **Note 4**). Mn-doped CdS core was first formed by fast mixing of Cd, Mn, and Na_2S microemulsions, and stirring for 15 min. This was followed by the slow addition (1.5–2 mL/min using peristaltic pump (*see* **Note 5**)) of Zn microemulsion under continuous stirring. An excess of sulfide ions added in the previous step were used to form the ZnS shell surrounding the CdS:Mn core.

3.3.2. Derivatization and Incorporation of Functional Features

This was achieved by first forming a silica shell around the Qdot core followed by an additional layer of silica containing chelating ligands. The silica shell was formed by the addition of 7.4 mL of TEOS to the microemulsion and stirring for ~30 min. The hydrolysis and condensation of TEOS were catalyzed by the addition of NH_4OH microemulsion (4.4 mL NH_4OH in 150 mL of 0.165 M AOT in heptane) to the above microemulsion. The reaction was allowed to go on for 24 h. Next 3.7 mL of TEOS and 0.74 mL of APTS were added to the microemulsion and the contents stirred for 15 min. Another microemulsion prepared by solubilizing chelating ligands and surface functionalization agents (2.22 mL THPMP and 1.11 mL TSPET in 10.66 mL water) in AOT (0.59 M in heptane, 50 mL) was added to the above microemulsion. This was followed by the addition of NH_4OH microemulsion (2.64 mL NH_4OH in 50 mL of 0.3 M AOT in heptane) and 24 h of stirring. Finally, Gd containing microemulsion (0.3608 g of Gd acetate in 5.28 mL H_2O was solubilized in 50 mL of 0.59 M AOT) was added to the above microemulsion and allowed to react for additional 24 h.

3.3.3. Extraction

The multimodal Qdots were extracted from the microemulsion following similar procedure as described in **Section 3.2.4**.

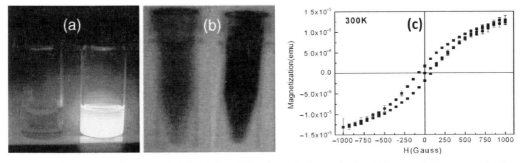

Fig. 5.4. (a) Fluorescence images of Q-dots (*right*) and DI water (*left*) obtained using 366 nm excitation source. (b) Fluoroscopy images of Q-dots (*right*) and Omnipaque, a commercial X-ray contrast agent (*left*) obtained at equal concentration using X-ray source. (c) Magnetization curve for Q-dots. Reprinted with permission from (35). Copyright 2005 American Chemical Society.

Figure 5.4 shows the fluorescence, X-ray contrast, and magnetic properties of the multimodal quantum dots.

3.4. Synthesis of MR-PAT Multimodal Contrast Agents

Traditionally, the contrast agents for PAT include near-infrared absorbing dyes (e.g., indocyanine green) and silica core gold shell nanoparticles. Our group has recently reported the synthesis of Gd-doped gold-speckled silica (GSS) nanoparticles as multimodal contrast agent for MRI and PAT using reverse micelles (37). One of the main differences of GSS nanoparticles as compared to other particles previously reported exists in the method and pattern of gold deposition on the silica particle surface (**Fig. 5.5**). In the current approach of using w/o microemulsions, the one-pot synthesis results in the discontinuous, irregular deposition of gold nanodomains on the silica surface previously doped with Gd giving rise to a speckled surface. Numerous metal–dielectric (gold–silica) interfaces created by this method result in the unique photothermal properties of these nanoparticles which have a characteristic broad absorption making these constructs effective PAT contrast agents. The incorporation of Gd in the silica matrix

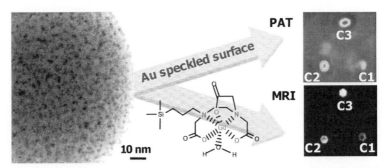

Fig. 5.5. Gold-speckled silica nanoparticles doped with gadolinium shell show both PAT and MRI contrasts. C1, C2, and C3 are in the increasing order of particle concentration in tissue-like phantom.

adds MR contrast. The synthesis of these particles in nonionic microemulsions is described below.

3.4.1. Synthesis of the Silica Core

The preparation of the core was carried out in the traditional way as described previously in **Section 3.2.1**.

3.4.2. Derivatization and Incorporation of Functional Features

The surface of the silica particles was modified with silane-chelating agents as described previously in **Section 3.2.2** by co-condensation of TSPET and TEOS with small modification. The reaction and stirring time were reduced to 4 h post-TSPET addition. As mentioned previously, the solution needed to be stirred vigorously after small intervals of time to enable the solubilization of high osmolality solution of TSPET. Thereafter, 125 µL of 0.5 M $HAuCl_4$ (prepared in degassed water) was added in small aliquots to the microemulsion and stirred for 30 min. The incubation of the silica nanoparticle and gold ions within the aqueous core allow the penetration of the ions within the pores of the silica matrix. The reduction of the gold ions was carried by the addition of 1.1 M solution of reducing agent dropwise to the microemulsion. A gradual darkening in the color of the solution was observed, turning finally to dark green/black. The solution was stirred overnight for ∼12 h.

3.4.3. Extraction and Washing Off the Particles

The particles were extracted and washed by using the method previously described in **Section 3.2.4**. The MR and PAT contrast-generating ability of the Gd-doped GSS nanoparticles in tissue-like phantom is shown in **Fig. 5.5**.

3.4.4. Surface Modification for Dispersion

The Gd-doped GSS nanoparticles had a discontinuous, irregular deposition of 1–5 nm gold nanodomains on the silica surface and tend to fall out of solution on standing. To improve the dispersion of the nanoparticles, the gold domains on the silica surface were pegylated using O-[2-(3-mercaptopropionylamino)ethyl]-O'-methylpolyethylene glycol (PEG-thiol 5,000 MW). Briefly, 10 mg of Gd-doped GSS particles were dispersed by sonication in 30 mL of degassed water. About 15 mg of PEG-thiol dissolved in 2 mL of degassed water was added to the GSS suspension under sonication. To prevent the oxidation of the thiol groups, N_2 gas was constantly bubbled through the suspension and the stirring was continued for 2 h. The particles were purified (to remove unbound PEG) by repeated centrifugation and redispersion in double deionized water.

3.5. Surface Modification for Active Targeting

In order to image/detect the tumor cells, delivery of nanoparticles to the tumor cite is essential. The multimodal nanoparticles described above, due to their small size, extravasate out of tumor microvasculature and deposit in the tumor interstitium (enhanced permeation and retention (EPR) effect). The targeting efficiency of these nanoparticles can further be enhanced by their surface functionalization with antibodies, peptides, aptamers, carbohydrates, and small molecules. Surface modification of particles for conjugation of targeting agents generally involves two steps. First, the particle surface is modified to obtain appropriate functional groups like amines, carboxyls, and thiols. Second, the nanoparticles are "bioconjugated" or attached to the bio-recognition molecules using suitable coupling reagents (38). For example, amine-modified Qdots were conjugated to TAT peptide (cell-penetrating peptide) using N-succinimidyl 3-(2-pyridyldithio)propionate (SPDP) chemistry (35). The in vivo bioimaging ability of the particles was demonstrated by injecting the TAT-conjugated Qdots through the right common carotid artery to the right part of the rat's brain. **Figure 5.6** shows the labeling of branches of the right middle cerebral artery.

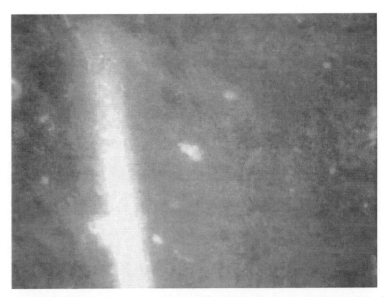

Fig. 5.6. The fluorescence image of cross section of rat brain showing the labeling of the branches of right middle cerebral artery with TAT-conjugated Qdots. Reprinted (in part) with permission from (35). Copyright 2005 American Chemical Society.

3.6. Conclusion and Future Directions

In summary, the microemulsion-based synthesis of multimodal nanoparticles (MR-Optical and MR-PAT), characterization, and functional evaluation as contrast agents was described. In addition to the multimodal imaging capabilities, therapeutic functionality (drug/gene delivery or photothermal therapy) may be implemented via these particles. For instance, in addition to photoacoustic imaging, the absorbance property of irregular gold nanodomains of GSS can also be utilized for the photothermal ablation of tumors. Development of these multifunctional nanoconstructs has great potential in the field of nanomedicine and nanodiagnostics. However, their biocompatibility, dispersion, and stability in biological medium need to be addressed before any direct clinical applications can be made.

4. Notes

1. Upon mixing the microemulsion solution should appear optically clear; if not then modifications to the protocol are necessary to ensure the production of monodisperse particles. Because of variations in the manufactured properties of TX-100, which is a polydisperse nonionic surfactant, we have noticed that, on occasion, additional water may need to be added to the microemulsion to induce clarity (e.g., 480 μL instead of 340 μL of water). Alternatively, the TX-100 surfactant concentration may be reduced to also induce clarity at the same water content. If difficulties are encountered, it is advised that simple titration experiments are performed to determine where the water-in-oil suspension transits from a whitish emulsion to a clear microemulsion. Because we are performing subsequent aqueous additions, it is advantageous to be at lower water loadings within the clear microemulsion regime. The amount of water that can be added to microemulsions is limited; after a certain threshold is reached microemulsions will revert back to thermodynamically unstable emulsions.

2. TSPET is a 45-wt% solution in water and it tends to form oligomers with time. Formation of oligomers in TSPET solution decreases its solubility in water and hence use of aged TSPET should be avoided in the synthesis.

3. A quick check to ensure that the surfactants have been sufficiently removed is to check for suspension foamability in water. In the presence of small amounts of TX-100 relatively stable, surfactant-induced foaming occurs with aerating mechanical agitation. Hence, one can determine if additional washing steps are necessary if a noticeable and relatively stable foam layer appears after vigorously shaking the washed nanoparticle suspension in water. It should also be noted that depending on the conditions used during synthesis, surfactants may leach out of the silica particles over time. Usually, after completing the initial washing steps, we will store the nanoparticles for 24 h and recheck for foamability. If foaming is noticed, the samples should be re-washed and then rechecked for surfactant leaching. Typically, subsequent leaching after the second washing procedure does not occur.

4. As previously noted, the microemulsions should be clear prior to continuing any subsequent addition. For AOT surfactant, we have noticed that aging of the surfactant can hinder the formation of clear microemulsions. Hence use of fresh surfactant solution is advised. Also, depending on manufacturer and impurities some modifications to the microemulsion formulation may be necessary in parallel to the advice given in **Note 1**.

5. Plasticizer-free silicone tubing is recommended. Leachants from lower grade peristaltic tubings can severely impact the synthesis of quantum dots.

Acknowledgments

The authors acknowledge the financial support of the Particle Engineering Research Center (PERC) at the University of Florida, the National Science Foundation (NSF Grant EEC-94-02989, NSF-NIRT Grant EEC-0506560), the National Institute of Health (RO1HL75258, R01HL78670), James and Esther King Biomedical Research Program (Grant 06NIR-05), Patricia Adams Cancer Nanotechnology Research Fund, and the Industrial Partners of the PERC for support of his research. Any opinions, findings, and conclusions or recommendations expressed in this material are those of the author(s) and do not necessarily reflect those of the National Science Foundation. NMR (MRI) data were obtained at the Advanced Magnetic Resonance Imaging and Spectroscopy (AMRIS) facility in the McKnight Brain Institute of the University of Florida. P.S. acknowledges Principal, St. Stephen's College, Delhi, India, for granting leave for research.

References

1. Frullano, L. and Meade, T. J. Multimodal M. R. I. contrast agents (2007) *J Biol Inorg Chem* **12**(7), 939–949.
2. Rudin, M. and Weissleder, R. Molecular imaging in drug discovery and development (2003) *Nat Rev Drug Discov* **2**(2), 123–131.
3. Tallury, P., Payton, K., and Santra, S. Silica-based multimodal/multifunctional nanoparticles for bioimaging and biosensing applications (2008) *Nanomedicine* **3**(4), 579–592.
4. Kim, J., Piao, Y., and Hyeon, T. Multifunctional nanostructured materials for multimodal imaging, and simultaneous imaging and therapy (2009) *Chem Soc Rev* **38**(2), 372–390.
5. Cheon, J. and Lee, J. H. Synergistically integrated nanoparticles as multimodal probes for nanobiotechnology (2008) *Accounts Chem Res* **41**(12), 1630–1640.
6. Mulder, W. J. M., Griffioen, A. W., Strijkers, G. J., Cormode, D. P., Nicolay, K., and Fayad, Z. A. Magnetic and fluorescent nanoparticles for multimodality imaging (2007) *Nanomedicine* **2**(3), 307–324.
7. Graves, E. E., Ripoll, J., Weissleder, R., and Ntziachristos, V. A submillimeter resolution fluorescence molecular imaging system for small animal imaging (2003) *Med Phys* **30**(5), 901–911.

8. Ntziachristos, V. and Weissleder, R. Charge-coupled-device based scanner for tomography of fluorescent near-infrared probes in turbid media (2002) *Med Phys* **29**(5), 803–809.
9. Kircher, M. F., Mahmood, U., King, R. S., Weissleder, R., and Josephson, L. A multimodal nanoparticle for preoperative magnetic resonance imaging and intraoperative optical brain tumor delineation (2003) *Cancer Res* **63**(23), 8122–8125.
10. Bremer, C. and Weissleder, R. Molecular imaging – in vivo imaging of gene expression: MR and optical technologies (2001) *Acad Radiol* **8**(1), 15–23.
11. Persigehl, T., Heindel, W., and Bremer, C. MR and optical approaches to molecular imaging (2005) *Abdom Imaging* **30**(3), 342–354.
12. Sosnovik, D. and Weissleder, R. (2005) Magnetic resonance and fluorescence based molecular imaging technologies. *Imaging Drug Discov Early Clin Trials* **62**, 83–115.
13. Esenaliev, R. O., Karabutov, A. A., and Oraevsky, A. A. Sensitivity of laser optoacoustic imaging in detection of small deeply embedded tumors (1999) *IEEE J Sel Top Quant Electron* **5**(4), 981–988.
14. Wang, X. D., Pang, Y. J., Ku, G., Xie, X. Y., Stoica, G., and Wang, L. H. V. Noninvasive laser-induced photoacoustic tomography for structural and functional in vivo imaging of the brain (2003) *Nat Biotechnol* **21**(7), 803–806.
15. Ku, G., Wang, X., Stoica, G., and Wang, L. V. Multiple-bandwidth photoacoustic tomography (2004) *Phys Med Biol* **49**(7), 1329–1338.
16. Ku, G., Fornage, B. D., Jin, X., Xu, M. H., Hunt, K. K., and Wang, L. V. Thermoacoustic and photoacoustic tomography of thick biological tissues toward breast imaging (2005) *Technol Cancer Res Treatment* **4**(5), 559–565.
17. Oraevsky, A. A., Ermilov, S. A., Conjusteau, A., et al (2007) Initial clinical evaluation of laser optoacoustic imaging system for diagnostic imaging of breast cancer. *Breast Canc Res Treat* **106**, S47.
18. Ku, G., Wang, X. D., Xie, X. Y., Stoica, G., and Wang, L. H. V. Imaging of tumor angiogenesis in rat brains in vivo by photoacoustic tomography (2005) *Appl Optics* **44**(5), 770–775.
19. Wang, X. D., Xie, X. Y., Ku, G. N., and Wang, L. H. V. (2006) Noninvasive imaging of hemoglobin concentration and oxygenation in the rat brain using high-resolution photoacoustic tomography. *J Biomed Optics* **11**(2), 024015.
20. Pileni, M. P. Reverse micelles as microreactors (1993) *J Physical Chem* **97**(27), 6961–6973.
21. Evans, D. F. and Wennerström, H. (1994) *The Colloidal Domain: Where Physics, Chemistry, Biology, and Technology Meet.* VCH Publishers, New York, NY.
22. Mittal, K. L. and Kumar, P. (1999) *Handbook of Microemulsion Science and Technology.* Marcel Dekker, New York.
23. Pileni, M. P. (1989) *Structure and Reactivity in Reverse Micelles.* Elsevier, Amsterdam; New York.
24. Fendler, J. H. (1982) *Membrane Mimetic Chemistry: Characterizations and Applications of Micelles, Microemulsions, Monolayers, Bilayers, Vesicles, Host-Guest Systems, and Polyions.* Wiley, New York.
25. Texter, J. (2001) *Reactions and Synthesis in Surfactant Systems.* Marcel Dekker, New York.
26. Rosano, H. L. and Clausse, M. (1987) *Microemulsion Systems.* M. Dekker, New York, NY.
27. Lopez-Quintela, M. A., Tojo, C., Blanco, M. C., Rio, L. G., and Leis, J. R. Microemulsion dynamics and reactions in microemulsions (2004) *Curr Opin Colloid Interface Sci* **9**(3–4), 264–278.
28. Sharma, P., Brown, S., Varshney, M., and Moudgil, B. (2008) Surfactant-Mediated Fabrication of Optical Nanoprobes. *Interfacial Proces Mol Aggregation Surfactants* **218**, 189–233.
29. Abarkan, I., Doussineau, T., and Smaihi, M. Tailored macro/micro structural properties of colloidal silica nanoparticles via microemulsion preparation (2006) *Polyhedron* **25**(8), 1763–1770.
30. Bagwe, R. P., Yang, C. Y., Hilliard, L. R., and Tan, W. H. Optimization of dye-doped silica nanoparticles prepared using a reverse microemulsion method (2004) *Langmuir* **20**(19), 8336–8342.
31. Santra, S., Wang, K. M., Tapec, R., and Tan, W. H. Development of novel dye-doped silica nanoparticles for biomarker application (2001) *J Biomed Optics* **6**(2), 160–166.
32. Schroedter, A. and Weller, H. Ligand design and bioconjugation of colloidal gold nanoparticles (2002) *Angewandte Chemie Int Ed* **41**(17), 3218–3221.
33. Santra, S., Yang, H., Dutta, D., et al (2004) TAT conjugated, FITC doped silica nanoparticles for bioimaging applications. *Chem Commun* **24**, 2810–2811.
34. Santra, S., Bagwe, R. P., Dutta, D., et al. Synthesis and characterization of fluorescent,

radio-opaque, and paramagnetic silica nanoparticles for multimodal bioimaging applications (2005) *Adv Mater* **17**(18), 2165–2169.

35. Santra, S., Yang, H. S., Holloway, P. H., Stanley, J. T., and Mericle, R. A. Synthesis of water-dispersible fluorescent, radio-opaque, and paramagnetic CdS: Mn/ZnS quantum dots: a multifunctional probe for bioimaging (2005) *J Am Chem Soc* **127**(6), 1656–1657.

36. Sharrna, P., Brown, S., Walter, G., Santra, S., and Moudgil, B. (2006) Nanoparticles for bioimaging. *Adv Colloid Interface Sci* **123**, 471–485.

37. Sharma, P., Brown, S. C., Bengtsson, N., et al. Gold-speckled multimodal nanoparticles for noninvasive bioimaging (2008) *Chem Mater* **20**(19), 6087–6094.

38. Hermanson, G. T. (2008) *Bioconjugate Techniques*. 2nd ed. Academic Press, New York.

Chapter 6

Gold Nanocages for Cancer Imaging and Therapy

Leslie Au, Jingyi Chen, Lihong V. Wang, and Younan Xia

Abstract

Gold nanocages are hollow nanostructures with porous walls that can be simply prepared via the galvanic replacement reaction between silver nanocubes and chloroauric acid. Their optical resonance peaks can be precisely tuned into the near-infrared region, in which the adsorption caused by blood or soft tissue is essentially negligible. Significantly, the strong absorption of gold nanocages makes them attractive as a novel class of contrast enhancement and photothermal agents for cancer detection and treatment. The well-established chemistry for gold also allows them to target specific cells by functionalizing their surface with various moieties such as antibodies, peptides, and DNAs. In this chapter, we focus on their use as a photothermal agent for the ablation of cancer cells and as a contrast agent for the in vivo noninvasive photoacoustic imaging of blood vessels and the sentinel lymph nodes in rats.

Key words: Localized surface plasmon resonance, hollow nanostructures, galvanic replacement reaction, silver nanocube, gold nanocage, contrast agent, photoacoustic imaging, photothermal therapy.

1. Introduction

Hollow nanostructures composed of noble metals have tunable optical properties and are finding use in a wide range of applications including catalysis (1), optical sensing (2), drug delivery (3), biomedical imaging (4–6), and photothermal therapy (7–10). The most versatile method for the synthesis of bimetallic hollow nanostructures is the galvanic replacement reaction (1, 11–18). In particular, the replacement reaction between silver nanocubes and chloroauric acid shown in equation [1] has been extensively explored (19) in the generation of gold nanocages with hollow interiors and porous walls.

$$3\text{Ag(s)} + \text{AuCl}_4^-(\text{aq}) \rightarrow \text{Au(s)} + 3\text{Ag}^+(\text{aq}) + 4\text{Cl}^-(\text{aq}) \quad [1]$$

By simply varying the amount of chloroauric acid added to a suspension of silver nanocubes (11–19), the localized surface plasmon resonance (LSPR) peak of the gold nanocages can be continuously and precisely tuned from 400 nm to the near-infrared region, where the attenuation of light by blood or soft tissue is essentially negligible. The extremely strong optical absorption associated with gold nanocages makes them a novel class of photothermal and contrast agent for biomedical applications (5, 8, 10). Specifically, gold nanocages are optimal contrast agents for photoacoustic imaging, which is sensitive to the optical absorption of biological tissue (20, 21). When the surface of the gold nanocages is modified with antibodies, peptides, or DNAs, they can actively target the specific receptors overexpressed on cancer cells. On the other hand, gold nanocages can passively accumulate at the cancer site via the enhanced permeability and retention (EPR) effect when the surface of the nanocages is modified with polyethylene glycol (PEG) which prolongs their circulation time and decreases their immunogenicity. As a result, both immuno and PEGylated gold nanocages are expected to find widespread use in the detection and treatment of cancer.

In this chapter, we focus on the preparation of gold nanocages, and their use in photothermal therapy and photoacoustic imaging. First, silver nanocubes are produced by a sulfide-mediated polyol process (22, 23), followed by their conversion to gold nanocages via the replacement reaction, and subsequently surface-modified with PEG or antibodies. Second, the photothermal effect of immuno gold nanocages on SK-BR-3 human breast cancer cells is qualitatively observed by fluorescence microscopy and quantitatively measured using flow cytometry. Finally, the PEGylated gold nanocages are applied as a contrast agent for photoacoustic imaging to better detect blood vessels and sentinel lymph nodes (SLN) in rats.

2. Materials

2.1. Preparation of Immuno Gold Nanocages

2.1.1. Chemicals for Silver Nanocube Synthesis

1. Ethylene glycol (EG) (Mallinckrodt Baker, Phillipsburg, NJ, cat. no. 9300) with low concentrations of iron and chloride ions (*see* **Note 1**).
2. Poly(vinyl pyrrolidone) (PVP), powder, $M_w \approx 55,000$ (Sigma-Aldrich, St. Louis, MO, cat. no. 856568), is dissolved at 20 mg/mL in EG (*see* **Note 2**).
3. $Na_2S \cdot 9H_2O$ (Mallinckrodt Baker, cat. no. 3910) or NaHS (Sigma-Aldrich, cat. no. 161527) is dissolved in EG at 3 mM (*see* **Note 3**).

4. AgNO$_3$, >99% (Sigma-Aldrich, cat. no. 209139) is dissolved in EG at 48 mg/mL (*see* **Note 4**).

5. Acetone (reagent grade).

6. Ethanol (reagent grade).

7. 18.1 MΩ·cm water which is referred to as pure water throughout this chapter.

2.1.2. Chemicals for Gold Nanocage Synthesis

1. Silver nanocubes as synthesized.

2. Chloroauric acid, >99.9% (HAuCl$_4$·3H$_2$O, Sigma-Aldrich, cat. no. 520918), is dissolved in pure water at 0.2 mM (*see* **Note 5**).

3. PVP, powder, $M_w \approx$ 55,000 or 29,000 (Sigma-Aldrich, cat. no. 856568 or 234257), is dissolved in pure water at 1 mg/mL.

4. Sodium chloride (NaCl) crystal, >99%.

2.1.3. Chemicals for Surface Modification

1. Gold nanocages suspended in 1 mL of pure water at 2 nM.

2. To increase the circulation time of gold nanocages, methoxy poly(ethylene glycol)-thiol (mPEG-SH), $M_w \approx$ 5,000, is dissolved in 1 mL of pure water at 1 mM. For the gold nanocages to target specific cells, orthopyridyl disulfide-poly(ethylene glycol)-succinimidyl carbonate (OPSS-PEG-SC), $M_w \approx$ 5,000 (Laysan Bio, Arab, AL), is dissolved in 1 mL of pure water at 1 mM (*see* **Note 6**).

3. Phosphate-buffered saline (PBS), pH = 7.4, 1×, liquid (Invitrogen, Carlsbad, CA, cat. no. 10010).

4. Mouse anti-HER2 (Invitrogen, cat. no. 28-0003Z) diluted in 1 mL of PBS at 40 μL/mL.

2.1.4. Equipment for the Synthesis

1. Stirring hotplate with a temperature controller.

2. Crystallization dish filled with silicone fluid (Thomas Scientific, Swedesboro, NJ, cat. no. 6428-R15).

3. Vial holder (custom-made for crystallization dish, *see* **Fig. 6.1a**) to fit 24-mL borosilicate vials (VWR, West Chester, PA, cat. no. 66011-143) (*see* **Note 7**) supported by rubber O-rings.

4. Teflon-coated magnetic stir bars (VWR, cat. no. 58949-010) (*see* **Note 8**).

5. 50-mL round bottom flask with bushing-type adaptor and septum for covering the bushing-type adaptor hole.

6. Poly(propylene) centrifuge tubes, capacity 50 mL.

7. Poly(propylene) micro-centrifuge tubes, capacity 1.5 mL.

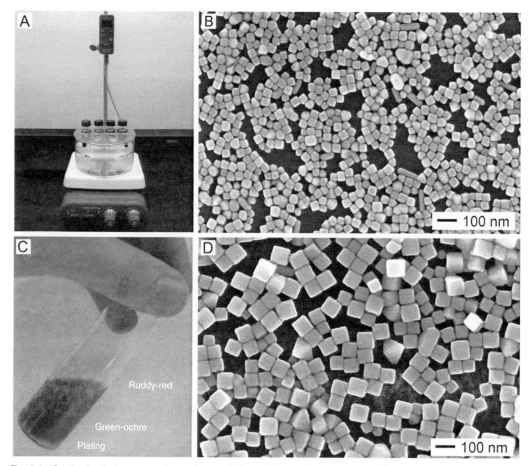

Fig. 6.1. Synthesis of silver nanocubes using a sulfide-mediated polyol process. (**a**) Photograph of the setup for silver nanocube synthesis; (**b**) SEM image of silver nanocubes with an average edge length of 45 nm that was obtained at 7 min into the reaction; (**c**) photograph of the reaction solution, which would display a green-ochre color with a ruddy-red meniscus; and (**d**) SEM image of silver nanocubes with an average edge length of 90 nm that was obtained when the reaction was prolonged to 20 min. Reproduced with permission from (22). Copyright 2007, Nature Publishing Group.

9. Programmable syringe pump with digital display (KD Scientific, Holliston, MA, cat. no. KDS100 230).
10. Disposable plastic syringe, 10 mL (BD Vacutainer, Franklin Lakes, NJ, cat. no. 309604 EMD) and poly(vinyl chloride) (PVC) tubing (VWR, cat. no. 60985-501) for reagent delivery and any necessary adaptors.

2.1.5. Instrumentation for Characterization of Gold Nanocages

1. UV–visible spectrometer.
2. Scanning electron microscope (SEM).
3. Transmission electron microscope (TEM).
4. Inductively coupled plasma mass spectrometer (ICP-MS).

2.2. Preparation for Photothermal Treatment In Vitro

2.2.1. Chemicals for Cell Culture

1. SK-BR-3 human breast cancer cells (ATCC, Manassas, VA, cat. no. HTB-30).
2. McCoy's 5a Medium Modified (ATCC, cat. no. 30-2007) containing 10% fetal bovine serum (Invitrogen, cat. no. 16000) and 1% streptomycin/penicillin (Invitrogen, cat. no. 15140).
3. Phosphate-buffered saline (PBS)
4. Trypsin, 0.25% (1×) with EDTA, liquid (Invitrogen, cat. no. 25200).
5. 96-well plate, tissue culture treated, flat bottom.

2.2.2. Equipment for Photothermal Treatment

1. Near-infrared femtosecond-pulsed laser (home-built Kerr-lens mode-locked Ti:sapphire laser) with a bandwidth of 54 nm, a pulsed repetition rate at 82 MHz, and a central wavelength tuned to match the absorption peak of the gold nanocages.
2. Appropriate lens and mirrors to focus and direct, respectively, the laser beam with a spot size of 2 mm in diameter on the sample.
3. Neutral density attenuator to adjust the power of the laser.
4. Power meter to measure the output power of the laser.

2.2.3. Qualitative Study of the Photothermal Effect

1. 1 mL of 2 nM immuno gold nanocages.
2. SK-BR-3 cells grown to 80–90% confluency in 96-well plates.
3. Calcein-AM and ethidium homodimer-1 (EthD-1) (Invitrogen, cat. no. L3224) or another viability/cytotoxicity kit for mammalian cells.
4. Fluorescence microscope.

2.2.4. Quantitative Study of the Photothermal Effect

1. 1 mL of 2 nM immuno gold nanocages.
2. SK-BR-3 cells grown to 80–90% confluency in 96-well plates.
3. Propidium iodide (PI) (Invitrogen, cat. no. P3566) is diluted to 1 µg/mL with pure water
4. Flow cytometer.

2.3. Preparation for Photoacoustic Imaging In Vivo

1. 2 mL of 2 nM gold nanocages (bare or with PEG on surface).
2. Sprague Dawley rats.
3. Q-switched Nd:YAG laser (LS-2137/2, LOTISII)-pumped tunable Ti:sapphire laser (LT-2211A, LOTIS TII)

with a full width at half maximum <15 ps, a pulse repetition rate of 10 Hz, a central wavelength tuned to match the absorption peak of gold nanocages, and incident energy density of <10 mJ/cm^2.

4. Unfocused ultrasonic transducer with a central frequency of 3.5–10 MHz and a –6 dB bandwidth of about 70%.
5. Hair-removal lotion.
6. Mixture of ketamine (85 mg/kg body weight) and xylazine (15 mg/kg body weight).
7. Vaporized isoflurane (1 L/min oxygen and 0.75% isoflurane, Euthanex Corp., Allentown, PA).
8. Pulse oximeter (NONIN Medical Inc., Plymouth, MN, 8600 V).
9. Saline (0.9%).
10. Pentobarbital.

3. Methods

3.1. Synthesis of Immuno Gold Nanocages

3.1.1. Synthesis of Silver Nanocubes

1. Preheat the oil bath to 150–155°C and set the spin rate between 260 and 350 rpm.
2. Pipette 6 mL of EG into each reaction vial and add a new or clean stir bar to each vial.
3. Suspend each vial with an O-ring as a support in the heated oil bath using the vial holder as shown in **Fig. 6.1a**. Place a cap loosely on top of each vial to allow water vapor to escape. Heat for 1 h and in the meantime prepare EG solutions of PVP, Na$_2$S or NaHS, and AgNO$_3$.
4. After the vials containing EG have been heated for 1 h, remove their caps and pipette 70–100 μL of the approximately 3 mM Na$_2$S or NaHS solution in EG into the vials (*see* **Note 9**). Place the caps loosely on top of the vials and wait for 8 min.
8. Remove the vial caps and pipette 1.5 mL of the PVP solution into each vial and wait for 1.5 min.
9. Pipette 0.5 mL of the AgNO$_3$ solution into each vial. Screw caps tight on top of the vials. A series of color changes should be observed. The solution darkens from a bright yellow to a deep orange after 3 min into the reaction due to the growth of small silver particles. Between 3 and 7 min, the cubes grow to 45 nm as shown in **Fig. 6.1b**, displaying a ruddy-red color at the meniscus, a green-ochre-colored reaction media, and some plating on the vial as shown in

Fig. 6.1c. Allowing the reaction to proceed for a slightly longer time, up to 20 min, will yield larger nanocubes with an average edge length of ~90 nm as shown in **Fig. 6.1d** and is characterized by a more ochre-colored appearance. However, substantially longer reaction times will result in the etching of silver cubes and/or rounding of their corners.

10. To quench the reaction, remove the reaction vials from the heated oil bath and place them in a water bath held at room temperature.

11. Once the reaction solution has cooled, transfer the content of each vial into a 50-mL centrifuge tube. Rinse each vial with acetone and transfer the washings into their appropriate centrifuge tube. Spin down the product at $2,000 \times g$ for 15–20 min. Remove and discard the supernatant (*see* **Note 10**).

12. Add approximately 2 mL of pure water to each centrifuge tube, sonicate to re-disperse the products, then transfer as much of each product to its own 1.5-mL centrifuge tube. Spin down the product at $9,000 \times g$ for 10 min. Remove and discard the supernatant.

13. Transfer any remaining product into its corresponding 1.5-mL centrifuge tube and fill the remaining of tube volume with pure water. Spin down the product at $9,000 \times g$ for 10 min. Remove and discard the supernatant.

14. Once each product has been consolidated to its corresponding centrifuge tube, re-disperse the product via sonication in pure water, spin down the product, and remove and discard the supernatant; repeat this washing process with pure water a total of three times.

15. To store the silver nanocubes, transfer the washed nanocubes to a scintillation vial and dilute to 4 mL with pure water (*see* **Note 11**). For a successful synthesis, this dilution corresponds to a concentration of approximately 6–8 nM for silver nanocubes of 40 nm in edge length as determined by ICP-MS and SEM imaging. A reaction yield of greater than 90% is typical.

16. To characterize the silver nanocubes with SEM, deposit approximately 1 μL of the silver nanocube suspension (prepared in Step 15) on a piece of silicon substrate and allow to dry under ambient conditions. Wash the dried sample in a flow cell with water for 30–60 min to remove excess PVP. Blow the sample dry with a quick burst of dry nitrogen. Image the sample by SEM within a few hours of preparation following your institution's operating procedures (typical conditions: 10 kV).

90   Au et al.

3.1.2. Synthesis of Gold Nanocages

1. Pipette 5 mL of the aqueous PVP solution into a 50-mL round bottom flask to which a clean stir bar has been added. Then pipette 100 μL of the as-obtained silver nanocubes into the PVP solution. Place the bushing-type adaptor on top of the round bottom flask, covering the adaptor's hole loosely with a rubber septum. Heat the suspension to a mild boil for approximately 10 min.

2. Load the $HAuCl_4$ solution into a disposable plastic syringe equipped with PVC tubing and place the syringe into a syringe pump. Remove the rubber septum from the adaptor. With the syringe pump, add a specific volume of the $HAuCl_4$ solution to the reaction flask at a rate of 0.75 mL/min. As the $HAuCl_4$ solution is added to the reaction flask, a series of color changes as shown in **Fig. 6.2a** will be observed and can be used to estimate the position of the absorption peak for the gold nanocages. Stop adding $HAuCl_4$ solution when the appropriate color is observed: e.g., blue, so the resonance peak will overlap with the Ti:sapphire laser with a center wavelength at 825 nm.

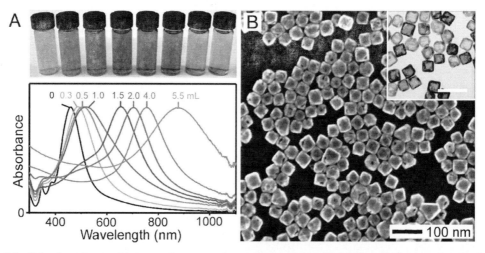

Fig. 6.2. Galvanic replacement between silver nanocubes and chloroauric acid. (**a**) The optical resonant peak of gold nanocages can be tuned to different wavelengths depending on the amount of chloroauric acid added; and (**b**) SEM and TEM (inset) images of typical gold nanocages obtained from this synthesis. The *scale bar* in the inset corresponds to 100 nm. Reproduced with permission from (22) and (23). Copyright 2007 and 2006, Nature Publishing Group and Elsevier.

3. Record the volume of $HAuCl_4$ solution added. Continue to reflux the reaction for an additional 10 min until its color becomes stable and then cool down the system to room temperature. Vigorous magnetic stirring should be maintained during the entire process.

4. Record a UV–visible spectrum from the reaction suspension to determine the absorption peak of the gold

nanocages. Repeat Steps 1–3, adjusting the volume of HAuCl$_4$ added to fine tune the resonance peak for your application (i.e., additional HAuCl$_4$ solution will further red-shift the resonance peak of the product). The reaction solution can be left under ambient conditions for several weeks without any observable changes to the quality of the gold nanocages.

5. To harvest the gold nanocages, transfer the product to a 50-mL centrifuge tube. Rinse the reaction flask with deionized water and add the washings to the centrifuge tube. During the galvanic replacement reaction, AgCl is generated, which precipitates out of the solution upon cooling of the reaction. The AgCl solid can be dissolved and removed with the addition of a saturated solution of NaCl. To achieve this, add NaCl crystals to the aqueous dispersion of gold nanocages until saturation is reached.

6. Centrifuge the mixture at $9,000 \times g$ for a minimum of 30 min. A pellet of gold nanocages should be obtained on top of the precipitated NaCl and a blue tinge will color the wall of the centrifuge tube. Remove and discard the supernatant containing the dissolved AgCl.

7. Re-disperse the gold nanocages in 20 mL of water to dissolve the excess NaCl crystals. Isolate the gold nanocages by centrifugation, followed by decantation. Perform this procedure a minimum of three more times to completely remove NaCl and excess PVP.

8. Re-disperse the gold nanocages in a 1:1 mixture of ethanol and pure water; sonication will likely be necessary to remove the gold nanocages from the wall of the centrifuge tube and disperse them into the solvent mixture. Transfer the dispersed nanocages to a 1.5-mL centrifuge tube. Collect the gold nanocages by centrifugation, followed by decantation. Store the nanocages in pure water until use (*see* **Note 12**). Approximately 10% of the gold nanocages are often lost during the washing process.

9. Acquire an SEM image of each product. Deposit approximately 1 μL of the gold nanocage suspension onto a piece of silicon wafer and allow the water to evaporate under ambient conditions. Wash the dried sample in a flow cell with water for 30–60 min to remove excess PVP. Allow the sample to dry. Image the sample using your instrument's operating procedures (typically: 10 kV).

10. Acquire a TEM image of each product. Deposit approximately 10 μL of the gold nanocage suspension on a carbon-coated copper TEM grid and allow to dry under ambient conditions. Wash the dried sample in a flow cell

3.1.3. Surface Modification of Gold Nanocages for Increasing the Circulation Time or Targeting Cancerous Cells

with water for 30–60 min to remove excess PVP. Allow the sample to dry. Image the sample using your instrument's operating procedures (typical conditions: 80–100 kV). **Figure 6.2b** shows the typical SEM and TEM (inset) images of gold nanocages produced via the replacement reaction between silver nanocubes and chloroauric acid.

1. Centrifuge the solution of gold nanocages to a pellet.
2. Re-suspend the gold nanocages in an aqueous solution of mPEG-SH or OPSS-PEG-SC and let it sit at room temperature in the dark for ~12 h.
3. Centrifuge the suspension at $9,000 \times g$ for 20 min. Remove excess mPEG-SH or OPSS-PEG-SC from the nanocages by discarding the supernatant after centrifugal separation.
4. Re-suspend the sample in PBS and centrifuge at $9,000 \times g$ for 10 min. Remove and discard the supernatant after centrifugal separation. For mPEG-SH sample, re-suspend it in 1 mL PBS and store until use at 4°C up to 2 weeks.
5. Re-suspend the gold nanocages PEGylated with OPSS-PEG-SC in an anti-HER2 solution and incubate overnight at 4°C. Then centrifuge the sample at $9,000 \times g$ for 5 min to remove the unbound antibody and re-disperse it in 1 mL of PBS. The final products are referred to as immuno gold nanocages throughout this chapter and could be stored at 4°C for up to 1 week. **Figure 6.3** summarizes this two-step process and demonstrates the specific targeting capability of the immuno gold nanocages for SK-BR-3 cells.

3.2. Photothermal Therapy with Gold Nanocages In Vitro

3.2.1. Cell Culture

1. Culture SK-BR-3 cells in modified McCoy's medium at 37°C in 5% CO_2 (v/v). Change the medium two–three times a week.
2. When cells approach confluency of 80–90%, harvest the cells and seed them onto another growth vessel (e.g., flask, petridish, or multiwell plate).

3.2.2. Photothermal Treatment

1. Incubate SK-BR-3 cells in 96-well plates (~90% confluency) with 12 μL of the immuno gold nanocages in growth medium for 3 h (with 1 h of gentle agitation) at 37°C in 5% CO_2 (v/v).
2. Irradiate the cells in the center of the wells using a near-infrared laser with a spot size of 2 mm in diameter as shown in **Fig. 6.4a**. Other parameters such as the duration of the irradiation and power density can be varied in a controllable fashion. The power can be adjusted with a neutral density attenuator and measured with a power meter.

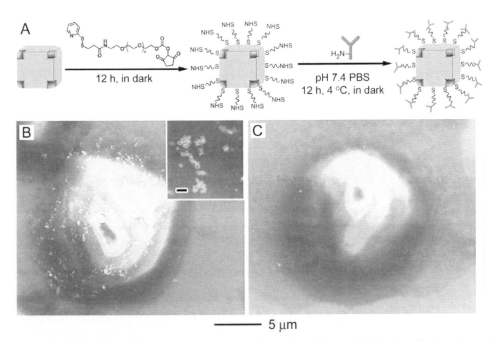

Fig. 6.3. Bioconjugation of gold nanocages for targeting SK-BR-3 cells. (**a**) Schematic illustration of the two-step protocol used to conjugate the antibody to the surface of a gold nanocage. In the first step, OPSS-PEG-SC (NHS-activated PEG) bonded to the gold nanocage by breaking its internal disulfide bond and forming a gold-thiolate linkage. In the second step, the PEG–NHS reacted with the primary amine of an antibody. To demonstrate the targeting capability of the immuno gold nanocages, SK-BR-3 cells were incubated with immuno gold nanocages for 3 h, followed by extensive washing with a buffer to remove the unbound nanocages. (**b**) SEM image showing the immuno gold nanocages selectively attached to the SK-BR-3 cell. The *inset* shows the nanocages at a higher magnification. Inset scale bar = 100 nm. In a control experiment, the same process was repeated for bare gold nanocages. (**c**) SEM image indicating that the bare gold nanocages did not attach to the SK-BR-3 cell. Reproduced with permission from (4). Copyright 2005, American Chemical Society.

3. After irradiation, incubate the cells in medium at 37°C until further analysis with qualitative or quantitative measurements.

3.2.3. Qualitative Study of the Photothermal Effect

1. Within 12 h of irradiation perform the staining protocol. Incubate the cells with calcein-AM and EthD-1 following the standard staining protocols.

2. Examine samples by fluorescence microscopy. The colorless calcein-AM will be enzymatically converted to green fluorescence calcein only in viable cells, while EthD-1 can penetrate through cells, stain DNAs, and emit red fluorescence only when the cell membrane has been irreversibly compromised (e.g., due to the photothermal damage as in this study). Typical images are shown in **Fig. 6.4(b–e)**.

3.2.4. Quantitative Study of the Photothermal Effect

1. Gently remove the cells from the growth vessel within 3 h of irradiation. First, rinse the cells with PBS and then incubate

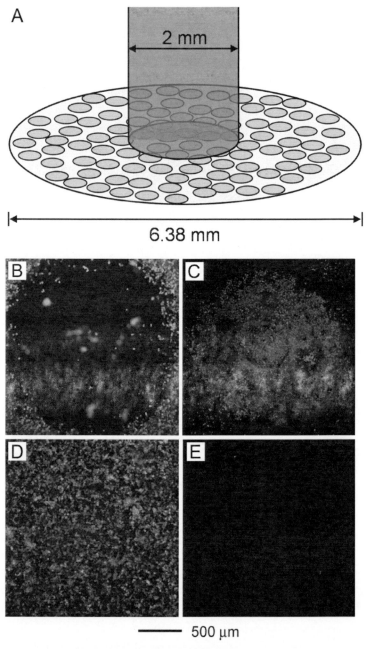

Fig. 6.4. Qualitative analysis of the photothermal effect of immuno gold nanocages on SK-BR-3 cells. (a) Illustration depicting the experimental setup. The cellular growth vessel had a diameter of 6.38 mm. The cells were irradiated with a Ti:sapphire laser with a spot size of 2 mm in diameter (∼10% of the growth area). SK-BR-3 breast cancer cells that were targeted with immuno gold nanocages and then irradiated at a power density of 1.5 W/cm^2 for 5 min. The sample showed a well-defined circular zone of dead cells as revealed by (b) calcein-AM assay (where bright spots indicates that the cells were alive), and (c) EthD-1 assay (where bright spots indicates that the cells were dead). In the control experiment, cells irradiated under the same conditions but without immuno gold nanocages maintained viability, as indicated by (d) calcein-AM fluorescence assay and (e) the lack of intracellular EthD-1 uptake. Reproduced with permission from (8) and (10). Copyright 2007 and 2008, American Chemical Society.

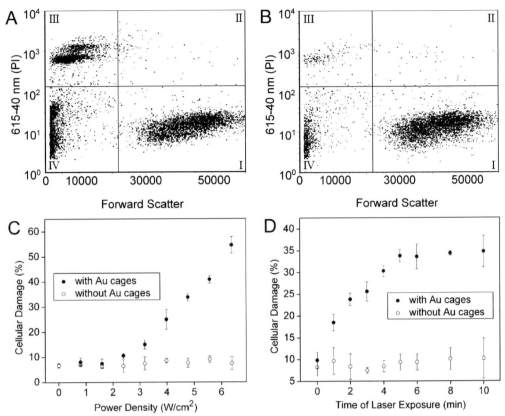

Fig. 6.5. Quantitative analysis of the photothermal effect of immuno gold nanocages on SK-BR-3 cells using flow cytometry. (a) A typical flow cytometry graph of SK-BR-3 cells treated with immuno gold nanocages and then irradiated for 5 min at a power density of 4.77 W/cm^2, showing four well-resolved populations when stained with PI. The populations in quadrants I–IV represented live cells, cells with compromised membrane integrity, dead cells, and background signal together with debris from ruptured cells. (b) In the control experiment, cells without gold nanocages were irradiated and stained with the same procedure. The population of dead cells for treatment with gold nanocages was much higher than without gold nanocages. Since quadrant IV did not representatively correspond to live or damaged cells, the percentage of cellular damage was normalized to quadrant I, II, and III. Plots of percentage of cellular damage against (c) laser power density for exposure time = 5 min and (d) time of laser exposure at power density = 4.7 W/cm^2. Reproduced with permission from (10). Copyright 2008, American Chemical Society.

with trypsin. Stop trypsinization process by adding some more growth media. Then, collect the suspensions of cells and PBS rinses in an appropriate tube for flow cytometry analysis.

2. Treat the cellular suspension (~400 μL) with 12 μL of PI and then inserted into the flow cytometer. Collect the PI fluorescent signal using a 625/25 BP filter and analyze data with an appropriate software. An example of the data is shown in **Fig. 6.5**.

3.3. Photoacoustic Imaging with Gold Nanocages In Vivo

1. Administer the dose of ketamine and xylazine intramuscularly to anesthetize the rats.

2. Remove hair from region of interest using a commercial hair-removal lotion before imaging.
3. Inject three successive dosages of 100 μL of 2 nM nanocages through the tail or saphenous vein to image blood vessels or inject intradermally 100 μL of 2 nM nanocage solution on left forepaw pad to image lymphatic vessels.
4. Image with the photoacoustic system following your system's standard procedures. During all image acquisitions, maintain anesthesia using vaporized isoflurane, monitor vitals using a pulse oximeter, and administer 8 mL of saline for hydration. Enhanced contrast with gold nanocages was observed for the blood vessels in the brain and SLN in rats as shown in **Fig. 6.6**.
5. After image acquisition, euthanize animals by injecting an overdose of pentobarbital. Perform all animal experiments in compliance with your institution's guidelines.

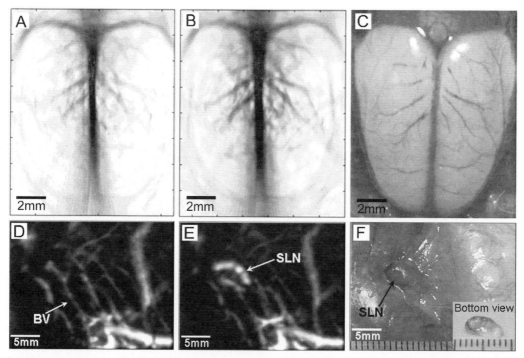

Fig. 6.6. Demonstration of in vivo noninvasive photoacoustic imaging of the cerebral cortex (**a–c**) and SLN (**d–f**) in rats using gold nanocages as an optical contrast agent. The photoacoustic images of the cerebral cortex acquired (**a**) before the injection of PEGylated nanocages and (**b**) about 2 h after the second injection of PEGylated nanocages via tail vein. (**c**) An open-skull photograph of the rat's cerebral cortex showed that the photoacoustic images agreed with the location of blood vessels. The photoacoustic images of the SLN acquired (**d**) before and (**e**) about 2 h after the intradermal injection of bare nanocages via forepaw pad. (**f**) Photograph, with skin and fatty tissue removed, indicates that the photoacoustic images matched the location of SLN. The lymphatic channel dyed with gold nanocages as *dark color* at the bottom of the SLN is shown in the *inset*. BV = blood vessels. Reproduced with permission from (20) and (21). Copyright 2007 and 2009, American Chemical Society.

4. Notes

1. Select Lot no.'s with low Fe and Cl contents; for example, Lot no.'s B25B15 with Cl < 1 ppm and Fe < 0.04 ppm, C42B27 with Cl < 0.1 ppm and Fe < 0.12 ppm, and C46B29 with Cl < 1 ppm and Fe < 0.2 ppm have all generated high-quality silver nanocubes. Also note that EG is very hydroscopic; we recommend replacing the bottles approximately every month or sealing a fresh bottle of EG with an air-tight dispenser (e.g., VWR Labmax Bottle-Top Dispenser) for repeated, reliable use.

2. It is beneficial to add the EG to the vial first, as the PVP will otherwise stick to the wall of the container and require additional time to dissolve. Also, the ratio of PVP to $AgNO_3$ is critical to the formation of high-quality silver nanocubes; correct for any PVP (or $AgNO_3$) over-additions by adding more EG.

3. The Na_2S or NaHS solutions are made fresh since volatile or gaseous sulfide species (e.g., H_2S) will evaporate with time.

4. Wrap the vial with aluminum foil and keep the solution in the dark. Ideally, use solution within 30 min after preparation.

5. $HAuCl_4$ solutions are light-sensitive; keep the solution vials wrapped with aluminum foil and store in the dark until use. High concentration of $HAuCl_4$ solutions (>5 mM) can be kept for up to 1 week when stored in the dark. Low concentrations of $HAuCl_4$ solutions (<2 mM) are good only the day it is made.

6. Aqueous solution of OPSS-PEG-SC used should be prepared just before the use to prevent extensive ester hydrolysis.

7. It is important to use VWR, cat. no. 66011-143, vials as switching to other vials has altered the shape of the final product, presumably due to differences in reaction mixing and the rate of EG dehydration.

8. It is important to use VWR, cat. no. 58949-010, stir bars (or those with exactly the same dimensions and shape) as other stir bars have altered the reaction, presumably due to differences in reaction mixing. To clean stir bars, scrub them with a coarse paper towel to remove any visible debris and sonicate them in acetone for a minimum of 15 min. The stir bars are then soaked in a 1:1 mixture of aqua regia and pure water for a minimum of 1 h. They are finally

rinsed with copious amounts of deionized water and dried in an oven until use.

9. Out of necessity, the silver nanocube synthesis is performed in tandem in four disposable glass vials to which reagents are simply pipetted into the vessels. It has been found that the preparation of silver nanocubes by this sulfide-mediated method is highly sensitive to the concentration of NaHS or Na_2S used. There is, however, an unavoidable uncertainty in the Na_2S concentration because this solid is extremely hydroscopic, with commercial sources containing unknown/inhomogeneous quantities of absorbed water. This problem is effectively eliminated by performing the synthesis in tandem with slightly different volumes of Na_2S solution being added to each reaction vial. Notably, once this procedure is learned, the reaction can be scaled-up by conducting the synthesis simultaneously in a greater number of vials; we routinely perform the synthesis simultaneously in 12 vials.

10. Adding more acetone (5–6 × the volume of the reaction solution) to wash the nanocubes will decrease the centrifuge time to 5 min.

11. Dried silver nanocubes will tarnish with time upon exposure to the sulfide species in air. To increase the shelf life of silver nanocubes, possibly to several years as we have found, store them in pure water in a well-sealed vial.

12. The isolation of nanocages must be completed in 1 day as storage of the gold nanocages in an aqueous NaCl solution can cause them to agglomerate. The gold nanocages can be dispersed in pure water and stored in the dark until further use without significantly changing their properties.

References

1. Kim, S. W., Kim, M., Lee, W. Y., and Hyeon, T. (2002) Fabrication of hollow palladium spheres and their successful application to the recyclable heterogeneous catalyst for Suzuki coupling reactions. *J Am Chem Soc* **124**, 7642–7643.
2. Sun, Y. and Xia, Y. (2002) Increased sensitivity of surface Plasmon resonance of gold nanoshells compared to that of gold solid colloids in response to environmental changes. *Anal Chem* **74**, 5297–5305.
3. Yavuz, M. S., Cheng, Y., Chen, J., Cobley, C. M., Zhang, Q., Rycenga, M., Xie, J., Kim, C., Song, K. H., Schwartz, A. G., Wang, L. V., and Xia, Y. (2009) Gold nanocages covered by smart polymers for controlled released with near-infrared light. *Nat Mat* DOI: 10. 1038/nmat2564.
4. Chen, J., Saeki, F., Wiley, B. J., Cang, H., Cobb, M. J., Li, Z.-Y., Au, L., Zhang, H., Kimmey, M. B., Li, X., and Xia, Y. (2005) Gold nanocages: bioconjugation and their potential use as optical imaging contrast agents. *Nano Lett* **5**, 473–477.
5. Chen, J., Wiley, B. J., Li, Z.-Y., Campbell, D., Saeki, F., Cang, H., Au, L., Lee, J., Li, X., and Xia, Y. (2005) Gold nanocages: engineering their structure for biomedical applications. *Adv Mater* **17**, 2255–2261.
6. Cang, H., Sun, T., Li, Z.-Y., Chen, J., Wiley, B. J., Xia, Y., and Li, X. (2005) Gold nanocages as contrast agents for

spectroscopic and conventional optical coherence tomography. *Opt Lett* **30**, 3048–3050.
7. Loo, C., Lin, A., Hirsch, L., Lee, M. H., Barton, J., Halas, N., West, J., and Drezek, R. (2004) Nanoshell-enabled photonics-based imaging and therapy of cancer. *Technol Cancer Res Treat* **3**, 33–40.
8. Chen, J., Wang, D., Xi, J., Au, L., Siekkinen, A., Warsen, A., Li, Z.-Y., Zhang, H., Xia, Y., and Li, X. (2007) Immuno gold nanocages with tailored optical properties for targeted photothermal destruction of cancer cells. *Nano Lett* **7**, 1318–1322.
9. Hirsch, L. R., Gobin, A. M., Lowery, A. R., Tam, F., Drezek, R. A., Halas, N. J., and West, J. L. (2006) Metal nanoshells. *Ann Biomed Eng* **34**, 15–22.
10. Au, L., Zheng, D., Zhou, F., Li, Z.-Y., Li, X., and Xia, Y. (2008) A quantitative study on the photothermal effect of immuno gold nanocages targeted to breast cancer cells. *ACS Nano* **2**, 1645–1652.
11. Sun, Y. and Xia, Y. (2002) Shape-controlled synthesis of gold and silver nanoparticles. *Science* **298**, 2176–2179.
12. Sun, Y., Mayers, B., and Xia, Y. (2003) Metal nanostructures with hollow interiors. *Adv Mater* **15**, 641–646.
13. Wiley, B. J., Sun, Y., Chen, J., Cang, H., Li, Z.-Y., Li, X., and Xia, Y. (2005) Shape-controlled synthesis of silver and gold nanostructures. *MRS Bull* **30**, 356–361.
14. Yang, J., Lee, J. Y., and Too, H. P. (2005) Core-shell Ag–Au nanoparticles from replacement reaction in organic medium. *J Phys Chem B* **109**, 19208–19212.
15. Chen, J., McLellan, J. M., Siekkinen, A., Xiong, Y., Li, Z.-Y., and Xia, Y. (2006) Facile synthesis of gold–silver nanocages with controllable pores on the surface. *J Am Chem Soc* **128**, 14776–14777.
16. Yin, Y., Erdonmez, C., Aloni, S., and Alivisatos, A. P. (2006) Faceting of nanocrystals during chemical transformation: from solid silver spheres to hollow gold octahedra. *J Am Chem Soc* **128**, 12671–12673.
17. Au, L., Lu, X., and Xia, Y. (2008) A comparative study of galvanic replacement reactions involving silver nanocubes and $AuCl_2^-$ or $AuCl_4^-$. *Adv Mater* **20**, 2517–2522.
18. Skrabalak, S., Chen, J., Au, L., Lu, X., Li, X., and Xia, Y. (2007) Gold nanocages for biomedical applications. *Adv Mater* **19**, 3177–3184.
19. Sun, Y. and Xia, Y. (2004) Mechanistic study on the replacement reaction between silver nanostructures and chloroauric acid in aqueous medium. *J Am Chem Soc* **126**, 3892–3901.
20. Yang, X., Skrabalak, S. E., Li, Z.-Y., Xia, Y., and Wang, L. V. (2007) Photoacoustic tomography of a rat cerebral cortex in vivo with gold nanocages as an optical contrast agent. *Nano Lett* **7**, 3798–3802.
21. Song, K. H., Kim, C., Cobley, C. M., Xia, Y., and Wang, L. V. (2009) Near-infrared gold nanocages as a new class of tracers for photoacoustic sentinel lymph node mapping on a rat model. *Nano Lett* **9**, 183–188.
22. Skrabalak, S. E., Au, L., Li, X., and Xia, Y. (2007) Facile synthesis of Ag nanocubes and Au nanocages. *Nat Protoc* **2**, 2182–2190.
23. Siekkinen, A. R., McLellan, J. M., Chen, J., and Xia, Y. (2006) Rapid synthesis of small silver nanocubes by mediation polyol reduction with a trace amount of sodium sulfide or sodium hydrosulfide. *Chem Phys Lett* **432**, 491–496.

Chapter 7

Nanoshells for Photothermal Cancer Therapy

Jennifer G. Morton, Emily S. Day, Naomi J. Halas, and Jennifer L. West

Abstract

Cancer is a leading cause of death in the United States and contributes to yearly rising health care costs. Current methods of treating cancer involve surgical removal of easily accessible tumors, radiation therapy, and chemotherapy. These methods do not always result in full treatment of the cancer and can in many cases damage healthy cells both surrounding the tissue area and systemically. Nanoshells are optically tunable core/shell nanoparticles that can be fabricated to strongly absorb in the near-infrared (NIR) region where light transmits deeply into tissue. When injected systemically, these particles have been shown to accumulate in the tumor due to the enhanced permeability and retention (EPR) effect and induce photothermal ablation of the tumor when irradiated with an NIR laser. Tumor specificity can be increased via functionalizing the nanoshell surface with tumor-targeting moieties. Nanoshells can also be made to strongly scatter light and therefore can be used in various imaging modalities such as dark-field microscopy and optical coherence tomography (OCT).

Key words: Nanoshells, cancer, photothermal therapy, tumor targeting, tumor imaging.

1. Introduction

Nanoshells are optically tunable nanoparticles consisting of a dielectric core and a thin metal shell. These particles can be designed to primarily scatter or absorb light based on the core and shell dimensions. A larger core results in greater scattering contribution to the total extinction while a smaller core typically induces primarily absorbing properties. The location of the peak extinction within the spectrum is dependent upon the ratio of the core radius to shell thickness, as demonstrated in **Fig. 7.1**.

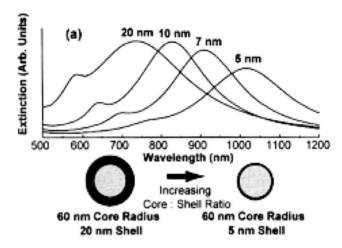

Fig. 7.1. The optical properties of nanoshells are dependent on the core size/shell thickness ratio. With a dielectric core of the same size, a thinner gold shell results in a red-shifted peak while a thicker shell pushes the peak to shorter wavelengths. (Reproduced from (1) with permission.)

A thinner shell induces a shift of peak extinction to the longer wavelengths, while a thicker shell produces a peak blueshift (1).

Due to their ability to either scatter or absorb light, nanoshells possess great potential in both imaging and therapeutic applications, specifically optical imaging and photothermal ablation of tumors. Other applications include tissue welding (2) and probes for antigen detection in whole blood (3). This review describes in detail the physical optical properties of nanoshells, their use in tumor therapeutic and imaging applications, and the steps involved in nanoshell synthesis.

1.1. Optical Properties of Nanoshells

Nanoshells are unique in that their peak absorbance can be preferentially placed by manipulating the core size and shell thickness. This property is described by the Mie theory, the solution for the Maxwell equations for a dilute colloidal system. Extending the Mie theory to nanoparticles with a metal shell involves specifying the boundary conditions at one additional interface, that of the core and shell. Because $r \ll \lambda$ for these nanoparticles, where r is the particle radius and λ is the wavelength of the incident electromagnetic field, the quasi-static approach can be used in order to simplify Mie theory calculations. In this model, the electromagnetic incident field does not vary spatially over the diameter of the metal shell and therefore the spatial variance is neglected in the calculations. The time dependence of the incident wave, however, is preserved. For further simplification, the nanoshells are assumed to be perfectly spherical and interactions between nanoparticles are neglected due to the low-nanoshell concentration (4).

Averitt et al. derived and described this quasi-static theory of nanoshells (4). The geometry of the nanoshell is shown in **Fig. 7.2** where r_1 is the core radius, r_2 is the total particle radius, and ε_1, ε_2, and ε_3 are the dielectric constants of the core, shell, and medium.

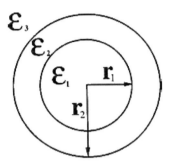

Fig. 7.2. The geometry of a nanoshell: r_1 is the core radius while r_2 is the total particle radius. ε_1, ε_2, and ε_3 are the dielectric constants of the core, shell, and medium. (Reproduced from (4) with permission.)

Applying the Mie scattering theory, the absorption cross-section of the nanoshells obtained is described by equation [**1**]

$$\sigma_{abs} = \frac{k}{\varepsilon_0}\mathrm{Im}\,(\alpha), \qquad [1]$$

where the polarizability (α), the tendency of charge distribution to be distorted by an external electric field, is described by equation [**2**]

$$\alpha = 4\pi\varepsilon_0 r_2^3 \left[\frac{\varepsilon_2\varepsilon_a - \varepsilon_3\varepsilon_b}{\varepsilon_2\varepsilon_a + 2\varepsilon_3\varepsilon_b}\right]. \qquad [2]$$

Combining equations [**1**] and [**2**], the absorption cross-section is given as

$$\sigma_{abs} = \frac{8\pi^2\sqrt{\varepsilon_3}}{\lambda} r_2^3 \mathrm{Im}\left(\frac{\varepsilon_2\varepsilon_a - \varepsilon_3\varepsilon_b}{\varepsilon_2\varepsilon_a + 2\varepsilon_3\varepsilon_b}\right), \qquad [3]$$

where

$$\varepsilon_a = \varepsilon_1(3 - 2P) + 2\varepsilon_2 P, \qquad [4]$$

$$\varepsilon_b = \varepsilon_1 P + \varepsilon_2(3 - P), \qquad [5]$$

and P, the shell volume to total particle volume ratio, is described by

$$P = 1 - \left(\frac{r_1}{r_2}\right)^3. \qquad [6]$$

Similarly, the scattering cross-section is described as

$$\sigma_{sca} = \frac{128\pi^5}{3\lambda^4} \varepsilon_3^2 r_2^6 \left| \frac{\varepsilon_2 \varepsilon_a - \varepsilon_3 \varepsilon_b}{\varepsilon_2 \varepsilon_a + 2\varepsilon_3 \varepsilon_b} \right|^2. \qquad [7]$$

Figure 7.3 shows the nanoshell extinction cross-sections using equations [2] and [6] where $r_2 = 4, 10, 17$. This demonstrates the dependency of the resonance wavelength on the ratio of core radius to total particle radius. For a given shell thickness, a larger particle diameter yields a peak plasmon resonance in the longer wavelengths.

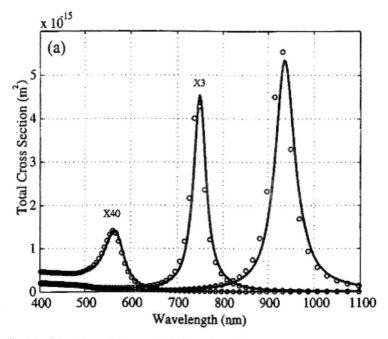

Fig. 7.3. Calculations of the nanoshell absorption and scattering cross-sections with a shell thickness of 2 and $r_2 = 4, 10, 17$ indicate that, for a given shell thickness, a larger core diameter yields a plasmon resonance shifted to longer wavelengths. (Reproduced from (4) with permission.)

The plasmon resonance of the electrons in the metal shell occurs at the point of maximum polarizability. From equation [7], it can be seen that this is when the denominator approaches zero ($\varepsilon_2 \varepsilon_a + 2\varepsilon_3 \varepsilon_b \to 0$). From equation [7] and the previous definitions, Averitt et al. developed the following expression describing the plasmon resonance as a function of wavelength if both the core and embedding medium are dielectrics:

$$\frac{r_1}{r_2} = \left[1 + \frac{3}{2} \frac{\varepsilon'(\lambda)(\varepsilon_1 + 2\varepsilon_3)}{[\varepsilon'_2(\lambda)]^2 - \varepsilon'_2(\lambda)(\varepsilon_1 + \varepsilon_3) + \{\varepsilon_1 \varepsilon_3 - [\varepsilon''_2(\lambda)]^2\}} \right]^{\frac{1}{3}}, \qquad [8]$$

when $r_2 \ll \lambda$, shell thickness ($r_2 - r_1$) is greater than a few atomic layers. This expression demonstrates the fact that the wavelength of plasmon resonance is dependent on the core/shell geometry of the particle (4).

Due to the tunability of the optical properties, the ability to control the core and shell dimensions is desirable. Oldenburg et al. developed a nanoshell with a dielectric silica core and a gold shell (1). The silica cores are made using the Stöber method in which tetraethyl orthosilicate is reduced in ammonium hydroxide (NH_4OH) in ethanol. The size of the silica particles is correlated with the amount of NH_4OH added to the solution, therefore providing control over core size. The shell is formed by reducing gold colloid particles on the surface of the core. The size of the shell is dependent on the relative amount of gold to silica cores during the reduction process, thereby providing control over the shell thickness.

1.2. Nanoshell-Assisted Photothermal Therapy

The tunability of nanoshells enables potential use in biological applications in that they can be designed to strongly absorb light in the near-infrared (NIR) region (650–900 nm). In this range, the absorption coefficients of water and hemoglobin are at their lowest, and therefore light is able to penetrate deeply into tissues (**Fig. 7.4**) (5).

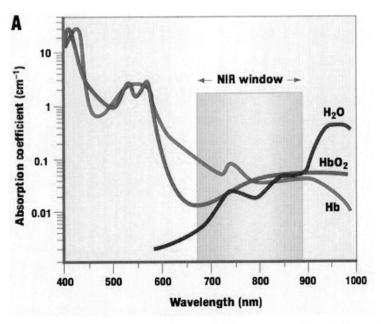

Fig. 7.4. In the NIR window, the absorption coefficients of water and hemoglobin are at their lowest, enabling light of wavelengths within this range to deeply penetrate tissue. (Reproduced from (5) with permission.)

When injected systemically, NIR-absorbing nanoshells have been shown to extravasate out of the leaky tumor vasculature where, when irradiated with an NIR laser, they generate heat, resulting in photothermal destruction of the tumor (6). This section describes the development of this method known as nanoshell-assisted photothermal therapy (NAPT).

The first use of nanoshells in photothermal ablation of tumors was shown by Hirsch et al. in 2003 (7). SKBr3 human breast epithelial carcinoma cells were incubated in vitro with nanoshells and then irradiated with NIR light. Cells without nanoshells were irradiated with the laser as a control. Calcein AM staining (**Fig. 7.5**) revealed a circle of cell death corresponding to the spot size of the laser in the nanoshell-treated cells and no death in the cells that were treated with the laser only. Fluorescein-dextran, a high molecular-weight dye impermeable to healthy cells, was shown to penetrate the membranes of the cells receiving the nanoshell/laser treatment. This implies that cell membrane destruction is a mechanism involved in cell death resulting from nanoshell/laser treatment.

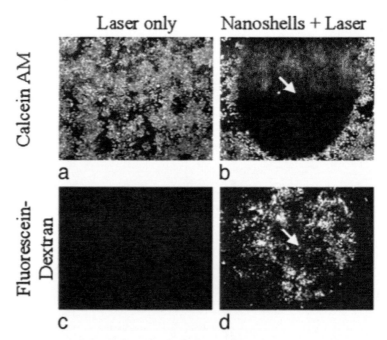

Fig. 7.5. Calcein AM staining shows cell death in those cells receiving nanoshell treatment (**a, b**). High molecular weight dye indicates membrane destruction as the mechanism of cell death (**c, d**). (Reproduced from (7) with permission.)

In addition to the previously mentioned study, nanoshell treatment of tumors in mice and the resultant heat profiles within the tumors were investigated (7). Mice were inoculated with canine TVT cells on both hind legs. After the tumors reached a diameter of 1 cm, nanoshells were injected interstitially into the tumor. Prior to injection, the nanoshell surfaces were functionalized with poly(ethylene glycol) thiol (PEG–SH) to provide steric stabilization and to minimize aggregation due to protein adsorption in the physiological environment. After 5–30 min of injection, the tumor sites were exposed to the NIR laser. Magnetic resonance thermal imaging (MRTI) was used to monitor the temperature distribution within the tumor during treatment. Nanoshell-treated tumors resulted in an average temperature increase of 37.4 ± 6.6°C, high enough to cause irreversible tissue damage, while nanoshell-free controls experienced an average temperature increase of only 9.1 ± 4.7°C. Gross pathology, silver staining, and histology of the tumors indicated edema, coagulation, cell shrinkage, and loss of nuclear staining in the same area as the localized nanoshells (**Fig. 7.6**) (7).

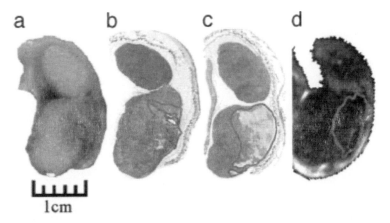

Fig. 7.6. Analysis of an excised tumor from a mouse receiving nanoshell-assisted photothermal therapy reveals that the area of tissue damage coincides with the area of localized nanoshells. (**a**) Gross pathology reveals hemorrhaging, (**b**) silver staining reveals the area of localized nanoshells, (**c**) hematoxylin/eosin staining reveals the area of tissue damage, and (**d**) MRTI calculations reveal the area of irreversible thermal damage. (Reproduced from (7) with permission.)

O'Neal et al. investigated NAPT in mice with delivery to the tumor site through the vasculature (6). Mice were inoculated subcutaneously with CT26 colon carcinoma tumor cells and when the tumor reached 3–5.5 mm diameter, PEGylated nanoshells were injected into the tail vein. To allow enough time for the nanoshells to accumulate in the tumor site, laser treatments were performed 6 h after nanoshell injection. Within 10 days of treatment, complete resorption of the tumors was observed in the nanoshell-treatment group (**Fig. 7.7**) and 90 days after treatment, all nanoshell-treated mice were healthy and tumor-free. Tumors in the control groups continued to grow rapidly and all mice were euthanized by day 19 due to excessive tumor growth.

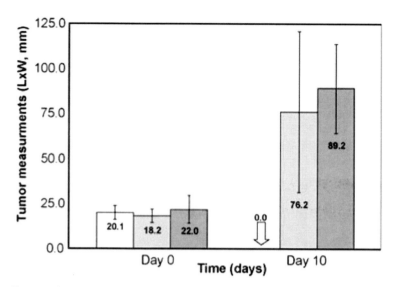

Fig. 7.7. Mean tumor size measured on treatment day (day 0) and 10 days post-treatment. All tumors receiving NAPT showed resorption after 10 days. (Reproduced from (6) with permission.)

1.2.1. Immunotargeted Nanoshells

In order to increase nanoshell specificity to the tumor site, targeting the nanoshells with antibodies against over-expressed cell-surface oncoproteins has been investigated (8). In order to target human epidermal growth factor receptor 2 (HER2), which is over-expressed on human breast cancer cells, nanoshells were targeted using the anti-HER2 antibody. HER2+ SKBr3 cells were incubated with antibody-functionalized nanoshells and then irradiated with an NIR laser. Nanoshells conjugated to anti-IgG, a nonspecific control antibody, served as a control. Following laser irradiation, the cells were stained with calcein AM, which indicated a circular area of cell death corresponding to the spot size of the laser for those cells incubated with targeted nanoshells. No cell death was observed for cells incubated with non-targeted nanoshells or for cells receiving only laser irradiation (**Fig. 7.8**).

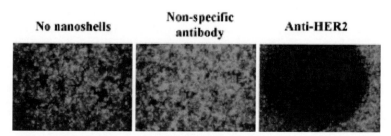

Fig. 7.8. Therapy of SKBr3 cells using HER2-targeted nanoshells. Calcein staining reveals cell death in cells receiving NIR-laser treatment following exposure to HER2-targeted nanoshells. (Reproduced from (8) with permission.)

1.3. Nanoshell-Assisted Imaging Techniques

As mentioned previously, nanoshells can be designed to strongly scatter light, which is of great use in optical imaging modalities. Their use in in vitro dark-field imaging of HER2 expression has been described (8–10). Nanoshells with a 120-nm core radius and a 35-nm shell thickness were conjugated to anti-HER2 and incubated with HER2+ SKBr3 cells, and then imaged under dark-field magnification (10). **Figure 7.9** demonstrates the contrast provided by targeted nanoshells as opposed to non-targeted or the absence of nanoshells.

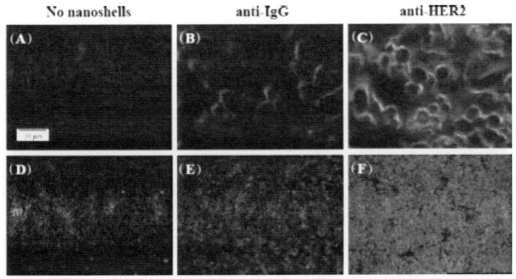

Fig. 7.9. (**a–c**) High magnification (×40) dark-field images of HER2+ SkBr3 cells incubated with no nanoshells, anti-IgG-labeled nanoshells, and HER2-targeted nanoshells. (**d–f**) Dark-field images (×10) of HER2+ cells. (Reproduced from (10) with permission.)

Nanoshells have also been investigated in the use of signal enhancement in optical coherence tomography (OCT). Loo et al. compared OCT images of saline, a suspension of 2 μm polystyrene microspheres, and a nanoshell (100-nm core radius, 20-nm shell thickness) suspension at a concentration of 1×10^9 NS/mL. Basing OCT intensity on a log scale where black = 255 and white = 0, the average intensity of saline was 247 while nanoshell intensity was 160, showing that nanoshells provided higher contrast (9).

Due to their ability to be designed to both scatter and absorb light, nanoshells can be used in combined imaging and therapy applications. This was first demonstrated with an in vitro study in which SKBr3 cells were incubated with HER2-targeted nanoshells followed by laser irradiation (820 nm, 0.008 W/m^2, 7 min) (8). Cell viability was then assessed via calcein staining and nanoshell binding was assessed through silver staining. The nanoshells bound to cells were viewed using dark-field

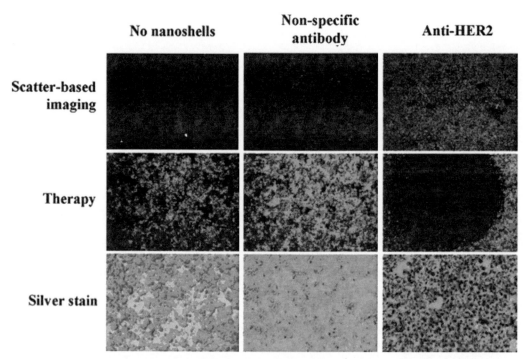

Fig. 7.10. Combined imaging and therapy of SKBr3 cells using HER2-targeted nanoshells. (*Top row*) Dark-field imaging. (*Middle row*) Calcein staining revealing cell death in nanoshell-treated cells. (*Bottom row*) Silver stain imaging of targeted nanoshells. (Reproduced from (8) with permission.)

microscopy. **Figure 7.10** shows increased contrast and cytotoxicity in cells resulting from targeted nanoshell/laser therapy compared to both cells treated with non-targeted nanoshells and laser irradiation and cells treated with laser only.

Gobin et al. investigated the application of nanoshells in combined imaging and therapy in vivo (11). Nanoshells were made with a core diameter of 119 nm and a shell thickness of 12 nm. Mice were subcutaneously inoculated with CT-26 cells on the right hind flank, forming a tumor. Tumors were allowed to grow to a diameter of 5 mm after which PEG-conjugated nanoshells were injected into the mice through the tail vein. PBS was injected into one group of the mice as a control. After allowing an accumulation time of 20 h, the tumors were imaged using OCT. Representative OCT images (**Fig. 7.11**) reveal significant increase in contrast intensity in tumors of mice treated with nanoshells and no contrast intensity increase in tumors of mice not receiving nanoshells. Quantification of this intensity increase is shown in **Fig. 7.12**.

Following OCT imaging, mice were randomly divided into three groups: treatment group (nanoshells + laser), sham group (PBS + laser), and control group (untreated). The tumors of the treatment and sham groups were irradiated with an NIR laser (808 nm, 4 W/cm^2, 3 min), after which tumor size and

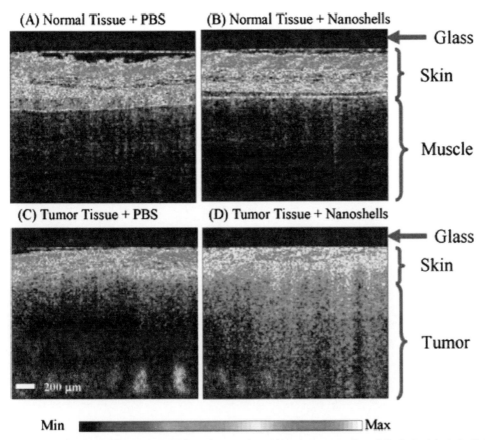

Fig. 7.11. Representative OCT images of skin/muscle areas (**a** and **b**) or tumor areas (**c** and **d**) of mice injected with PBS (**a** and **c**) or nanoshells (**b** and **d**). Increase in contrast between normal tissue and tumor tissue is apparent in mice with nanoshells but not those injected with PBS. (Reproduced from (11) with permission.)

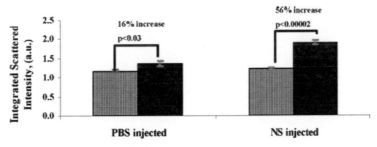

Fig. 7.12. Quantification of OCT image intensity reveals a significant difference in intensity between normal (*gray bar*) and tumor tissue (*black bar*) of mice injected with nanoshells and no significant difference between the intensity of tissues in those mice injected with PBS. (Reproduced from (11) with permission.)

animal survival were monitored for the next 7 weeks. Twelve days after treatment, all but two tumors in the treatment group had regressed while tumors of those mice in the sham and control

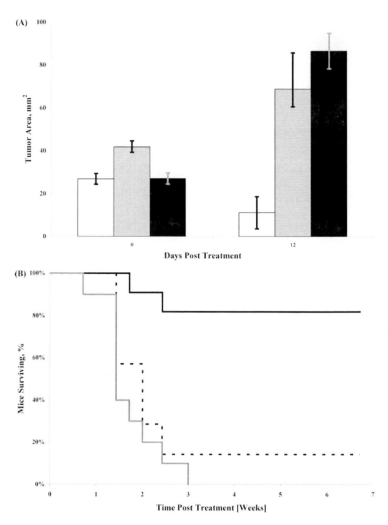

Fig. 7.13. (a) Tumor size before treatment and 12 days after treatment for treatment group (*white bar*), sham group (*gray bar*), and control group (*black bar*). Tumor size decreased for those mice receiving nanoshells + laser treatment but increased in those receiving PBS + laser and those receiving no treatment. (b) Kaplan–Meier survival curve indicates survival of 80% of those mice receiving nanoshells + laser treatment 7 weeks after treatment (*black line*). (Reproduced from (11) with permission.)

groups continued to grow (**Fig. 7.13A**). By day 21 after treatment, survival of the treatment group was significantly greater than either the sham or control groups (**Fig. 7.13B**).

There are many advantages to using nanoshells in treatment of tumors as opposed to current treatment methods. The peak optical absorption of nanoshells can be tuned to the NIR region and can therefore absorb light and generate heat when irradiated with an NIR laser. Due to the low absorption and high transmittance of light in the NIR range in tissues, irradiation does not cause damage to the skin or surrounding tissue. This therefore provides a safe noninvasive method of photothermal ablation of tumors.

Current chemotherapeutic therapy involves systemically administering DNA-damaging drugs, often destroying healthy cells. The facile conjugation of biomolecules to the nanoshell surface enables tumor-specific targeting of the nanoshells. The nanoshells can be targeted to molecules on the surface of the tumor cells (8). This tumor-specific targeting enables more rapid accumulation of the nanoshells within the tumor (6). Laser irradiation of the tumor containing targeted nanoshells results in localized tumor cell death.

The combined scattering and absorbing properties of nanoshells enable them to be used in combined imaging and therapy applications (8, 9, 11). Subsequently, nanoshells can be used simultaneously as an imaging contrast agent and therapeutic agent. Following injection of the nanoshells, tumors can be localized through scatter-based imaging methods and then immediately irradiated for tumor photothermal ablation. This is potentially advantageous to the patient due to more rapid therapy upon tumor localization.

2. Materials

2.1. Silica–Gold Nanoshell Synthesis

1. Concentrated ammonium hydroxide (NH_4OH, 28%).
2. Ethanol (EtOH, 200 proof).
3. Tetraethyl orthosilicate (TEOS, Aldrich 99.999%).
4. 3-Aminopropyltriethoxysilane (APTES, Aldrich, 99%).
5. Tetrakis(hydroxymethyl)phosphonium chloride (THPC, Aldrich).
6. Sodium chloride (NaCl, 1 M).
7. A 29.7 mM (1%) solution of hydrogen tetrachloroaurate(III) ($HAuCl_4$, Alfa Aesar, 99.999%) dissolved in deionized (DI) water.
8. Potassium carbonate (K_2CO_3).
9. Formaldehyde (37%).

2.2. Antibody Conjugation to Nanoshells

1. OPSS–PEG–NHS (Creative PEGWorks).
2. 100 mM sodium bicarbonate (pH 8.5).
3. Mouse monoclonal antihuman HER2 antibody (purified without BSA and Azide) (NeoMarkers).

3. Methods

3.1. Silica–Gold Nanoshell Synthesis

3.1.1. Silica Core Formation (Stöber Method)

1. Set up small (~80 mL) glass beakers with stir bars on stir plates. Add 45 mL EtOH to each beaker.
2. Add (NH$_4$OH) to EtOH, varying the volume between 2.5 mL and 3.1 mL to achieve particle sizes in the range of 80–140 nm (*see* **Note 1**).
3. While rapidly stirring, add 1.5 mL (TEOS) to each beaker and stir rapidly for 1 min.
4. Reduce the stirring rate and allow the mixture to stir for a period of at least 8 h. Cover the beakers with parafilm to prevent EtOH from evaporating.
5. Centrifuge the particle suspension twice (1900×*g*, 30 min), resuspending particles in fresh 100% EtOH each time (*see* **Note 2**).
6. Determine the size and polydispersity of silica nanoparticles using a scanning electronic microscope (SEM). Only those particles with a polydispersity of less than 10% should be used in subsequent steps.

3.1.2. Functionalization of the Silica Cores

1. While rapidly stirring, add 200 µL APTES to each batch of cores and let stir for a period of at least 8 h.
2. While stirring, boil the cores at a constant volume of EtOH for 1 h. Prevent the suspension from drying up by adding EtOH periodically.
3. Centrifuge twice (1900×*g*, 30 min) and resuspend in the appropriate amount of fresh EtOH to achieve a weight percent of 4.
4. Silica cores should be stored in a tightly closed plastic container (such as a polystyrene centrifuge tube) on the bench top until use.

3.1.3. Gold Colloid Formation

1. Prepare a stock solution of THPC by adding 400 µL of THPC to stirring 33 mL of DI water (*see* **Note 3**).
2. Add 4 mL of THPC stock and 1.2 mL of 1 M NaOH to stirring 180 mL chilled DI water (18°C) and allow the solution to stir for 5 min.
3. Increase the stirring rate of the solution and quickly add 6.75 mL of 1% HAuCl$_4$ to the solution. Remove beaker from stir plate immediately upon the appearance of a visible color change (2–5 s).
4. Pour colloid into tightly closed plastic container and let age at 4°C for 10 days.

3.1.4. Seed Growth

1. Add 1 mL of functionalized silica cores at 4 wt% and 9 mL of 1 M NaCl to 180 mL THPC solution.
2. Let react at 4°C for 3 days.
3. Centrifuge seed particles twice (1300×g, 15 min), resuspending in DI water each time.
4. Dilute seed particles with DI water to have an extinction of 0.1 units at a wavelength of 530 nm.

3.1.5. Shell Formation

1. Prepare potassium carbonate stock solution: 200 mL water, 50 mg K_2CO_3, 3 mL 1% $HAuCl_4$. Let age in the dark at room temperature for a minimum of 12 h.
2. Perform optimization ratio sweeps at a 1-mL volume:
   a. Add 1 mL K_2CO_3 solution to five UV–Vis cuvettes.
   b. Add diluted seed to each cuvette. Vary the volume of seed between 100 and 500 µL.
   c. Lay out cuvette caps on the bench top and add 10 µL formaldehyde to the inside of each cuvette.
   d. Quickly place the cap on top of a cuvette and vortex at the highest setting for a few seconds or until a color change is visible.
   e. Repeat Step 2d for each cuvette.
   f. Record UV–Vis spectrum of each small volume of nanoshells. Determine which ratio gives an absorbance peak nearest to 800 nm.
3. Scale-up the optimum ratio to make a larger batch of nanoshells.
   a. Mix seed and K_2CO_3 at the appropriate volume ratios.
   b. While rapidly stirring, add formaldehyde at a volume of 10 µl per 1 mL K_2CO_3 solution.
   c. Stir for an additional 2 min. Verify the completion of the reaction by recording the UV–Vis spectrum.
4. Divide nanoshells into 20 mL volumes and centrifuge one time (700×g, 20 min), resuspending in DI water.
5. Use nanoshells within 24 h.

3.2. Antibody Conjugation to Nanoshells

To provide a flexible linkage, antibodies can be tethered onto the nanoparticle surface via a heterobifunctional poly(ethylene glycol) (PEG) linker that consists of an NHS group at one end and an OPSS group at the other. The NHS fragment acts as a leaving group where primary amines on antibodies can then react with the PEG molecule. The sulfur groups in the OPSS segment bind strongly with gold atoms on the particle surface, enabling assembly of the PEG–antibody complex onto nanoshells. Here, we describe preparation of the OPSS–PEG–antibody followed by subsequent conjugation to nanoshells.

3.2.1. Prepare OPSS–PEG–Antibody

1. Every step of this procedure should be performed on ice.
2. Dissolve antibody in 100 mM sodium bicarbonate (pH 8.5) to desired concentration.
3. Thaw OPSS–PEG–NHS on ice, let then come to room temperature. Avoid opening when the vial is still cold as this could lead to collection of condensation which lowers the reactivity. After weighing the desired amount of PEG (*see* **Note 4**), run argon over the vial for 30 s and quickly recap to help remove moisture from ambient air which will eventually spoil the PEG.
4. Prepare the OPSS–PEG–NHS in 100 mM sodium bicarbonate (pH 8.5) to a concentration that is 10–20 times higher than that of the antibody. Once the PEG is dissolved in buffer, work quickly since the NHS groups have a short half-life in aqueous solution.
5. Add one part PEG to nine parts antibody. Vortex.
6. Allow reaction to proceed at least for 2 h at 4°C. Store product frozen in working aliquots.

3.2.2. Attach OPSS–PEG–Antibody to Nanoshells

1. Suspend nanoshells in water to the desired concentration. Typically, performing the reactions with particles concentrated to $OD^{800} = 1.5$ gives satisfactory results.
2. Thaw OPSS–PEG–antibody on ice and then add appropriate amount to nanoshell solution. Generally, adding OPSS–PEG–antibody to place 0.02 antibody/nm^2 on the surface gives good results. (For SiO_2 nanoshells with a 150 nm diameter, this corresponds to about 1500 antibodies per nanoshell in the reacting solution.)
3. Allow reaction to proceed at 4°C for 1–4 h.
4. Add 1 μL of 10 mM PEG–SH for every 2 mL of nanoshells at an $OD^{800} = 1.5$. Let reaction proceed at 4°C overnight.
5. To remove unbound antibody and PEG–SH, centrifuge nanoshells to form a pellet, remove the supernatant, and suspend the particles in the necessary buffer for their intended use.

4. Notes

1. Because of the potential variability in particle size between batches with the same volume of NH_4OH, it is best to make two batches of each NH_4OH to EtOH ratio.

2. The best results are found when the particle suspensions are centrifuged in 20–25 mL volumes in 50 mL polystyrene centrifuge tubes. Following centrifugation, the supernatant may have a slight milky color due to the smaller particles not having yet packed into the pellet. If this is present, continue centrifuging in 10-min increments until the supernatant is mostly clear. Discard the supernatant, resuspend in fresh ethanol, and continue with the second centrifuge step.

3. When preparing all reagents, only DI water should be used.

4. The PEG–SH used to stabilize the nanoshells has a molecular weight of 5,000 Da. Smaller PEG chains may not provide sufficient stabilization, and larger PEG chains could interfere with antibody activity.

References

1. Oldenburg, S. J., et al. (1998) Nanoengineering of optical resonances. *Chem Phys Lett* **288**, 243–247.
2. Gobin, A. M., et al. (2005) Near infrared laser-tissue welding using nanoshells as an exogenous absorber. *Lasers Surg Med* **37**, 123–129.
3. Hirsch, L. R., et al. (2003) A whole blood immunoassay using gold nanoshells. *Analytical Chem* **75**, 2377–2381.
4. Averitt, R. D., Westcott, S. L., and Halas, N. J. (1999) Linear optical properties of gold nanoshells. *J Optical Soc Am B Optical Phys* **16**, 1824–1832.
5. Weissleder, R. (2001) A clearer vision for in vivo imaging. *Nat Biotechnol* **19**, 316–317.
6. O'Neal, D. P., et al. (2004) Photo-thermal tumor ablation in mice using near infrared-absorbing nanoparticles. *Cancer Lett* **209**, 171–176.
7. Hirsch, L. R., et al. (2003) Nanoshell-mediated near-infrared thermal therapy of tumors under magnetic resonance guidance. *PNAS* **100**, 13549–13554.
8. Loo, C., et al. (2005) Immunotargeted nanoshells for integrated cancer imaging and therapy. *Nano Lett* **5**, 709–711.
9. Loo, C., et al. (2004) Nanoshell-enabled photonics-based imaging and therapy of cancer. *Technol Cancer Res Treatment* **3**, 33–40.
10. Loo, C., et al. (2005) Gold nanoshell bioconjugates for molecular imaging in living cells. *Optics Lett* **30**, 1012–1014.
11. Gobin, A. M., et al. Near-infrared resonant nanoshells for combined optical imaging and photothermal cancer therapy. *Nano Lett* **7**, 1929–1934.

Chapter 8

Gold Nanorods: Multifunctional Agents for Cancer Imaging and Therapy

Alexander Wei, Alexei P. Leonov, and Qingshan Wei

Abstract

Gold nanorods (GNRs) are strongly absorbing at near-infrared (NIR) frequencies and can be employed as multifunctional agents for biological imaging and theragnostics. GNRs can support nonlinear optical microscopies based on two-photon-excited luminescence and can enhance the contrast of biomedical imaging modalities such as optical coherence tomography and photoacoustic tomography. GNRs are also efficient at mediating the conversion of NIR light energy into heat and can generate localized photothermal effects. However, future clinical applications will require the rigorous removal of CTAB, a micellar surfactant used in GNR synthesis, and reliable methods of surface functionalization for cell-selective targeting and for minimizing nonspecific uptake into cells. This can be accomplished by using polystyrenesulfonate (PSS) as a sorbent for removing CTAB, and in situ dithiocarbamate formation for introducing chemisorptive ligands onto GNR surfaces.

Key words: Gold, biomedical imaging, nonlinear optical microscopy, photothermal effects, surface functionalization, targeting.

1. Introduction

Recent developments in nanomaterials synthesis have enabled colloidal gold particles to be engineered into nanostructures with tunable surface plasmon resonances, with strong optical activity at visible and near-infrared (NIR) wavelengths (1). Gold nanoparticles ($d < 100$ nm) with plasmon resonances in the NIR region are currently being employed as contrast agents for optical biomedical imaging modalities such as optical coherence tomography (OCT), photoacoustic tomography (PAT), and nonlinear optical microscopies (2). The NIR spectrum between 750 and 1,300 nm provides a "biological window" for optical imaging, as shorter wavelengths are extinguished by hemoglobin or other endogenous pigments, and longer wavelengths are strongly attenuated by water (3).

Gold nanorods (GNRs) are especially attractive as NIR-resonant contrast agents: their synthesis is relatively straightforward and reproducible, and their plasmon resonances can be tuned as an approximately linear function of their aspect ratios. GNRs support a higher NIR absorption cross section per unit volume than most other nanostructures and have narrower linewidths than nanospheres at comparable resonance frequencies (4). The efficient NIR absorption has enabled GNRs to produce novel modes of contrast for nonlinear optical microscopy, and also various types of optical imaging modalities for deeper penetration into biological tissue. With respect to nonlinear optical effects, GNRs have large two-photon absorption cross sections in the NIR and can be excited with ultrafast laser pulses to produce a luminescence that can be detected at the single-particle level (5–7). Two-photon luminescence (TPL) imaging of GNRs can be performed under confocal conditions with submicron spatial resolution and has been employed in vitro for visualizing cell uptake (8) and for the targeted labeling of tumor cells (9, 10) and bacterial spores (11), and in vivo for noninvasive imaging of GNRs passing through subcutaneous blood vessels (5) (**Fig. 8.1**).

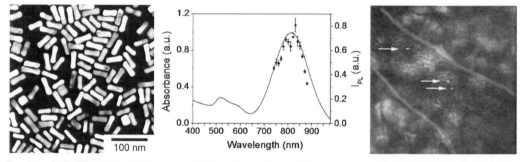

Fig. 8.1. *Left*, TEM image of NIR-resonant GNRs, 14 × 50 nm (24). Reprinted with permission from the American Chemical Society. *Center*, absorbance spectrum of GNRs (*solid line*) superimposed on TPL excitation data (*circles*), both having maxima near 820 nm. *Right*, in vivo TPL image of GNRs (indicated by *arrows*) passing through a blood vessel in a mouse ear, a few minutes after a tail vein injection (5). Blood vessel walls enhanced for clarity.

With respect to biomedical imaging, GNRs can support various OCT modalities with millimeter penetration depths and nanorod detection limits in the picomolar range (12). Recently, GNRs have been shown to produce contrast in an excised sample of human breast invasive ductal carcinoma, using a spectroscopic mode of OCT (13). GNRs can also generate optoacoustic contrast for photoacoustic tomography (PAT), an emerging imaging technique analogous to ultrasound (14). Pulsed NIR laser irradiation above a threshold power results in photo-induced cavitation effects (see below), and the low diffusion of propagating acoustic waves allows a depth resolution of up to several centimeters in biological tissue. GNR-enhanced PAT imaging has recently been demonstrated in vivo using a rat model.

GNRs are more than just passive imaging agents; most of the absorbed NIR photons are actually converted into heat (15). When exposed to higher laser fluencies, GNRs can mediate intense photothermal effects and inflict localized injury on nearby cells (9, 10, 16, 17) and tissues (18). This has provided lift to one of the more exciting concepts in nanomedicine in which therapeutic effects are integrated with diagnostic imaging, often popularly described by the portmanteau *theragnostics* (19). Two types of photothermal effects have been established: at the macroscopic level, the dissipated heat can induce a hyperthermic response in nearby cells, typically resulting in necrosis (16–18). The hyperthermic response is nonspecific but localized and can be controlled by the dosimetry of NIR irradiation. At the microscopic level, photothermally excited nanoparticles can raise the temperature of its immediate environment by hundreds to thousands degrees, resulting in superheating and cavitation (20, 21). The photoacoustic effects are generated on a timescale of nano- to microseconds and can deliver a mechanical form of cell injury if the GNRs are directly attached. We have recently established that membrane-bound GNRs can mediate tumor cell necrosis by compromising cell membrane integrity, which leads to an influx of calcium and a disruption of intracellular homeostasis (**Fig. 8.2**) (10).

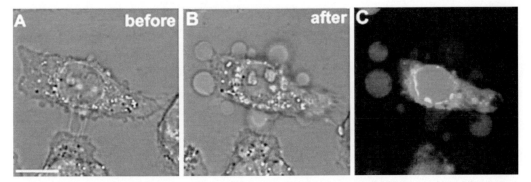

Fig. 8.2. (*color online*) (**A, B**) Folate-conjugated GNRs (*positive contrast, red*) targeted to the membranes of KB cells, before and after a 1-min exposure to a scanning NIR laser (12 J/cm^2). (**C**) Membrane perforation followed by blebbing could be visualized by ethidium bromide (*red*) and a fluorescent dye indicating free intracellular Ca^{2+} (*negative contrast, green*) (10). Reprinted with permission from Wiley–VCH.

In vivo demonstrations of GNRs as theragnostic agents are now emerging (18) and serve as important milestones on the trajectory toward clinical application. However, much depends on the ability to produce uniform GNRs on a batch scale, and to establish an appropriate surface coating protocol to navigate them through preclinical evaluations. With respect to synthesis, GNRs of well-defined size and aspect ratio are most often prepared by a seeded growth approach in aqueous solutions of cetyltrimethylammonium bromide (CTAB), a micellar surfactant (22, 23). This practical and popular method can be finely tuned by changes in stoichiometry (23) and by introducing chemical additives (24) for further control over growth kinetics. In particular, the presence of Ag ion has been found to be critical for producing uniform GNRs in high yield (25, 26) and is thought to selectively passivate high-energy facets of the GNRs during anisotropic growth (27). The synthesis of GNRs in micellar CTAB solutions is also scalable and has been performed on a gram scale with narrow size dispersity (28) and excellent shape control (29).

With respect to GNR surface coatings and functionalization, numerous methods have been introduced and are sufficient to support biological studies in a laboratory setting (*see* **Fig. 8.3** for selected examples). However, in order to be considered eligible for in vivo clinical studies, such coatings must at minimum meet the following criteria: (i) dispersion stability in blood and other physiological fluids, (ii) resistance against nonspecific cell uptake and protein adsorption, (iii) amenable to ligand functionalization for site-selective targeting and/or cell uptake, (iv) sufficiently

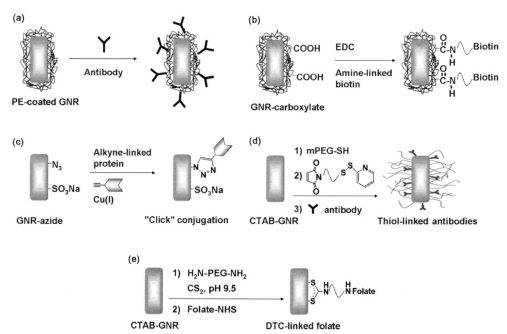

Fig. 8.3. Some surface functionalization and bioconjugation methods applied toward GNRs. (**a**) Electrostatic adsorption onto polyelectrolyte (PE)-coated GNRs (16); (**b**) covalent attachment via carbodiimide coupling (38); (**c**) "click" bioconjugation (39, 40); (**d**) chemisorption using thiols (11, 41); (**e**) chemisorption using in situ dithiocarbamate (DTC) formation (9, 10).

long circulation lifetimes to allow efficient delivery to the region of interest, and (v) low cytotoxicity and inflammatory response. Meeting these criteria implies that the coated GNRs should be robust against chemical degradation while under biological exposure, to avoid compromising its ability to meet the criteria above. Consequently, the surface chemistry of GNRs requires at least as much attention and development as their synthesis, if they are to be deployed in clinically relevant settings.

The biomedical applications involving GNRs are further challenged by the presence of CTAB, the micellar surfactant used in GNR synthesis. CTAB has a poor biocompatibility profile, with in vitro toxicological studies yielding IC_{50} values in the low micromolar range (30–32). In addition, CTAB-coated GNRs are susceptible to nonspecific uptake even at very low surfactant levels (8). These problems require the rigorous purification of GNR formulations prior to biomedical testing; however, attempts to strip CTAB from GNRs are often met with a loss of dispersion stability. We have recently established a protocol to remove CTAB by introducing sodium polystyrenesulfonate (PSS, 70 kDa) as an adsorbent and detergent, one which permits GNR detoxification without rapid flocculation (33). CTAB-laden PSS can be exchanged with fresh polyelectrolyte to produce biocompatible, CTAB-depleted GNRs with no significant cytotoxicity up to 85 μg/mL, the highest level evaluated (**Fig. 8.4**). This purification protocol sets the stage for pursuing robust methods of GNR surface functionalization, without concern for contamination by CTAB.

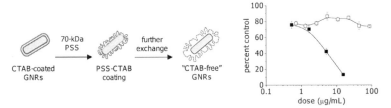

Fig. 8.4. (color online) Left, schematic describing protocol for removing CTAB from GNRs using 70-kDa PSS (33). Right, Cytotoxicity profile using KB cells of PSS-coated GNRs contaminated with CTAB (■) and after further exchange with unadulterated PSS (□). Reprinted with permission from the American Chemical Society.

2. Materials

2.1. Synthesis

1. Deionized (DI) water using an ultrafiltration system (Milli-Q, Millipore) with a measured resistivity above 18 MΩ.cm and passed through a 0.22-μm filter to remove particulate matter is used.

2. Seed solution: CTAB (SigmaUltra, > 99%, *see* **Note 1**) is dissolved in DI water at 0.2 M; gold chloride (HAuCl$_4$) is dissolved in DI water at 0.5 mM; sodium borohydride (NaBH$_4$) is dissolved in DI water at 10 mM.

3. Growth and quenching solutions: CTAB (SigmaUltra, > 99%, *see* **Note 1**) is dissolved in DI water at 0.2 M; HAuCl$_4$ is dissolved in DI water at 1 mM; silver nitrate (AgNO$_3$) is dissolved in DI water at 4 mM; ascorbic acid is dissolved in deionized water at 78.8 mM; sodium sulfide (Na$_2$S) is dissolved in DI water at 4 mM.

2.2. Purification

1. Sodium PSS (Aldrich, M_w 70 kDa) is dissolved in DI water as a 1% w/v solution. A 73-µg/mL PSS solution is prepared by diluting 51 µL of a 1% solution in 7 mL of aqueous NaOH at pH 10.

2. Cellulose membrane filters (nominal molecular weight limit, 100 kDa).

2.3. Surface Functionalization

1. *O,O'*-bis(2-aminoethyl)octadecaethylene glycol (Fluka) is dissolved in DI water as a 10-mM solution and adjusted by base titration to a pH of 9.5 (one-pot procedure), or dissolved in methanol as a 58-mM solution (two-step procedure).

2. Carbon disulfide (CS$_2$) is distilled from CaH$_2$, then dispersed in DI water as a saturated (28 mM) solution.

3. Folic acid is dissolved in anhydrous dimethyl sulfoxide (DMSO) as a 5% w/v solution; triethylamine, dicyclohexylcarbodiimide, and *N*-hydroxysuccinimide (Aldrich) were used as supplied.

3. Methods

3.1. Seeded Growth of Gold Nanorods

1. Preparation of gold nanoparticle seeds: 5 mL of a 0.2-M CTAB solution is combined with 5 mL of a 0.5-mM HAuCl$_4$ solution at room temperature. About 0.6 mL of a 10-mM NaBH$_4$ solution is cooled to 0°C in an ice bath for 10 min, then injected into the reaction mixture. The solution, which turned dark brown, is swirled by hand for at least 3 min. A portion of this solution is used within 2 h for Step 2 (*see* **Note 2**).

2. Conditions for seeded growth (*see* **Note 3**): Approximately 400 mL of a GNR growth solution is prepared by combining 200 mL of a 0.2-M CTAB solution, 200 mL of a

1-mM HAuCl$_4$ solution, 9.6 mL of a 4-mM AgNO$_3$ solution, and 2.8 mL of a 78.8-mM solution of ascorbic acid. This is treated with 0.48 mL of a freshly prepared solution of Au nanoparticle seeds, then allowed to stand at room temperature for up to 50 min. The reaction mixture gradually turned from colorless to a deep purplish-brown.

3. Sulfide-arrested growth: The solution above is treated with 100 mL of a 4-mM Na$_2$S solution, yielding a 500-mL suspension of GNRs with an absorption maximum near 800 nm (*see* **Notes 4, 5**) and an optical density (O.D.) close to 1. The GNR suspension is subjected to centrifugation at 24,000×*g* for 20 min using a fixed-angle rotor and the CTAB-saturated supernatant was removed by decantation. The residual GNRs are resuspended in 23 mL water to yield a highly concentrated sample (O.D. ca. 16.8, based on 1/20 dilution).

3.2. Detoxification of Gold Nanorods

1. Stabilization with PSS: 8 mL of a highly concentrated suspension of CTAB-stabilized GNRs (O.D. 16.8) is combined with 8 mL of chloroform and agitated for 1 min with a vortex mixer to produce an emulsion. The phases are separated by centrifugation at 1,000×*g* for 4 min, and the aqueous phase is carefully removed and treated with 0.45 mL of a 1% w/v solution of 70-kDa PSS. Additional CTAB is removed by washing the aqueous GNR suspension three more times with 8 mL of chloroform, every 3 h. The PSS-treated GNR suspension is diluted with fresh water to 200 mL, then concentrated to 2 mL using a stirred ultrafiltration cell (Millipore, Model 8010) outfitted with a regenerated cellulose membrane having a nominal molecular weight limit (NMWL) of 100 kDa. The GNRs are subjected to two more cycles of membrane ultrafiltration, with starting volumes of 200 mL and final volumes of 2–7 mL. The final dialyzed suspensions of PSS-treated GNRs may be diluted with phosphate-buffered saline (PBS) solution (pH 7.4) without loss of dispersion stability and were stable at room temperature for at least 30 days.

2. Detoxification by PSS exchange (*see* **Notes 6, 7**): 7 mL of PSS-treated GNRs (O.D. 16.6) is subjected to centrifugation at 6,000×*g* for 5 min to strip the CTAB-contaminated PSS coating from the GNR surface. The supernatant is decanted and the GNRs were re-dispersed in 7 mL of a 73-µg/mL solution of 70-kDa PSS. The centrifugation–redispersion cycle is repeated twice to yield PSS-coated GNR suspensions depleted of CTAB. These GNR dispersions exhibit moderate levels of stability in PBS (*see* **Note 8**), but do not exhibit any appreciable cytotoxicity based on a standard MTT viability assay (33).

3.3. Functionalization of GNRs with Oligoethyleneglycol–Folate Conjugate

1. Attachment of amine-terminated oligoethyleneglycol chains by in situ dithiocarbamate (DTC) formation (one-pot procedure): 3 mL of an aqueous suspension of PSS-stabilized GNRs (O.D. 1) is treated while stirring with 1 mL of a 10-mM solution of O,O'-bis(2-aminoethyl)-octadecaethylene glycol adjusted to pH 9.5, followed by 0.1 mL of a saturated aqueous solution of CS_2. The mixture is stirred for 12 h, then subjected to membrane dialysis with a molecular weight cutoff (MWCO) of 6,000–8,000 for 2 h in 200 mL water.

2. Attachment of amine-terminated oligoethyleneglycol chains by in situ dithiocarbamate (DTC) formation (two-step procedure) (see **Note 9**): (a) 190 µL of a 58-mM methanolic solution of O,O'-bis(2-aminoethyl)octadecaethylene glycol is treated with 10 µL of a 110-mM solution in CS_2, then agitated with a vortex mixer, and allowed to stand for 1 h to yield a 5.5-mM solution of the corresponding mono-DTC derivative with excess diamine. This is diluted 100-fold with aqueous NaOH at pH 10 to yield 20 mL of a 55-µM solution of the mono-DTC derivative. (b) 21 mL of an aqueous suspension of PSS-stabilized GNRs (O.D. 14.4) is adjusted to pH 10 by dropwise addition of 1 M NaOH, then treated with 110 µL of a 55-µM solution of the mono-DTC derivative. The suspension is agitated with a vortex mixer and allowed to stand overnight, then subjected twice to membrane dialysis for 2 h in 200 mL water, with a molecular weight cutoff (MWCO) of 6,000–8,000 (see **Note 10**).

3. Synthesis of N-hydroxysuccinimidyl (NHS)-folate (34): 100 mL of a 5% solution of folic acid in anhydrous DMSO is treated with 2.5 mL of triethylamine and 4.7 g of dicyclohexylcarbodiimide, followed by 2.6 g of N-hydroxysuccinimide. The reaction mixture is stirred for 12 h at room temperature, then filtered to remove the dicyclohexylurea byproduct. The reaction mixture is diluted with 500 mL of diethyl ether, then filtered again to collect the precipitated NHS-folate, which is washed with additional ether and dried under vacuum to yield 3.8 g of a yellow powder. Some of the NHS-folate is redissolved in dry DMSO to form a 40-µM solution.

4. Conjugation of amine-functionalized GNRs with folic acid: 1 mL of a dispersion of GNRs functionalized with DTC-anchored O,O'-bis(2-aminoethyl)octadecaethylene glycol (O.D. 10) is adjusted to pH 9.5 with 1 M NaOH, then treated with 0.1 mL of a 40-µM solution of NHS-folate in DMSO. The mixture is agitated with a vortex mixer and allowed to stand for 12 h, then subjected to membrane dialysis for 12 h in 900 mL deionized water (see **Note 10**).

4. Notes

1. The source and purity of CTAB are known to have an influential role on the kinetics of GNR growth (35). We have tested seven different sources of CTAB, and found five of these to be compatible with the GNR synthesis described in **Section 3.1**. The other two sources of CTAB appear to accelerate the rate of gold chloride reduction, with poor control over particle shape; reasons for loss of control have recently been ascribed to the presence of iodide above trace levels (42).

2. The diameter of the seed particles are typically 3 – 4 nm, according to TEM size analysis (22). However, the average particle size is age dependent and can increase due to Ostwald ripening. Therefore, it is recommended to use freshly prepared nanoparticles for GNR growth.

3. All glassware should be cleaned with aqua regia (75% conc. HCl, 25% conc. HNO_3) and rinsed with filtered DI water prior to use, to maximize GNR formation and uniformity. Plastic centrifuge tubes can be used as received.

4. Plasmon resonance peaks typically appear at NIR wavelengths (800–900 nm) 15–20 min after seed addition and reach their maximum absorbance intensities after 50–60 min. During this period, the resonance peaks often shift toward shorter wavelengths (see below). In addition, GNR formation can be quite sensitive to both nucleation and growth conditions, and it is not uncommon for the plasmon resonance peaks to vary from batch to batch. GNR batches prepared and isolated under apparently identical conditions can differ in their absorbance maxima by as much as 30 nm.

5. The addition of Na_2S is recommended to prevent a shift in GNR absorbance maxima from NIR to visible wavelengths, due to a slow growth in the lateral direction (i.e., the GNR width). This "optical drift" occurs because the plasmon resonance wavelength has an approximately linear relationship with the GNR aspect ratio, which is highest at the early stages of growth but decreases with reaction time due to changes in growth kinetics. Simply isolating GNRs from the reaction solution by centrifugation is not sufficient to arrest growth, as significant amounts of gold ion are still associated with the CTAB layers. Quenching the reaction with millimolar concentrations of Na_2S prevents further lateral growth by reducing residual gold ions, both in solution and in association with CTAB. It should also

be noted that higher concentrations of Na_2S can have the opposite effect on GNR plasmon resonance, i.e., cause a significant shift toward *longer* wavelengths. These shifts are acute and also beneficial for NIR imaging and excitation and have been attributed to the formation of metal sulfides (particularly Ag_2S) on the GNR surface (24, 36).

6. The PSS-treated GNRs in Step 1 of **Section 3.2** are contaminated with residual CTAB and exhibit a remarkably high level of cytotoxicity, higher than that observed from CTAB-stabilized GNRs (33). This is because the polyelectrolyte coating (presumed to be a PSS–CTAB complex) can gradually leach from the GNR surface and compromise the membrane integrity of afflicted cells. It is thus necessary to remove CTAB-contaminated PSS from GNR dispersions.

7. For short-term in vitro and in vivo studies, it is possible to use freshly prepared PSS-coated GNRs for surface functionalization and subsequent targeted delivery, if care is taken to remove excess CTAB and desorbed polyelectrolyte prior to administration. However, the long-term stability of such functionalized GNRs cannot be assumed.

8. The dispersion stability of PSS-treated GNRs is dependent on the amount of residual CTAB. For instance, the CTAB-depleted and essentially nontoxic GNRs described in Step 2 of **Section 3.2** have a half-life of approximately 24 h in PBS solution when dispersed with PSS and much less than that in serum. Therefore, PSS is most beneficial as a detergent for removing CTAB. Substituting PSS with chemisorptive forms of polyethylene glycol has proven to be useful for in vitro studies involving cell uptake (8) and also in vivo GNR biodistribution studies (37).

9. The one-pot surface functionalization of GNRs with amine-terminated oligoethyleneglycol chains by in situ DTC formation is convenient, but the two-step procedure is cleaner and may provide better control over surface coverage. In particular, the surface ligand density can be adjusted by using higher concentrations of *O,O'*-bis (2-aminoethyl)octadecaethylene glycol, mono-DTC.

10. For GNR functionalization on a larger scale, stirred ultrafiltration can be performed in lieu of membrane dialysis.

Acknowledgments

We gratefully acknowledge financial support from the National Institutes of Health (EB-001777) and the Oncological Sciences Center at Purdue University. We thank Dr. Stephan Stern and Dr. Anil Patri (Nanomaterials Characterization Laboratory, SAIC-Frederick) for cytotoxicity evaluations and additional materials characterization, supported under NCI contract N01-CO-12400, and Prof. Ji-Xin Cheng and his group members (Purdue University) for valuable collaborative research and scientific discussions.

References

1. Liao, H., Nehl, C. L., and Hafner, J. H. (2006) Biomedical applications of plasmon resonant metal nanoparticles. *Nanomedicine* 1, 201–208.
2. Tong, L., Wei, Q., Wei, A., and Cheng, J. -X. (2009) Gold nanorods as contrast agents for biological imaging: surface conjugation, two-photon luminescence, and photothermal effects. *Photochem Photobiol* 85, 21–32.
3. Weissleder, R. (2001) A clearer vision for in vivo imaging. *Nat Biotechnol* 19, 316–317.
4. Jain, P. K., Lee, K. S., El-Sayed, I. H., and El-Sayed, M. A. (2006) Calculated absorption and scattering properties of gold nanoparticles of different size, shape, and composition: applications in biological imaging and biomedicine. *J Phys Chem B* 110, 7238–7248.
5. Wang, H., Huff, T. B., Zweifel, D. A., He, W., Low, P. S., Wei, A., and Cheng, J. -X. (2005) In vitro and in vivo two-photon luminescence imaging of single gold nanorods. *Proc Natl Acad Sci USA* 102, 15752–15756.
6. Imura, K., Nagahara, T., and Okamoto, H. (2005) Near-field two-photon-induced photoluminescence from single gold nanorods and imaging of plasmon modes. *J Phys Chem B* 109, 13214–13220.
7. Bouhelier, A., Bachelot, R., Lerondel, G., Kostcheev, S., Royer, P., and Wiederrecht, G. P. (2005) Surface plasmon characteristics of tunable photoluminescence in single gold nanorods. *Phys Rev Lett* 95, 267405.
8. Huff, T. B., Hansen, M. N., Zhao, Y., Cheng, J. -X., and Wei, A. (2007) Controlling the cellular uptake of gold nanorods. *Langmuir* 23, 1596–1599.
9. Huff, T. B., Tong, L., Zhao, Y., Hansen, M. N., Cheng, J. -X., and Wei, A. (2007) Hyperthermic effects of gold nanorods on tumor cells. *Nanomedicine* 2, 125–132.
10. Tong, L., Zhao, Y., Huff, T. B., Hansen, M. N., Wei, A., and Cheng, J. -X. (2007) Gold nanorods mediate tumor cell death by compromising membrane integrity. *Adv Mater* 19, 3136–3141.
11. He, W., Henne, W. A., Wei, Q., Zhao, Y., Doorneweerd, D. D., Cheng, J. -X., Low, P. S., and Wei, A. (2008) Two-photon luminescence imaging of *Bacillus* spores using peptide-functionalized gold nanorods. *Nano Res* 2, 450–456.
12. Oldenburg, A. L., Hansen, M. N., Zweifel, D. A., Wei, A., and Boppart, S. A. (2006) Plasmon-resonant gold nanorods as low-albedo contrast agents for optical coherence tomography. *Opt Express* 14, 6724–6738.
13. Oldenburg, A. L., Hansen, M. N., Ralston, T. S., Wei, A., and Boppart, S. A. (2009) Imaging gold nanorods in excised human breast carcinoma by spectroscopic optical coherence tomography. *J. Mater Chem* 19, 6407–6411.
14. Eghtedari, M., Oraevsky, A., Copland, J. A., Kotov, N., Conjusteau, A., and Motamedi, M. (2007) High sensitivity of in vivo detection of gold nanorods using a laser optoacoustic imaging system. *Nano Lett* 7, 1914–1918.
15. Chou, C. -H., Chen, C. -D., and Wang, C. R. C. (2005) Highly efficient, wavelength-tunable, gold nanoparticle based optothermal nanoconvertors. *J Phys Chem B* 109, 11135–11138.
16. Huang, X., El-Sayed, I. H., Qian, W., and El-Sayed, M. A. (2006) Cancer cell imaging and photothermal therapy in the near-infrared region by using gold nanorods. *J Am Chem Soc* 128, 2115–2120.
17. Takahashi, H., Niidome, T., Nariai, A., Niidome, Y., and Yamada, S. (2006) Gold nanorod-sensitized cell death: microscopic observation of single living cells irradiated by pulsed near-infrared laser light in the presence of gold nanorods. *Chem Lett* 35, 500–501.
18. Dickerson, E. B., Dreaden, E. C., Huang, X., El-Sayed, I. H., Chu, H., Pushpanketh, S., McDonald, J. F., and El-Sayed, M. A. (2008) Gold nanorod assisted near-infrared plasmonic photothermal therapy (PPTT) of squamous cell carcinoma in mice. *Cancer Lett* 269, 57–66.
19. Cuenca, A. G., Jiang, H., Hochwald, S. N., Delano, M., Cance, W. G., and Grobmyer,

S. R. (2006) Emerging implications of nanotechnology on cancer diagnostics and therapeutics. *Cancer* **107**, 459–466.
20. Pitsillides, C. M., Joe, E. K., Wei, X., Anderson, R. R., and Lin, C. P. (2003) Selective cell targeting with light-absorbing microparticles and nanoparticles. *Biophys J* **84**, 4023–4032.
21. Zharov, V. P., Galitovskaya, E. N., Johnson, C., and Kelly, T. (2005) Synergistic enhancement of selective nanothermolysis with gold nanoclusters: potential for cancer therapy. *Lasers Surg Med* **37**, 219–226.
22. Jana, N. R., Gearheart, L., and Murphy, C. J. (2001) Seed-mediated growth approach for shape-controlled synthesis of spheroidal and rod-like gold nanoparticles using a surfactant template. *Adv Mater* **13**, 1389–1393.
23. Murphy, C. J., Gole, A. M., Hunyadi, S. E., and Orendorff, C. J. (2006) One-dimensional colloidal gold and silver nanostructures. *Inorg Chem* **45**, 7544–7554.
24. Zweifel, D. A. and Wei, A. (2005) Sulfide-arrested growth of gold nanorods. *Chem Mater* **17**, 4256–4261.
25. Nikoobakht, B. and El-Sayed, M. A. (2003) Preparation and growth mechanism of gold nanorods (nrs) using seed-mediated growth method. *Chem Mater* **15**, 1957–1962.
26. Sau, T. K. and Murphy, C. J. (2004) Seeded high yield synthesis of short Au nanorods in aqueous solution. *Langmuir* **20**, 6414–6420.
27. Liu, M. Z. and Guyot-Sionnest, P. (2005) Mechanism of silver(I)-assisted growth of gold nanorods and bipyramids. *J Phys Chem B* **109**, 22192–22200.
28. Jana, N. R. (2005) Gram-scale synthesis of soluble, near-monodisperse gold nanorods and other anisotropic nanoparticles. *Small* **1**, 875–882.
29. Khanal, B. P. and Zubarev, E. R. (2008) Purification of high aspect ratio gold nanorods: complete removal of platelets. *J Am Chem Soc* **130**, 1263–1264.
30. Cortesi, R., Esposito, E., Menegatti, E., Gambari, R., and Nastruzzi, C. (1996) Effect of cationic liposome composition on in vitro cytotoxicity and protective effect on carried DNA. *Int J Pharm* **139**, 69–78.
31. Mirska, D., Schirmer, K., Funari, S., Langner, A., Dobner, B., and Brezesinski, G. (2005) Biophysical and biochemical properties of a binary lipid mixture for DNA transfection. *Colloids Surf B* **40**, 51–59.
32. Takahashi, H., Niidome, Y., Niidome, T., Kaneko, K., Kawasaki, H., and Yamada, H. (2006) Modification of gold nanorods using phosphatidylcholine to reduce cytotoxicity. *Langmuir* **22**, 2–5.
33. Leonov, A. P., Zheng, J., Clogston, J. D., Stern, S. T., Patri, A. K., and Wei, A. (2008) Detoxification of gold nanorods by treatment with polystyrenesulfonate. *ACS Nano* **2**, 2481–2488.
34. Lee, R. J. and Low, P. S. (1994) Delivery of liposomes into cultured KB cells via folate receptor-mediated endocytosis. *J Biol Chem* **269**, 3198–3204.
35. Smith, D. K. and Korgel, B. A. (2008) The importance of the CTAB surfactant on the colloidal seed-mediated synthesis of gold nanorods. *Langmuir* **24**, 644–649.
36. Liu, M. Z. and Guyot-Sionnest, P. (2006) Preparation and optical properties of silver chalcogenide coated gold nanorods. *J Mater Chem* **16**, 3942–3945.
37. Niidome, T., Yamagata, M., Okamoto, Y., Akiyama, Y., Takahashi, H., Kawano, T., Katayama, Y., and Niidome, Y. (2006) PEG-modified gold nanorods with a stealth character for in vivo applications. *J Control Release* **35**, 500–501.
38. Gole, A. and Murphy, C. J. (2005) Biotin-streptavidin-induced aggregation of gold nanorods: tuning rod-rod orientation. *Langmuir* **21**, 10756–10762.
39. Oyelere, A. K., Chen, P. C., Huang, X., El-Sayed, I. H., and El-Sayed, M. A. (2007) Peptide-conjugated gold nanorods for nuclear targeting. *Bioconjug Chem* **18**, 1490–1497.
40. Gole, A. and Murphy, C. J. (2008) Azide-derivatized gold nanorods: functional materials for "Click" chemistry. *Langmuir* **24**, 266–272.
41. Liao, H. and Hafner, J. H. (2005) Gold nanorod bioconjugates. *Chem Mater* **17**, 4636–4641.
42. Smith, D. K., Miller, N. R., and Korgel, B. A. (2009) Iodide in CTAB prevents gold nanorod formation. *Langmuir* **25**, 9518–9524.

Chapter 9

Polymeric Micelles: Polyethylene Glycol-Phosphatidylethanolamine (PEG-PE)-Based Micelles as an Example

Rupa R. Sawant and Vladimir P. Torchilin

Abstract

One of the renowned nanosized pharmaceutical carriers for delivery of poorly soluble drugs, especially, in cancer, is micelles, which are self-assembled colloidal particles with a hydrophobic core and hydrophilic shell. Among the micelle-forming compounds, micelles made of polyethylene glycol-phosphatidylethanolamine (PEG-PE) have gained more attention due to some attractive properties such as good stability, longevity, and ability to accumulate in the areas with an abnormal vasculature via the enhanced permeability and retention effect (into the areas with leaky vasculature, such as tumors). Additionally these micelles can be made "targeted" by attaching specific targeting ligand molecules to the micelle surface or can be comprised of stimuli-responsive amphiphilic block copolymers. Addition of second component such as surfactant or another hydrophobic material to the main micelle forming material further improves the solubilizing capacity of micelles without compromising their stability. Micelles carrying various contrast agents may become the imaging agents of choice in different imaging modalities. Here, we have discussed various protocols for preparation and evaluation of PEG-PE-based micelles.

Key words: Drug delivery, cancer, polymeric micelles, mixed micelles, polyethylene glycol-phosphatidylethanolamine, immunomicelles, monoclonal antibody, paclitaxel, iron oxide nanoparticles.

1. Introduction

Polymeric micelles have rapidly gained interest as nanocarrier systems for cancer therapeutic applications due to their small size (10–100 nm), in vivo stability, ability to solubilize water-insoluble anticancer drugs, and prolonged blood circulation times

(1, 2). The typical core–shell structure of polymeric micelles is formed by self-assembly of amphiphilic block copolymers consisting of hydrophilic and hydrophobic monomer units in aqueous media (1). The major driving force behind self-association of amphiphilic polymers is the decrease in free energy of the system due to removal of hydrophobic fragments from the aqueous surroundings with the formation of a micelle core stabilized with hydrophilic blocks exposed to water (3, 4). At low concentration in an aqueous medium, these exist as separate units. However, as their concentration is increased, aggregation takes place. The concentration of monomeric amphiphile at which micelles form is called the critical micelle concentration (CMC).

When used as drug carriers in aqueous media, micelles solubilize molecules of poorly soluble non-polar pharmaceuticals within the micelle core. Polar molecules can be adsorbed on the micelle surface, and substances with intermediate polarity distribute along surfactant molecules in intermediate positions. The micellar solubilization of drug results in an increased water solubility of sparingly soluble drug (5–7), improves its bioavailability (7), reduces toxicity and other adverse effects (8), enhances permeability across physiological barriers, and shows some positive changes in biodistribution (4, 9).

Beyond solubilizing hydrophobic drugs, block copolymer micelles can target their payload to specific tissues actively or passively. Passive targeting is due to the small micellar size which permits spontaneous penetration into the interstitium of body compartments with relatively leaky vasculatures (e.g., tumors and infarcts) by the enhanced permeability and retention (EPR) effect (1, 2, 8). Active targeting can be achieved by surface attachment of target-specific molecules (1, 2). Ideally, the core compartment of a pharmaceutical polymeric micelle should demonstrate high loading capacity, controlled release profile of the incorporated drug, and good compatibility between the core-forming block and the incorporated drug. The micelle corona is responsible for providing an effective steric protection for the micelle and determines the micelle hydrophilicity, the charge, the length and surface density of hydrophilic blocks, and the presence of reactive groups suitable for further micelle derivatization, such as attachment of targeting moieties (1). **Figure 9.1** shows a typical scheme of micelle formation from an amphiphilic molecule, its loading with a poorly soluble drug, and some ways to further modify the micelle to improve its performance as a pharmaceutical carrier.

Within the structure of an amphiphilic polymer, monomer units with different hydrophobicities can be combined randomly, represented by two conjugated blocks each consisting of the same type (A–B type copolymers), or be made from alternating blocks with different hydrophobicity (A–B–A type copolymers). Alternatively, the hydrophilic backbone chain of a

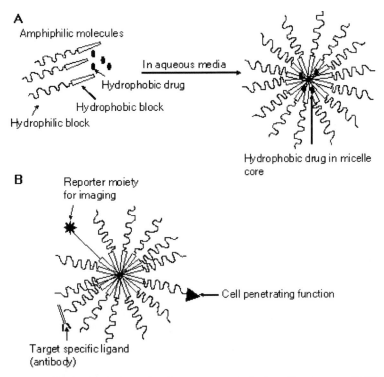

Fig. 9.1. Pharmaceutical micelles. Spontaneous micelle formation from amphiphilic molecules in aqueous media and loading with hydrophobic drug (a), multifunctional pharmaceutical micelle (b).

polymer can be grafted with hydrophobic blocks (graft copolymers) (1, 10). The shell is responsible for micelle stabilization and interaction with plasma proteins and cell membranes. It usually consists of poly(ethyleneglycol) (PEG) blocks with a molecular weight from 1 to 15 kDa. Other polymers such as poly(N-isopropylacrylamide) (11) and poly(alkylacrylic acid) (12) impart temperature or pH sensitivity to the micelles. The hydrophobic core generally consists of a biodegradable polymer such as poly(β-benzyl-L-aspartate) (13–16), poly(D,L-lactide) (17) or poly(ε-caprolactone) (18, 19) or non-biodegradable polymer such as polystyrene or poly(methyl methacrylate) (20). The core may also consist of a water-soluble polymer (e.g., poly(aspartic acid)) which is rendered hydrophobic by chemical conjugation of a hydrophobic drug (21). In some cases, phospholipid residues can also be used as hydrophobic core forming compounds (1, 22, 23). Polylactone-PEG double and triple block copolymers (24) have been suggested as micelle-forming polymers as well as poly(2-ethyl-2-oxazoline-block-poly(ε-caprolactone)), which forms 20 nm micelles with good load of paclitaxel (25). Chitosan grafted with hydrophobic groups such as palmitoyl has become popular for pharmaceutical micelles preparation due to its high biocompatibility (26). Dendrimeric micelles, such as biaryl-based ones, have also been suggested (27). New materials for pharmaceutical micelles include new copolymers of PEG (28) and completely new macromolecules, such as scorpion-like polymers (29) and other star-like and core–shell constructs (30). Examples of drug loaded into various polymeric micelles are presented in Table 9.1.

Table 9.1
Examples of block copolymers used to prepare drug-loaded micelles

Block copolymer	Drugs incorporated
Pluronics	Doxorubicin (31), haloperidol (32), ATP (33)
Polycaprolactone-b-PEG	FK506, L-685,818 (34)
Polycaprolactone-b-methoxy-PEG	Indomethacin (35)
Poly(N-isopropylacrylamide)-b-PEG	Miscellaneous (36)
Poly(γ-benzyl-L-glutamate)-b-PEG	Clonazepam (37)
Poly(β-benzyl-L-aspartate)-b-PEG	Doxorubicin (15, 38), indomethacin (39), KRN (40, 41), amphotericin B (42)
Poly(L-lysine)-b-PEG	DNA (43, 44)
PEG-PE	Dequalinium (45), soya bean trypsin inhibitor (46), camptothecin (47), paclitaxel (48), porphyrin (48), vitamin K_3 (49)
Poly(D,L-lactide)-b-methoxy-PEG	Paclitaxel (50), testosterone, griseofulvin (51)
Poly(N-vinyl-2-pyrrolidone)-b-poly(D,L-lactide)	Indomethacin (52)
Poly(N-isopropylacrylamide)-based micelles (pH-sensitive)	Phthalocyanine (53)
Poly(L-histidine)-b-PEG (folate-targeted)	Doxorubicin (54)
Chitosan grafted with palmitoyl	Ibuprofen (26), puerarin (55)

A typical protocol for the preparation of drug-loaded polymeric micelles from amphiphilic copolymers without involving the electrostatic complex formation includes the following steps. Solutions of an amphiphilic polymer and a drug of interest in miscible volatile organic solvents are mixed, and organic solvents are evaporated to form a polymer/drug film. The film obtained is then hydrated in the presence of an aqueous buffer, and the micelles are formed by intensive shaking. If the amount of a drug exceeds the solubilization capacity of micelles, the excess drug precipitates in a crystalline form and is removed by filtration. The loading efficiency for different compounds varies from 1.5 to 50% by weight. This value apparently correlates with the hydrophobicity of a drug.

The use of lipid moieties as hydrophobic blocks capping hydrophilic polymer (such as PEG) chains can provide additional advantages for particle stability when compared with conventional amphiphilic polymer micelles due to the presence of two fatty acid acyls, which can contribute considerably to an increase in the hydrophobic interactions between the polymeric chains in the micelle core (22). The chemical structure of PEG-PE is shown in **Fig. 9.2**. All versions of PEG-PE conjugates form micelles with a spherical shape, uniform size distribution (7–35 nm), and very low CMC values (in a high nanomolar to low micromolar range) because of strong hydrophobic interactions between the double acyl chains of the phospholipid residues (**Table 9.2**). These micelles are structured in such a way that the outer PEG corona, known to be highly water soluble and highly hydrated, serves as an efficient steric protector in biological media. On the other hand, the phospholipid residues, which represent the micelle core, are extremely hydrophobic and can

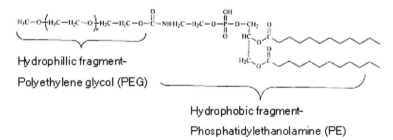

Fig. 9.2. Chemical structure of PEG-PE.

Table 9.2
CMC values and particle diameter of PEG-PE micelles

Micelle-forming conjugate	CMC (M)	Particle size (nm)
PEG$_{750}$-DSPE	1×10^{-5}	7–15
PEG$_{2000}$-DSPE	1×10^{-5}	7–20
PEG$_{5000}$-DSPE	6×10^{-6}	10–40
PEG$_{2000}$-DOPE	9×10^{-6}	7–20
PEG$_{5000}$-DOPE	7×10^{-6}	10–35

solubilize various poorly soluble drugs including paclitaxel, camptothecin, porphyrin, tamoxifen, and vitamin K_3 (47–49). Micelles prepared from PEG-PE conjugates with shorter versions of PEG are more efficient carriers of poorly soluble drugs because of their greater hydrophobic-to-hydrophilic phase ratio and can be loaded with drug more efficiently on a weight-to-weight basis.

The PEG-PE micelles demonstrate good stability, longevity, and ability to accumulate in the areas with an abnormal vasculature via the EPR effect (22, 56). Since transport across the tumor vasculature depends somewhat on the particular type of tumor (57), the use of micelles as drug carriers can be particularly useful for tumors, whose vasculature has a low cutoff size (below 200 nm). Thus, 15–20 nm PEG-PE micelles effectively delivered a model protein drug to a solid tumor with a very low cutoff size (Lewis lung carcinoma) in mice (46), while even small 100 nm long-circulating liposomes did not show an increased accumulation of liposome-encapsulated drug (58). Other recent data also clearly indicate enhanced uptake of PEG-PE-based micelles by other experimental tumors (59) in mice as well as into ischemic areas of the heart in rabbits with experimental myocardial infarction (60).

Various attempts have been made to further increase the solubilization efficiency of micelles by forming mixed micelles with the addition of another surfactant or hydrophobic material. One should expect that these mixed micelles will allow for the better solubilization of poorly soluble drugs because of some loosening of the micelle core (e.g., with egg phosphatidyl choline) (23) or an increased volume of the lipophilic core of mixed micelles (e.g., with D-α-tocopheryl polyethylene glycol 1,000 succinate/vitamin E/Pluronic) (61–63).

PEG-lipid micelles have also gained attention as a carrier for contrast agents due to their small size which allows for better penetration to the target to be visualized (1). In the case of loading with superparamagnetic iron oxide nanoparticles (SPIONs), SPION-micelles exhibited better MRI T2 signal compared to similar concentrations of plain SPIONs due to the inhibition of aggregation of plain SPION.

Further, PEG-PE micelles can also be tumor-targeted by attachment of the anticancer nucleosome-specific monoclonal antibody 2C5 (mAb 2C5) to their outer shell, which recognizes the surface of a broad variety of tumor cells via tumor cell surface bound nucleosomes (23, 63–65). These immunomicelles have been prepared by using PEG-PE conjugates with the free PEG terminus activated with a *p*-nitrophenylcarbonyl (pNP) group (66). Diacyllipid fragments of such a bifunctional PEG derivative firmly incorporate into the micelle core, while the water-exposed pNP group, stable at pH values below 6, interacts with amino groups of various ligands (antibodies and their fragments or peptides) at pH values above 7.5 yielding a stable urethane (carbamate) bond. To prepare immunomicelles, the corresponding antibody is simply incubated with the drug-loaded pNP-PEG-PE-containing micelles at a pH around 8. It was shown that the mAb 2C5-immunomicelles were capable of bringing higher amounts of paclitaxel to tumors compared to paclitaxel-loaded non-targeted micelles or free drug formulations (23).

Micelles from PEG-PE conjugates can be prepared and loaded with poorly soluble anticancer drugs such as paclitaxel using a simple protocol and characterized for size distribution, drug solubilization efficiency, CMC, and in vitro cytotoxicity. These micelles can additionally be modified with mAb 2C5 antibody using a functionalized PEG-PE (59, 67).

2. Materials

2.1. Preparation of Drug-Loaded Micelles

1. Polyethyleneglycol-phosphatidylethanolamine (PEG$_{2000}$-PE) (Avanti Polar Lipids, Alabaster, AL) stored at –80°C.
2. Paclitaxel (Sigma, St. Louis, MO) dissolved in methanol at 10 mg/mL and stored at –20°C.
3. 4-(2-Hydroxyethyl)-1-piperazine-ethanesulfonic acid (HEPES) buffered saline (HBS): 5 mM HEPES, 141 mM NaCl, pH 7.4. Stored at room temperature.

2.2. Preparation of Drug-Loaded Mixed Micelles

1. Egg phosphatidylcholine (ePC) (Avanti Polar Lipids, Alabaster, AL) stored at –80°C.
2. D-α-Tocopheryl polyethylene glycol 1000 succinate (TPGS) (Eastman Chemicals, USA), dissolved in chloroform at 10 mg/mL and stored at –20°C.

2.3. Preparation of SPION-Micelles

1. SPION, synthesized using a thermal decomposition method developed by Hyeon et al. (68).

2.4. Preparation of Drug-Loaded Immunomicelles

1. *p*-Nitrophenylcarbonyl-PEG$_{3400}$-dioleoyl phosphatidylethanolamine (pNP-PEG-PE) synthesized inhouse (66).
2. Citrate-buffered saline (CBS): 5 mM Na-citrate, 141 mM NaCl, pH 5.0. Stored at room temperature.
3. The mAb 2C5 produced in ascites via the I.P. injection of 1.5 × 10^6 hybridoma cells/mL into pristine primed BALB/c 4-week-old male mice. The production and the purification of the mAb 2C5 were carried out by Harlan

Bioproducts (Indianapolis, IL) using the cell line from our laboratory.

4. Phosphate buffer: 100 mM disodium phosphate heptahydrate, 0.72 mM monosodium phosphate monohydrate, pH 9.0. Stored at room temperature.

2.5. ELISA

1. Tris-buffered saline (TBS): 50 mM Tris, 150 mM NaCl, pH 7.4. Stored at room temperature.
2. TBS containing 0.05% w/v Tween-20 (TBST). Stored at 2–8°C.
3. TBS containing 0.05% w/v Tween-20 and 2 mg/mL casein (TBST-Cas). Stored at 2–8°C.
4. Poly-L-lysine (PLL, MW 30–70 kDa) solution in TBS at 40 µg/mL. Stored at 2–8°C.
5. Nucleosome solution (the water-soluble fraction of calf thymus nucleohistone, Worthington Biochemical, Lakewood, NJ) in TBST-Cas at 40 µg/mL. Stored at 2–8°C.
6. Standard mAb 2C5 in TBST-Cas at 10 µg/mL. Stored at 2–8°C.
7. Goat anti-mouse IgG peroxidase conjugates (ICN Biomedical, Aurora, OH) in TBST-Cas 1:5,000 dilution and prepared fresh. Original stored at –20°C.
8. Enhanced Kblue® TMB peroxidase substrate (Neogen, Lexington, KY). Stored at 2–8°C.

2.6. In Vitro Cytotoxicity

1. Sterile 96-well plates (Corning, Inc., Corning, NY).
2. Dulbecco's Modified Eagle's Medium (DMEM) (CellGro, Kansas City, MO) supplemented with 10% fetal bovine serum (FBS, HyClone, Ogden, UT), 1 mM Na-pyruvate, 50 U/mL penicillin, and 50 µg/mL streptomycin (CellGro, Kansas City, MO).
3. Cell Titer 96® A$_{queous}$ One solution (Promega, Madison, WI). Stored at –20°C.

3. Methods

Micelles are prepared by the lipid film hydration method and loaded with various poorly soluble drugs or diagnostic agents. In addition, these micelles may contain a second component to form mixed micelles. The protocol for attachment of antibody requires PEG-PE with the free PEG terminus activated with pNP. Micelles are prepared from PEG-PE with the addition of a small

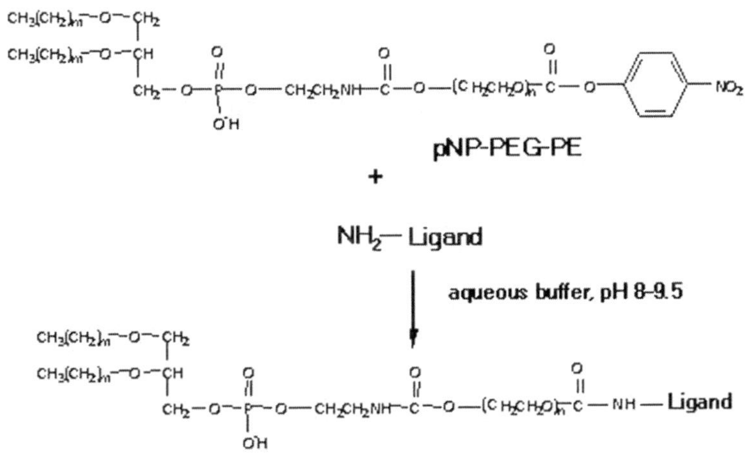

Fig. 9.3. Antibody attachment to pNP-PEG-PE via the pNP group.

fraction of pNP-PEG-PE. The PE residues form the micelle core, whereas pNP groups allow for fast and efficient attachment of amino group containing ligands via the formation of a urethane (carbamate) bond (**Fig. 9.3**).

It is important to characterize these micelles for size, CMC, and drug solubilization efficiency. To verify the immunological activity of micelle-attached mAb 2C5, a standard ELISA is used. Ultimately it is important to evaluate the in vitro cytotoxicity of drug-loaded micelles and immunomicelles against various cancer cells.

3.1. Preparation of Drug-Loaded Micelles

1. To prepare drug-loaded micelles, add drug dissolved in a suitable organic solvent (e.g., chloroform, methanol, acetonitrile) to the solution of PEG-PE in chloroform in a round bottom flask. In a typical case, for paclitaxel-loaded micelles, 0.2 mg of paclitaxel per 14.5 mg of PEG_{2000}-PE.

2. Remove the solvents on a rotary evaporator followed by freeze-drying.

3. Hydrate the dried film with 5 mM HBS, pH 7.4, at a PEG-PE concentration of 5 mM followed by vortexing for 5–10 min.

4. Remove the non-incorporated drug by filtration of the micelle suspension through a 0.2 μm polycarbonate membrane filter.

3.2. Preparation of Drug-Loaded Mixed Micelles

Prepare mixed micelles with one component being PEG-PE and a second component being surfactant (e.g., TPGS, Pluronic) or another lipid (e.g., ePC) or a hydrophobic material such as vitamin E.

1. To prepare drug-loaded mixed micelles, add drug dissolved in suitable organic solvents to a mixture of PEG-PE and one of the components mentioned above in chloroform in appropriate molar ratios (*see* **Note 1**). In a typical case, 1 mg of paclitaxel per 22 mg of lipid (PEG_{2000}-PE and TPGS, 1:1 molar ratio).

   Further procedure is the same as described in **Section 3.1**

3.3. Preparation of SPION-Micelles

1. Add SPION in hexane to a PEG-PE solution in chloroform. In a typical case, 0.25 mg of SPION per 10 mg of PEG-PE.
2. Remove organic solvents by rotary evaporation followed by freeze-drying.
3. Hydrate the dried film with 2 mL of 5 mM HBS, pH 7.4, with vortexing for 5 min followed by bath sonication for 5 min.

3.4. Preparation of Immunomicelles

1. To attach mAb 2C5 to micelles to obtain immunomicelles, supplement a chloroform solution of PEG-PE with 5 mol% of the reactive component, pNP-PEG-PE, in a round bottom flask (*see* **Note 2**).
2. Add the required amount of drug solution to this mixture and remove the organic solvents by rotary evaporation followed by freeze-drying.
3. Hydrate the dried film with 5 mM CBS, pH 5.0, to obtain net final concentration of 20 mg/mL lipid.
4. To 0.5 mL of the resultant mixture, add 0.3 mL of 2.94 mg/mL of a 2C5 solution in 100 mM phosphate buffer, pH 9.0, with vortexing. Adjust the pH of the mixture to pH 8.5 with 1 M NaOH to allow for the reaction between protein (antibody) amino groups and pNP groups of pNP-PEG-PE to yield immunomicelles.
5. Incubate the mixture for 3 h at room temperature.
6. Dialyze the drug-loaded immunomicelles against 1 L of 5 mM HBS, pH 7.4, using cellulose ester membranes with a cutoff size of 250 kDa.

3.5. In Vitro Evaluation of Micelles

3.5.1. Size Distribution Analysis

Measure the micelle size (hydrodynamic diameter) by dynamic light scattering (DLS) using a N4 Plus Submicron Particle System (Coulter Corporation, Miami, FL). Dilute the micelle suspension with deionized water to a concentration to provide a light scattering intensity of 5×10^4 to 1×10^6 counts/s. A typical size distribution of micelles is shown in **Fig. 9.4**.

3.5.2. CMC Determination

Estimate the CMC values of micelles/mixed micelles by standard pyrene method. The pyrene method is considered to be one of the most sensitive and precise techniques for CMC determination. It

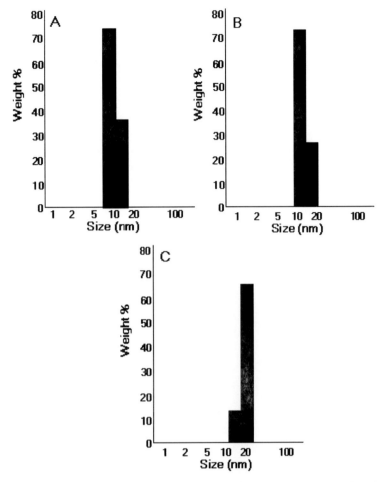

Fig. 9.4. Micelle size and size distribution of empty PEG_{2000}-PE micelles (**a**), paclitaxel-loaded PEG_{2000}-PE micelles (**b**), and paclitaxel-loaded PEG_{2000}-PE/TPGS micelles (**c**).

is based on the fact that some fluorescent probes, such as pyrene, have a tendency to associate with micelles rather than with the water phase, and their fluorescence changes depend on the surroundings. Below the CMC, the marker (pyrene) is solubilized in a polar solvent (water) only to a very small extent. However, in the presence of micelles a hydrophobic, non-polar micelle core solubilizes pyrene. Following the fluorescence intensity of a corresponding marker at different concentrations of an amphiphilic polymer, one can see the increase in fluorescence intensity as micelles begin to appear in the system and the marker becomes associated with the micelle core.

1. Prepare tubes containing 1 mg of pyrene crystals.
2. To these crystals, add 10^{-4} to 10^{-7} M micellar solution of PEG-PE in 5 mM HBS, pH 7.4.

3. Incubate the mixture for 24 h with shaking at room temperature.

4. Remove free pyrene by filtration through a 0.2 μm polycarbonate membrane filter.

5. Measure the fluorescence of the filtered samples at an excitation wavelength of 339 nm and emission wavelength of 390 nm using an F-2000 fluorescence spectrometer (Hitachi, Japan).

The graph for CMC determination of PEG-PE micelles is shown in **Fig. 9.5**.

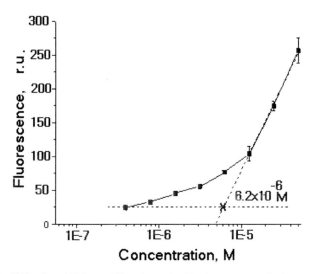

Fig. 9.5. CMC value of PEG_{5000}-PE as determined by the pyrene method.

3.5.3. Drug Solubilization Efficiency

Measure the amount of drug in micellar phase after disruption of micelles with suitable organic solvents. In the case of paclitaxel-loaded micelles, the amount micellar solubilized paclitaxel is measured after dilution of micelles with an acetonitrile and water mixture (70:30) and analyzed by reversed-phase HPLC (62). The drug solubilization efficiency of mixed micelles made of PEG_{2000}-PE/TPGS (1:1 molar ratio) was found to be 3.5% w/w compared to only 1.2% w/w as was found for the micelles prepared of PEG_{2000}-PE alone, i.e., the addition of TPGS actually improves paclitaxel solubilization by mixed micelles (62).

3.5.4. Magnetic Resonance Relaxation Rate of Plain SPION and SPION-Micelles

When used as a contrast agent for magnetic resonance imaging (MRI), SPION increases the relaxation rate of water and has the greatest effect on the T2 (spin–spin) relaxation rate. However, this change in the relaxation rate depends on the size of the SPION, degree of aggregation, surface coating thickness, etc. Measure the in vitro relaxation parameters of both plain SPION (i.e., SPION dispersed in HBS, pH 7.4) and SPION-micelle samples with a benchtop 5 mHz RADX NMR Proton Spin Analyzer at room temperature in HBS, pH 7.4, at different SPION concentrations. The in vitro relaxation rate comparison of plain SPION and SPION-micelles is shown in **Fig. 9.6**. PEG-PE-based polymeric micelles prevented the SPION from aggregation and hence the T2 relaxation rate was much greater in the case of SPION-micelles when compared with plain SPION at the same concentration.

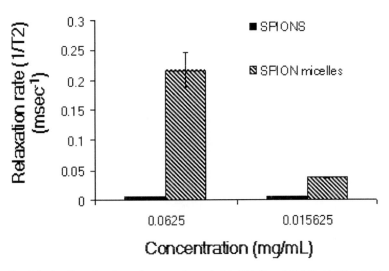

Fig. 9.6. In vitro relaxation rate comparison of plain SPION and SPION-micelles at different concentrations of SPION.

3.5.5. Specific Activity of Micelle-Attached mAb 2C5

1. To the microplate add 50 μL/well of a 40 μg/mL PLL solution in TBS and incubate overnight at 4°C.
2. Discard the PLL solution and to each well add 200 μL of TBST-Cas for 1 h at room temperature (to prevent non-specific binding).
3. Discard TBST-Cas and wash the wells three times with 200 μL of TBST.
4. To each well add 50 μL of a 40 μg/mL nucleosome solution in TBST-Cas for 1 h at room temperature.
5. Discard the nucleosome solution and wash the wells three times with 200 μL of TBST.
6. Incubate the wells with different concentrations of native mAb 2C5 and mAb 2C5 modified micelles for 1 h at room temperature.
7. Discard the samples and wash the wells three times with 200 μL of TBST.

8. Incubate with 50 µL/well of a 1:5,000 dilution of goat anti-mouse IgG peroxidase conjugate in TBST-Cas for 1 h at room temperature.

9. Discard the goat anti-mouse IgG peroxidase and wash the wells three times with 200 µL of TBST.

10. Incubate with 100 µL of enhanced Kblue® TMB peroxidase substrate for 15 min.

11. Read the microplate at a dual wavelength of 620 nm with the reference filter at 492 nm using a Labsystems Multiscan MCC/340 microplate reader installed with GENESIS-LITE windows-based microplate software.

A result for the ELISA of immunomicelles is shown in **Fig. 9.7**.

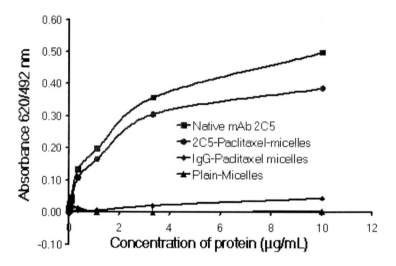

Fig. 9.7. Immunoreactivity of 2C5-PEG-PE micelles by ELISA.

3.5.6. Cytotoxicity Assay

Estimate the in vitro cytotoxicity of drug-loaded micelles using the 3-(4,5-dimethylthiazol-2yl)-2,5-diphenyl-tetrazolium bromide (MTT) method.

1. Plate the cells at 5×10^3 per well in 96-well plate in DMEM and incubate for 24 h at 37°C, 5% CO_2.

2. Replace the medium with media containing free drug dissolved in DMSO or drug-loaded micelles or mAb 2C5-immunomicelles for 72 h. In a typical case, a paclitaxel solution with concentration of 40 ng/mL or a dispersion of micelle or immunomicelles containing paclitaxel at equal concentration.

3. Wash each well thrice with DMEM.

4. Add 100 μL of DMEM to each well followed by 20 μL of Cell Titer 96® A$_{queous}$ One solution and incubate for 3 h at 37°C, 5% CO_2.

5. Measure the absorbance of the degraded MTT at 492 nm using an ELISA reader until the signal intensity of control untreated cells reached a value of 0.7–1 units of absorbance (typically 3 h in our case).

The result of the cytotoxicity test is shown in **Fig. 9.8**. The immunomicelles were significantly more toxic than both controls.

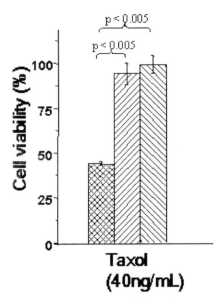

Fig. 9.8. In vitro cytotoxicity of taxol and micellar taxol with MCF7 mammary adenocarcinoma cells.

4. Notes

1. We have prepared and evaluated various mixed micelles in the following ratios. For micelles comprised of PEG-PE and TPGS, 1:1 or 1:2 molar ratio can be used. Also mixed micelles can be prepared with PEG-PE and vitamin E in an 89:11 molar ratio and PEG-PE and ePC in a 1:4 molar ratio.

2. Usually, about 30% of added 2C5 attaches to micelles containing 2 mol% of pNP-PEG-PE. From this yield it can be calculated that up to 10 antibody molecules bind to a single

micelle. Protein binding to micelles without pNP-PEG-PE is negligible. Also antibody attachment yield may be increased by increasing molar fraction of pNP-PEG-PE in micelles. The yield may reach as high as 50% when micelles contain 8 mol% of pNP-PEG-PE. Excessive amounts of pNP-PEG-PE, however, may cause over-modification of a protein molecule leading to its inactivation.

Acknowledgments

This work was in part supported by the NIH grant RO1 EB001961 to Vladimir P. Torchilin.

References

1. Torchilin, V. P. (2001) Structure and design of polymeric surfactant-based drug delivery systems. *J Control Release* **73**, 137–172.
2. Torchilin, V. P. (2007) Micellar nanocarriers: pharmaceutical perspectives. *Pharm Res* **24**, 1–16.
3. Martin, A. (Ed.) (1993) Physical Pharmacy, Lippincott, Williams and Wilkins, Philadelphia.
4. Kwon, G. S. and Okano, T. (1999) Soluble self-assembled block copolymers for drug delivery. *Pharm Res* **16**, 597–600.
5. Lin, S. Y. and Kawashima, Y. (1985) The influence of three poly(oxyethylene)poly(oxypropylene) surface-active block copolymers on the solubility behavior of indomethacin. *Pharm Acta Helv* **60**, 339–344.
6. Lin, S. Y. and Kawashima, Y. (1987) Pluronic surfactants affecting diazepam solubility, compatibility, and adsorption from i.v. admixture solutions. *J Parenter Sci Technol* **41**, 83–87.
7. Kabanov, A. V., Batrakova, E. V., and Alakhov, V. Y. (2002) Pluronic block copolymers as novel polymer therapeutics for drug and gene delivery. *J Control Release* **82**, 189–212.
8. Maeda, H., Wu, J., Sawa, T., Matsumura, Y., and Hori, K. (2000) Tumor vascular permeability and the EPR effect in macromolecular therapeutics: a review. *J Control Release* **65**, 271–284.
9. Yokoyama, M., Miyauchi, M., Yamada, N., Okano, T., Sakurai, Y., Kataoka, K., and Inoue, S. (1990) Characterization and anticancer activity of the micelle-forming polymeric anticancer drug adriamycin-conjugated poly(ethylene glycol)-poly(aspartic acid) block copolymer. *Cancer Res* **50**, 1693–1700.
10. Jones, M. and Leroux, J. (1999) Polymeric micelles – a new generation of colloidal drug carriers. *Eur J Pharm Biopharm* **48**, 101–111.
11. Chung, J. E., Yokoyama, M., Yamato, M., Aoyagi, T., Sakurai, Y., and Okano, T. (1999) Thermo-responsive drug delivery from polymeric micelles constructed using block copolymers of poly(N-isopropylacrylamide) and poly(butylmethacrylate). *J Control Release* **62**, 115–127.
12. Chen, W. -Y., Su, C. -K., Patrickios, C. S., Hertler, W. R., and Hatton, T. A. (1995) Effect of block size and sequence on the micellization of ABC triblock methacrylic acid polyampholytes. *Macromolecules* **28**, 8604–8611.
13. Kawano, K., Watanabe, M., Yamamoto, T., Yokoyama, M., Opanasopit, P., Okano, T., and Maitani, Y. (2006) Enhanced antitumor effect of camptothecin loaded in long-circulating polymeric micelles. *J Control Release* **112**, 329–332.
14. Watanabe, M., Kawano, K., Yokoyama, M., Opanasopit, P., Okano, T., and Maitani, Y. (2006) Preparation of camptothecin-loaded polymeric micelles and evaluation of their incorporation and circulation stability. *Int J Pharm* **308**, 183–189.
15. Kataoka, K., Matsumoto, T., Yokoyama, M., Okano, T., Sakurai, Y., Fukushima, S., Okamoto, K., and Kwon, G. S. (2000) Doxorubicin-loaded poly(ethylene

glycol)-poly(beta-benzyl-L-aspartate) copolymer micelles: their pharmaceutical characteristics and biological significance. *J Control Release* **64**, 143–153.

16. Lavasanifar, A., Samuel, J., and Kwon, G. S. (2002) Poly(ethylene oxide)-block-poly(L-amino acid) micelles for drug delivery. *Adv Drug Deliv Rev* **54**, 169–190.

17. Pierri, E. and Avgoustakis, K. (2005) Poly(lactide)-poly(ethylene glycol) micelles as a carrier for griseofulvin. *J Biomed Mater Res A* **75**, 639–647.

18. Savic, R., Azzam, T., Eisenberg, A., and Maysinger, D. (2006) Assessment of the integrity of poly(caprolactone)-b-poly(ethylene oxide) micelles under biological conditions: a fluorogenic-based approach. *Langmuir* **22**, 3570–3578.

19. Forrest, M. L., Won, C. Y., Malick, A. W., and Kwon, G. S. (2006) In vitro release of the mTOR inhibitor rapamycin from poly(ethylene glycol)-b-poly(epsilon-caprolactone) micelles. *J Control Release* **110**, 370–377.

20. Inoue, T., Chen, G., Nakamae, K., and Hoffman, A. S. (1998) An AB block copolymer of oligo(methyl methacrylate) and poly(acrylic acid) for micellar delivery of hydrophobic drugs. *J Control Release* **51**, 221–229.

21. Yokoyama, M., Kwon, G. S., Okano, T., Sakurai, Y., Seto, T., and Kataoka, K. (1992) Preparation of micelle-forming polymer-drug conjugates. *Bioconjug Chem* **3**, 295–301.

22. Lukyanov, A. N. and Torchilin, V. P. (2004) Micelles from lipid derivatives of water-soluble polymers as delivery systems for poorly soluble drugs. *Adv Drug Deliv Rev* **56**, 1273–1289.

23. Gao, Z., Lukyanov, A. N., Chakilam, A. R., and Torchilin, V. P. (2003) PEG-PE/phosphatidylcholine mixed immunomicelles specifically deliver encapsulated taxol to tumor cells of different origin and promote their efficient killing. *J Drug Target* **11**, 87–92.

24. Lin, W. J., Juang, L. W., and Lin, C. C. (2003) Stability and release performance of a series of pegylated copolymeric micelles. *Pharm Res* **20**, 668–673.

25. Cheon Lee, S., Kim, C., Chan Kwon, I., Chung, H., and Young Jeong, S. (2003) Polymeric micelles of poly(2-ethyl-2-oxazoline)-block-poly(epsilon-caprolactone) copolymer as a carrier for paclitaxel. *J Control Release* **89**, 437–446.

26. Jiang, G. B., Quan, D., Liao, K., and Wang, H. (2006) Novel polymer micelles prepared from chitosan grafted hydrophobic palmitoyl groups for drug delivery. *Mol Pharm* **3**, 152–160.

27. Ambade, A. V., Savariar, E. N., and Thayumanavan, S. (2005) Dendrimeric micelles for controlled drug release and targeted delivery. *Mol Pharm* **2**, 264–272.

28. Prompruk, K., Govender, T., Zhang, S., Xiong, C. D., and Stolnik, S. (2005) Synthesis of a novel PEG-block-poly(aspartic acid-stat-phenylalanine) copolymer shows potential for formation of a micellar drug carrier. *Int J Pharm* **297**, 242–253.

29. Djordjevic, J., Barch, M., and Uhrich, K. E. (2005) Polymeric micelles based on amphiphilic scorpion-like macromolecules: novel carriers for water-insoluble drugs. *Pharm Res* **22**, 24–32.

30. Arimura, H., Ohya, Y., and Ouchi, T. (2005) Formation of core-shell type biodegradable polymeric micelles from amphiphilic poly(aspartic acid)-block-polylactide diblock copolymer. *Biomacromolecules* **6**, 720–725.

31. Venne, A., Li, S., Mandeville, R., Kabanov, A., and Alakhov, V. (1996) Hypersensitizing effect of Pluronic L61 on cytotoxic activity, transport, and subcellular distribution of doxorubicin in multiple drug-resistant cells. *Cancer Res* **56**, 3626–3629.

32. Kabanov, A. V., Chekhonin, V. P., Alakhov, V., Batrakova, E. V., Lebedev, A. S., Melik-Nubarov, N. S., Arzhakov, S. A., Levashov, A. V., Morozov, G. V., Severin, E. S., et al. (1989) The neuroleptic activity of haloperidol increases after its solubilization in surfactant micelles. Micelles as microcontainers for drug targeting. *FEBS Lett* **258**, 343–345.

33. Slepnev, V. I., Kuznetsova, L. E., Gubin, A. N., Batrakova, E. V., Alakhov, V., and Kabanov, A. V. (1992) Micelles of poly(oxyethylene)-poly(oxypropylene) block copolymer (Pluronic) as a tool for low-molecular compound delivery into a cell: phosphorylation of intracellular proteins with micelle incorporated [gamma-32P]ATP. *Biochem Int* **26**, 587–595.

34. Allen, C., Yu, Y., Maysinger, D., and Eisenberg, A. (1998) Polycaprolactone-b-poly(ethylene oxide) block copolymer micelles as a novel drug delivery vehicle for neurotrophic agents FK506 and L-685,818. *Bioconjug Chem* **9**, 564–572.

35. Shin, I. G., Kim, S. Y., Lee, Y. M., Cho, C. S., and Sung, Y. K. (1998) Methoxy poly(ethylene glycol)/epsilon-caprolactone amphiphilic block copolymeric micelle containing indomethacin. I. Preparation and characterization. *J Control Release* **51**, 1–11.

36. Chung, J. E., Yokoyama, M., Aoyagi, T., Sakurai, Y., and Okano, T. (1998) Effect

of molecular architecture of hydrophobically modified poly(N-isopropylacrylamide) on the formation of thermoresponsive core-shell micellar drug carriers. *J Control Release* **53**, 119–130.
37. Jeong, Y. I., Cheon, J. B., Kim, S. H., Nah, J. W., Lee, Y. M., Sung, Y. K., Akaike, T., and Cho, C. S. (1998) Clonazepam release from core-shell type nanoparticles in vitro. *J Control Release* **51**, 169–178.
38. Kwon, G. S., Yokoyama, M., Okano, T., Sakurai, Y., and Kataoka, K. (1993) Biodistribution of micelle-forming polymer-drug conjugates. *Pharm Res* **10**, 970–974.
39. La, S. B., Okano, T., and Kataoka, K. (1996) Preparation and characterization of the micelle-forming polymeric drug indomethacin-incorporated poly(ethylene oxide)-poly(beta-benzyl L-aspartate) block copolymer micelles. *J Pharm Sci* **85**, 85–90.
40. Yokoyama, M., Fukushima, S., Uehara, R., Okamoto, K., Kataoka, K., Sakurai, Y., and Okano, T. (1998) Characterization of physical entrapment and chemical conjugation of adriamycin in polymeric micelles and their design for in vivo delivery to a solid tumor. *J Control Release* **50**, 79–92.
41. Yokoyama, M., Satoh, A., Sakurai, Y., Okano, T., Matsumura, Y., Kakizoe, T., and Kataoka, K. (1998) Incorporation of water-insoluble anticancer drug into polymeric micelles and control of their particle size. *J Control Release* **55**, 219–229.
42. Yu, B. G., Okano, T., Kataoka, K., and Kwon, G. (1998) Polymeric micelles for drug delivery: solubilization and haemolytic activity of amphotericin B. *J Control Release* **53**, 131–136.
43. Katayose, S. and Kataoka, K. (1997) Water-soluble polyion complex associates of DNA and poly(ethylene glycol)-poly(L-lysine) block copolymer. *Bioconjug Chem* **8**, 702–707.
44. Katayose, S. and Kataoka, K. (1998) Remarkable increase in nuclease resistance of plasmid DNA through supramolecular assembly with poly(ethylene glycol)-poly(L-lysine) block copolymer. *J Pharm Sci* **87**, 160–163.
45. Weissig, V., Lizano, C., and Torchilin, V. P. (1998) Micellar delivery system for dequalinium – a lipophilic cationic drug with anticarcinoma activity. *J Liposome Res* **8**, 391–400.
46. Weissig, V., Whiteman, K. R., and Torchilin, V. P. (1998) Accumulation of protein-loaded long-circulating micelles and liposomes in subcutaneous Lewis lung carcinoma in mice. *Pharm Res* **15**, 1552–1556.
47. Li, M., Chrastina, A., Levchenko, T., and Torchilin, V. P. (2005) Micelles from poly(ethylene glycol)-phosphatidyl ethanolamine conjugates (PEG–PE) as pharmaceutical nanocarriers for poorly soluble drug camptothecin. *J Biomed Nanotechnol* **1**, 190–195.
48. Gao, Z., Lukyanov, A. N., Singhal, A., and Torchilin, V. P. (2002) Diacyl polymer micelles as nanocarriers for poorly soluble anticancer drugs. *Nano Letters* **2**, 979–982.
49. Wang, J., Mongayt, D. A., Lukyanov, A. N., Levchenko, T. S., and Torchilin, V. P. (2004) Preparation and in vitro synergistic anticancer effect of vitamin K3 and 1,8-diazabicyclo[5,4,0]undec-7-ene in poly(ethylene glycol)-diacyllipid micelles. *Int J Pharm* **272**, 129–135.
50. Ramaswamy, M., Zhang, X., Burt, H. M., and Wasan, K. M. (1997) Human plasma distribution of free paclitaxel and paclitaxel associated with diblock copolymers. *J Pharm Sci* **86**, 460–464.
51. Hagan, S. A., Coombes, A. G. A., Garnett, M. C., Dunn, S. C., Davies, M. C., Illum, L. L., and Davis, S. S. (1996) Polylactide-poly-(ethylene glycol) copolymers as drug delivery systems, 1. Characterization of water dispersible micelle-forming systems. *Langmuir* **12**, 2153–2161.
52. Benahmed, A., Ranger, M., and Leroux, J. C. (2001) Novel polymeric micelles based on the amphiphilic diblock copolymer poly(N-vinyl-2-pyrrolidone)-block-poly(D,L-lactide). *Pharm Res* **18**, 323–328.
53. Dufresne, M. H., Garrec, D. L., Sant, V., Leroux, J. C., and Ranger, M. (2004) Preparation and characterization of water-soluble pH-sensitive nanocarriers for drug delivery. *Int J Pharm* **277**, 81–90.
54. Lee, E. S., Na, K., and Bae, Y. H. (2003) Polymeric micelle for tumor pH and folate-mediated targeting. *J Control Release* **91**, 103–113.
55. Weiping, S., Changqing, Y., Yanjing, C., Zhiguo, Z., and Xiangzheng, K. (2006) Self-assembly of an amphiphilic derivative of chitosan and micellar solubilization of puerarin. *Colloids Surf B Biointerfaces* **48**, 13–16.
56. Lukyanov, A. N., Gao, Z., Mazzola, L., and Torchilin, V. P. (2002) Polyethylene glycol-diacyllipid micelles demonstrate increased accumulation in subcutaneous tumors in mice. *Pharm Res* **19**, 1424–1429.
57. Hobbs, S. K., Monsky, W. L., Yuan, F., Roberts, W. G., Griffith, L., Torchilin, V. P., and Jain, R. K. (1998) Regulation of transport pathways in tumor vessels: role of tumor type and microenvironment. *Proc Natl Acad Sci USA* **95**, 4607–4612.

58. Parr, M. J., Masin, D., Cullis, P. R., and Bally, M. B. (1997) Accumulation of liposomal lipid and encapsulated doxorubicin in murine Lewis lung carcinoma: the lack of beneficial effects by coating liposomes with poly(ethylene glycol). *J Pharmacol Exp Ther* **280**, 1319–1327.

59. Torchilin, V. P., Lukyanov, A. N., Gao, Z., and Papahadjopoulos-Sternberg, B. (2003) Immunomicelles: targeted pharmaceutical carriers for poorly soluble drugs. *Proc Natl Acad Sci USA* **100**, 6039–6044.

60. Lukyanov, A. N., Hartner, W. C., and Torchilin, V. P. (2004) Increased accumulation of PEG–PE micelles in the area of experimental myocardial infarction in rabbits. *J Control Release* **94**, 187–193.

61. Li, L. and Tan, Y. B. (2008) Preparation and properties of mixed micelles made of Pluronic polymer and PEG–PE. *J Colloid Interface Sci* **317**, 326–331.

62. Dabholkar, R. D., Sawant, R. M., Mongayt, D. A., Devarajan, P. V., and Torchilin, V. P. (2006) Polyethylene glycol-phosphatidylethanolamine conjugate (PEG–PE)-based mixed micelles: some properties, loading with paclitaxel, and modulation of P-glycoprotein-mediated efflux. *Int J Pharm* **315**, 148–157.

63. Sawant, R. R., Sawant, R. M., and Torchilin, V. P. (2008) Mixed PEG–PE/vitamin E tumor-targeted immunomicelles as carriers for poorly soluble anti-cancer drugs: improved drug solubilization and enhanced in vitro cytotoxicity. *Eur J Pharm Biopharm* **70**, 51–57.

64. Skidan, I., Dholakia, P., and Torchilin, V. (2008) Photodynamic therapy of experimental B-16 melanoma in mice with tumor-targeted 5,10,15,20-tetraphenylporphin-loaded PEG–PE micelles. *J Drug Target* **16**, 486–493.

65. Roby, A., Erdogan, S., and Torchilin, V. P. (2006) Solubilization of poorly soluble PDT agent, meso-tetraphenylporphin, in plain or immunotargeted PEG–PE micelles results in dramatically improved cancer cell killing in vitro. *Eur J Pharm Biopharm* **62**, 235–240.

66. Torchilin, V. P., Levchenko, T. S., Lukyanov, A. N., Khaw, B. A., Klibanov, A. L., Rammohan, R., Samokhin, G. P., and Whiteman, K. R. (2001) p-Nitrophenylcarbonyl-PEG–PE-liposomes: fast and simple attachment of specific ligands, including monoclonal antibodies, to distal ends of PEG chains via p-nitrophenylcarbonyl groups. *Biochim Biophys Acta* **1511**, 397–411.

67. Lukyanov, A. N., Gao, Z., and Torchilin, V. P. (2003) Micelles from polyethylene glycol/phosphatidylethanolamine conjugates for tumor drug delivery. *J Control Release* **91**, 97–102.

68. Hyeon, T., Lee, S. S., Park, J., Chung, Y., and Na, H. B. (2001) Synthesis of highly crystalline and monodisperse maghemite nanocrystallites without a size-selection process. *J Am Chem Soc* **123**, 12798–12801.

Chapter 10

Fluorescent Silica Nanoparticles for Cancer Imaging

Swadeshmukul Santra

Abstract

In recent years, fluorescent silica nanoparticles (FSNPs) received immense interest in cancer imaging. FSNPs are a new class of engineered optical probes consisting of silica NPs loaded with fluorescent dye molecules. These probes exhibit some attractive features, such as photostability and brightness, which allow sensitive imaging of cancer cells. In general, FSNPs are chemically synthesized in solution using appropriate silane-based precursors. Fluorescent dye molecules are entrapped during the synthesis process. The synthetic process involves hydrolysis and condensation reactions of silane precursors. Stöber's sol–gel and water-in-oil (W/O) microemulsion methods are two popular chemical methods that have been used for synthesizing FSNPs. Silica matrix is capable of carrying hundreds of fluorescent dye molecules in each FSNP, resulting in bright fluorescence. In FSNPs, fluorescent molecules are somewhat protected by the surrounding silica layer, resulting in good photostability. For cancer cell imaging, surface modification of FSNPs is often necessary to obtain appropriate surface functional groups to improve NP aqueous dispersibility as well as bioconjugation capability. Using conventional bioconjugate chemistry, cancer cell-specific biomolecules are then attached to the surface-modified FSNPs. For targeting cancer cells, the FSNPs are often conjugated to specific biomolecules such as antibodies, aptamers, and folic acid. In this chapter, different approaches for the FSNP design will be discussed and some representative protocols for FSNP synthesis will be provided. We will also discuss FSNP surface modification and bioconjugation techniques that are useful for cancer cell imaging.

Key words: Fluorescent silica nanoparticles, silica nanoparticle, surface modification, bioconjugation, cancer imaging, Stöber synthesis, water-in-oil microemulsion.

1. Introduction

In the past several years, FSNPs have received strong interest in various cancer imaging applications (1–10). The FSNPs offer several features that are either absent in pure fluorescent molecules or very competitive to existing polymeric fluorescent NPs (11–13) and fluorescent semiconductor quantum dots (14–22). These features of FSNPs are described as follows. First, the silica matrix is capable of hosting fluorescent agents of various kinds such as organic and metallorganic fluorescent dyes. It has been demonstrated that FSNPs of different fluorescent colors can be chemically synthesized by incorporating dyes of different emission wavelengths (23, 24). Second, silica is an optically transparent matrix that allows excitation and emission of light to pass through, allowing FSNP fluorescence detection. Third, the fluorescence excitation and emission characteristics of the incorporated dyes within FSNPs do not usually alter. This is because of the inert nature of the silica matrix. Fourth, each FSNP, depending on their size, can carry hundreds of fluorescent molecules. This capability of FSNPs drastically improves the sensitivity of target detection. If a target is tagged to a single FSNP, as opposed to a single fluorescent dye, the signal-to-noise ratio is expected to become very large. Fifth, FSNP is water dispersible. This is because of co-existence of hydrophilic surface silanol (–Si–OH) and deprotonated silanol (–Si–O$^-$) groups at neutral pH. Sixth, FSNPs are quite photostable (10, 25). There is an increase in the photostability of fluorescent dyes as they remain protected by the surrounding silica layer. It is expected that such protection will prevent diffusion of oxygen molecules (dissolved oxygen which generates reactive oxygen species) from the surrounding aqueous environment. As a result of this protection, photochemical oxidation of fluorescent dyes by the reactive oxygen species (which leads to non-fluorescent species) is expected to be minimal. Seventh, the silica matrix is quite stable, i.e., resistant to pH, temperature, swelling, and microbial attack. Eighth, FSNP surfaces could be post-coated with appropriate silane reagents to obtain suitable functional groups for bioconjugation purposes. Ninth, silica is considered as a biocompatible material (26, 27). Lastly, FSNPs are easy to synthesize from alkoxysilane reagents that are readily available.

2. Materials

2.1. Fluorescent Silica Nanoparticle Synthesis

All the chemicals for the FSNP synthesis (as described under **Section 3**) were reagent grade and they were used as received.

1. Tris(2,2′-bipyridyl)dichlororuthenium(II) hexahydrate (RuBpy) (Sigma-Aldrich, USA)
2. Fluorescein isothiocyanate (FITC) (Acros Organics, USA)
3. Tetraethyl orthosilicate (TEOS) (Fluka, USA)
4. 3-Aminopropyltriethoxysilane (APTS) (Sigma-Aldrich, USA)

5. 3-Trihydroxysilylpropyl methylphosphonate (THPMP) (Gelest, Inc., Morrisville, USA)
6. Cyanogen bromide (CNBr) (Alfa Aesar, USA)
7. Triton X-100 (TX-100) (Sigma-Aldrich, USA)
8. Dioctyl sulfosuccinate (Aerosol OT or AOT) (Acros Organics, USA)
9. *n*-Hexanol (Acros Organics, USA)
10. *n*-Heptane (Fisher Scientific, USA)
11. Cyclohexane (Fisher Scientific, USA)
12. Ammonium hydroxide (NH_4OH, 28–30 wt%) and hydrochloric acid were purchased (Sigma-Aldrich, USA)
13. Tetramethylrhodamine (TMR)-dextran (MW 3000) (Invitrogen, USA).
14. Distilled, deionized water (EASYpure LF, Barnstead) was used in the preparation of all aqueous solutions.

3. Methods

A general strategy of FSNP synthesis involves incorporation of fluorescent (organic or metallorganic) dye molecules inside silica matrix (10, 25, 28–33). There are two synthesis routes reported in the literature for making FSNPs: Stöbers' sol–gel method and reverse microemulsion or water-in-oil (W/O) microemulsion method.

In a typical Stöbers' method, alkoxysilane compounds (e.g., tetraethyl orthosilicate (TEOS), tetramethyl orthosilicate (TMOS), a variety of TEOS or TMOS derivatives) are allowed to undergo base-catalyzed hydrolysis and condensation reactions in an ammonia–ethanol–water mixture containing appropriate fluorescent dyes or fluorescent dye-conjugated silane precursor. This method has the capability to produce moderately monodispersed FSNPs in the size ranging from a few tens of nanometers to several hundreds of nanometers (25, 34).

The W/O microemulsion (**Fig. 10.1**) is an isotropic, single-phase system consisting of surfactant, oil (bulk phase), and water (as droplets). In this system, water droplets are coated with surfactant molecules and they are stabilized in the oil phase. These water droplets act as a nano-reactor template for the synthesis of FSNPs. This W/O microemulsion method is capable of producing highly monodispersed FSNPs because of the confined environment of the nano-reactor. Similar to Stöbers' synthesis, alkoxysilanes are allowed to hydrolyze and condense in the presence of fluorescent

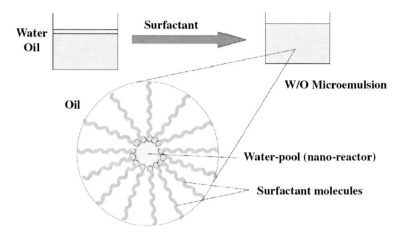

Fig. 10.1. Schematic representation of a W/O microemulsion system.

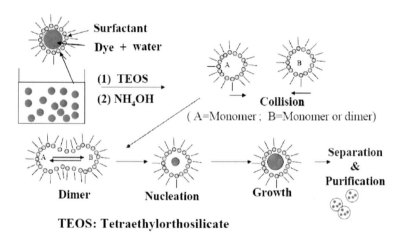

Fig. 10.2. Schematic representation of nucleation and growth processes of FSNPs in W/O microemulsion.

dyes or dye-conjugated silane precursors for producing FSNPs in a controlled manner. **Figure 10.2** shows a schematic representation of the nucleation and growth processes of FSNPs.

In a typical FSNP design, fluorescent dyes are incorporated within the amorphous silica matrix. Due to the hydrophilic and porous nature of the silica, it is challenging to incorporate hydrophobic dye molecules within the silica matrix. An attempt to incorporate hydrophilic dye molecules during the FSNP synthesis procedure results in leakage of dye molecules to the surrounding media over time. Therefore, appropriate design of FSNPs is very important. Several approaches have been undertaken to incorporate fluorescent molecules within the FSNPs as mentioned below.

Electrostatic incorporation of metallorganic fluorescent dyes within silica NPs. In this approach, positively charged metallorganic fluorescent dyes are trapped within the negatively charged silica NP matrix via electrostatic forces of attraction. Silica NPs synthesized via base catalysis are monodispersed (i.e., uniform in size) and porous. The NP surface (as well as NP pores) are highly hydrophilic because of the presence of a large number of silanol groups. At neutral pH, the majority of these silanol groups remain deprotonated. As a result, zeta potential value (which measures NP surface charge) is negative, typically ranging from –40 to –60 mV. Because of this negative surface property, silica can capture positively charged metal ions containing fluorescent dyes such as Tris(2,2′-bipyridyl)osmium(II)bis(hexafluorophosphate) (23) and RuBpy (10, 23) during the formation of FSNPs.

Water-soluble polymer-assisted incorporation of organic fluorescent dyes within silica NPs. In this approach, fluorescently tagged polymers are entrapped within the silica NP matrix during the NP synthesis. This approach takes advantage of the high quantum efficiency of organic fluorescent dyes for sensitive bioimaging and bioanalysis applications. It is, however, very challenging to incorporate hydrophobic organic fluorophores within hydrophilic silica NPs. Zhao and coworkers (35) demonstrated an approach where the TMR (an organic fluorescent dye) covalently linked to low molecular weight (MW = 3000), water-soluble dextran polymers was trapped inside the silica NP matrix.

Incorporation of organic fluorescent dyes within organically modified silica NPs. In this approach, organically modified hybrid silica NPs with hydrophobic cores are used to trap hydrophobic fluorescent dyes via hydrophobic–hydrophobic interactions. Tapec and coworkers (36) synthesized rhodamine 6G (R6G, a hydrophobic dye) dye-loaded FSNPs using this approach where the hybrid silica NPs were synthesized using two silane reagents, TEOS (a hydrophilic silane) and phenyl-triethoxysilane (PTES, a hydrophobic silane). As expected, R6G loading efficiency was directly proportional to the PTES amount.

Incorporation of organic fluorescent dyes into silica NPs via covalent binding. In this approach a fluorescent molecule is first covalently attached to an appropriate silane reagent to obtain fluorescently tagged silane (FTS). The FTS is then reacted with another silane reagent during the silica NP synthesis process. Santra and coworkers (9) synthesized FITC-loaded silica NPs using this approach. In a typical procedure, amine-reactive FITC was reacted with APTS forming a stable fluorescent conjugate, FITC–APTS. The FITC–APTS conjugate, TEOS, and a water-dispersible silane reagent, THPMP, were hydrolyzed and condensed in the presence of NH_4OH in ethanol to produce FITC-loaded FSNPs (9).

For imaging cancer cells, it is desirable to modify FSNP surfaces for attaching cancer-specific targeting molecules (e.g., antibodies, peptides, folic acids). The FSNP surface modification involves the following steps. First, the FSNP surface is modified to obtain appropriate functional groups such as amines, carboxyls, thiols. Second, using suitable coupling reagents, FSNPs are attached to the cancer-specific targeting molecules. A few general bioconjugation techniques are briefly discussed below. Some of these techniques could potentially be used for attaching cancer cell-specific targeting molecules including antibodies, aptamers, and vitamin folates.

3.1. Ternary W/O Microemulsion Synthesis of 30 nm Size RuBpy-Loaded FSNPs (34)

1. A ternary (surfactant/oil/water) W/O microemulsion is prepared first by dissolving 0.1 M AOT in 10 mL of heptane, followed by addition of 90 μL of aqueous solution of 0.1 M RuBpy dye, 100 μL of TEOS, and 60 μL of NH_4OH (29.6 wt%) (*see* **Note 1**).

2. The reaction is allowed to continue for 24 h. The FSNPs are isolated by destabilizing the W/O microemulsion system using either acetone or ethanol, followed by centrifuging and washing with ethanol and water several times to remove any surfactant molecules.

3.2. Quaternary W/O Microemulsion Synthesis of 50 nm Size RuBpy-Loaded FSNPs (10)

1. A quaternary (surfactant/co-surfactant/oil/water) W/O microemulsion is prepared first by mixing 1.77 mL of TX-100, 7.7 mL of cyclohexane, 1.6 mL of *n*-hexanol, and 400 μL of water.

2. Aqueous solution of RuBpy (80 μL, 0.1 M) is then added followed by the addition of 100 μL of TEOS. The hydrolysis and condensation reactions are then initiated by adding 100 μL of aqueous NH_4OH (25–28 wt%). The FSNPs are purified following the above procedure (**Fig. 10.3**).

3.3. W/O Microemulsion Synthesis of 60 nm Size TMR–Dextran-Loaded FSNPs (35)

1. A quaternary W/O microemulsion is prepared by mixing 1.77 mL TX-100, 7.5 mL of cyclohexane, 1.8 mL on *n*-hexanol, and 0.48 mL of 1.0 mM aqueous TMR–dextran solution in hydrochloric acid (pH 1.5–2.0).

2. The TEOS of 100 μL is then added followed by stirring for 30 min (*see* **Note 2**). The hydrolysis and condensation reactions are initiated by adding 60 μL of NH_4OH (29.6 wt%). The FSNPs are purified following the above procedure.

3.4. Stöbers' Synthesis of ~135 nm Size FSNPs in Ethanol–Water Mixture (9)

1. The APTS–FITC conjugate (a fluorescently labeled silane precursor) is first prepared by combining 69 mg APTS and 5.25 mg FITC together in 1.0 mL of absolute ethanol under dry nitrogen atmosphere, and the mixture was stirred magnetically for 12 h (*see* **Note 3**).

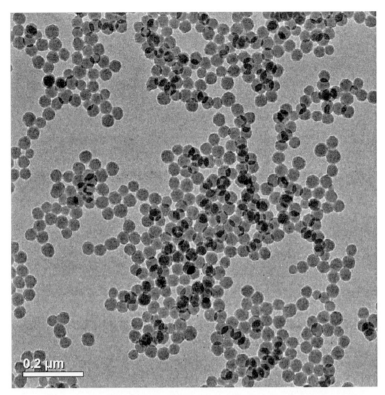

Fig. 10.3. A typical TEM image of RuBpy-loaded highly monodispersed FSNPs synthesized using a W/O microemulsion method. The ternary W/O microemulsion system consisted of cyclohexane (oil), TX-100 (surfactant), n-hexanol (co-surfactant), and water. Average particle size was calculated to be ~50 nm.

2. The FITC-loaded FSNPs are synthesized by the Stöber method. Typically, 800 µL of NH_4OH is combined with 10 mL of absolute ethanol in a 20-mL round-bottom flask with magnetic stirring.

3. After 5 min, 400 µL of TEOS and 200 µL of the FITC–APTS conjugate are added, followed by the addition of 60 µL of THPMP. Magnetic stirring is continued for 24 h. The FSNPs were purified by washing several times with ethanol–water mixture.

3.5. Surface Bioconjugation Strategies of FSNPs Using Carbodiimide Coupling Chemistry

1. This is one of the most common bioconjugation techniques to immobilize biomolecules such as proteins, peptides, and antibodies on the surface of FSNPs. The FSNPs could be surface modified with either carboxyl groups (–COOH) or primary amines (–NH_2).

2. Carboxylated FSNPs are prepared by chemically treating the surface of the FSNPs with a carboxylated silane reagent. Amine-containing biomolecules are then covalently attached

to the carboxyl functionalized FSNP using traditional carbodiimide coupling chemistry (37).

3. Aminated FSNPs are obtained via surface modification with an amine-containing silane reagent (e.g., APTS). Again, using traditional carbodiimide coupling chemistry aminated FSNPs are attached to carboxylated biomolecules (e.g., antibodies) or carboxyl group containing small molecules (e.g., folic acid).

3.6. Surface Bioconjugation Strategies of FSNPs Using Cyanogen Bromide Coupling Chemistry

1. Using this technique, FSNPs with natural surface silanol groups (Si–OH) are activated by the cyanogen bromide reagent, forming a reactive –OCN derivative of FSNPs.

2. The surface-reactive FSNPs are then reacted with the amine groups of protein molecules, forming a stable conjugate. Using this bioconjugate chemistry, FSNPs are attached to the cancer cell-specific antibodies (10).

3.7. Bioconjugation via Disulfide Bonding

1. The FSNP surface is modified with mercapto silane reagent to obtain sulfhydryl-modified FSNPs. These FSNPs then could be conjugated to disulfide-linked oligonucleotides via disulfide bond formation (36). Following this method, DNA aptamers could be easily attached to FSNPs.

3.8. Bioconjugation with Avidin–Biotin Binding

1. Avidin is a protein molecule that contains four specific binding pockets for biotin molecules. There exists a strong binding affinity between avidin and biotin molecules, which is comparable to covalent binding. Avidin-coated FSNPs could be attached to biotinylated biomolecules such as antibodies, proteins (38).

3.9. Cancer Imaging with FSNPs Using Antibody-Mediated Specific Targeting

Santra and coworkers reported the application of 60 nm size RuBpy dye-loaded FSNPs for labeling human leukemia cells (10). The surface silanol group of the FSNPs was chemically activated using CNBr coupling chemistry that formed an amine-reactive surface functional group (Si–OCN). The primary amine group of the human leukemia cell-specific CD10 monoclonal antibody was reacted to the activated FSNPs, forming antibody-conjugated FSNPs. Successful labeling of leukemia cells was confirmed via fluorescence microscopy. Control FSNPs without CD10 antibodies did not label leukemia cells. He and coworkers reported (8) antibody-mediated specific recognition of HepG liver cancer cells using FITC-conjugated FSNPs. The FSNPs were synthesized in W/O microemulsion using FITC–APTS conjugates and TEOS silane reagents. These FSNPs were surface immobilized with anti-human liver cancer monoclonal antibody HAb18. The antibody-coated FSNPs were able to efficiently label HepG liver cancer cells.

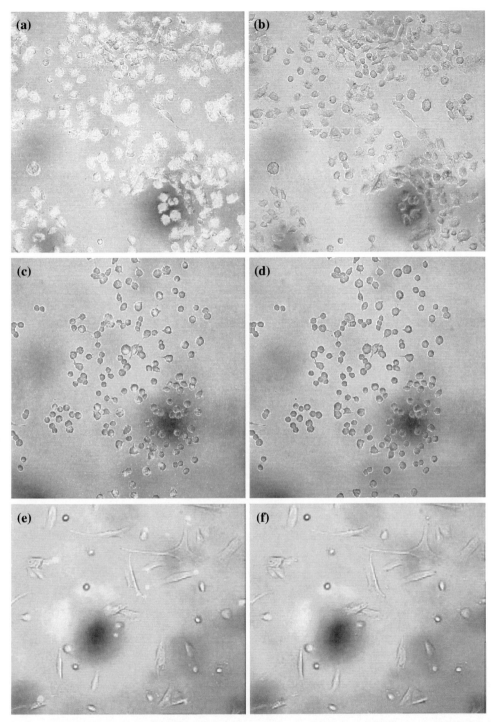

Fig. 10.4. Cell labeling experiments with folate-conjugated, 135-nm-sized, FITC-loaded FSNPs. Laser scanning confocal images of folate–FSNP treated (**a, b**) and amine-modified FSNP (control NP) treated (**c, d**) human lung adenocarcinoma (A-549) cells. These images clearly showed efficient uptake of folate-conjugated FSNPs by the A-549 cells. No significant labeling was observed when folate–FSNPs were treated with human dermal fibroblast cells (images **e** and **f**, control cells). *Right panel* shows transmission image and *left panel* shows transmission plus fluorescence image; scale bar: 100 μm.

3.10. Folic Acid (Folate)-Mediated Specific Targeting of FSNPs

Neoplasms such as breast adenocarcinoma (39), lung adenocarcinoma (40, 41), oral carcinoma (39), and pituitary adenoma (42) overexpress folate receptors because they proliferate rapidly. Folate receptors are, therefore, considered as one of the significant tumor biomarkers for these neoplasms (43). Santra and coworkers successfully labeled A549 (human lung cancer cells) (44, 45) (**Fig. 10.4a** and **b**) using folic acid-conjugated FITC-conjugated FSNPs. Control experiments with amine-functionalized nanoparticles (control FSNPs without folic acid, **Fig. 10.4c** and **d**) and with human dermal fibroblast cells (**Fig. 10.4e** and **f**, control cell line) did not result in effective cell labeling, suggesting that folate-conjugated FSNPs could be used for specific labeling of A549 cells. Similar cell labeling experiments also showed folate receptor overexpression in SCC9 (human oral carcinoma) cells (9) and suitability of using FSNPs for cancer cell labeling.

3.11. Aptamer-Mediated Specific Targeting of FSNPs

Aptamers are a novel class of ligands consisting of short strands of DNA/RNA for sds-specific recognition of a variety of targets including proteins and small molecules (46). Aptamer-based technology offers significant advantages over antibodies and peptides, including high affinity, excellent specificity, and lack of immunogenicity (46). Using aptamer-conjugated FSNPs, CCRF-CEM acute human leukemia cells were successfully targeted and detected using fluorescence microscopy or flow cytometry (1, 2).

4. Notes

1. All the syntheses described in the protocol were carried out at room temperature.
2. The water-to-surfactant molar ratio was kept constant at 10.
3. The FITC–APTS conjugate solution was protected from light during the reaction and storage to prevent photobleaching of FITC.

Acknowledgments

This work has been partly supported by the grants, NSF CBET-63016011, NSF-NIRT EEC-0506560, and NIH 2P01HL059412-11A1. The author acknowledges Professor Weihong Tan and his research group (Department of Chemistry, University of Florida) for their contribution in the area of fluorescent dye-loaded silica nanoparticle technology. The author also acknowledges the kind help of Christine Malgoza for proofreading this manuscript.

References

1. Herr, J. K., Smith, J. E., Medley, C. D., Shangguan, D. H., and Tan, W. H. (2006) Aptamer-conjugated nanoparticles for selective collection and detection of cancer cells. *Anal Chem* **78**, 2918–2924.
2. Smith, J. E., Medley, C. D., Tang, Z. W., Shangguan, D., Lofton, C., and Tan, W. H. (2007) Aptamer-conjugated nanoparticles for the collection and detection of multiple cancer cells. *Anal Chem* **79**, 3075–3082.
3. Trehin, R., Figueiredo, J. L., Pittet, M. J., Weissleder, R., Josephson, L., and Mahmood, U. (2006) Fluorescent nanoparticle uptake for brain tumor visualization. *Neoplasia* **8**, 302–311.
4. Bagwe, R. P., Zhao, X. J., and Tan, W. H. (2003) Bioconjugated luminescent nanoparticles for biological applications. *J Dispers Sci Technol* **24**, 453–464.
5. Santra, S., Xu, J. S., Wang, K. M. and Tan, W. H. (2004) Luminescent nanoparticle probes for bioimaging. *J Nanosci Nanotechnol* **4**, 590–599.
6. Tan, W. H., Wang, K. M., He, X. X., Zhao, X. J., Drake, T., Wang, L., and Bagwe, R. P. (2004) Bionanotechnology based on silica nanoparticles. *Med Res Rev* **24**, 621–638.
7. Yao, G., Wang, L., Wu, Y. R., Smith, J., Xu, J. S., Zhao, W. J., Lee, E. J., and Tan, W. H. (2006) FloDots: luminescent nanoparticles. *Anal Bioanal Chem* **385**, 518–524.
8. He, X. X., Duan, J. H., Wang, K. M., Tan, W. H., Lin, X., and He, C. M. (2004) A novel fluorescent label based on organic dye-doped silica nanoparticles for HepG liver cancer cell recognition. *J Nanosci Nanotechnol* **4**, 585–589.
9. Santra, S., Liesenfeld, B., Dutta, D., Chatel, D., Batich, C. D., Tan, W. H., Moudgil, B. M., and Mericle, R. A. (2005) Folate conjugated fluorescent silica nanoparticles for labeling neoplastic cells. *J Nanosci Nanotechnol* **5**, 899–904.
10. Santra, S., Zhang, P., Wang, K. M., Tapec, R., and Tan, W. H. (2001) Conjugation of biomolecules with luminophore-doped silica nanoparticles for photostable biomarkers. *Anal Chem* **73**, 4988–4993.
11. Brigger, I., Dubernet, C., and Couvreur, P. (2002) Nanoparticles in cancer therapy and diagnosis. *Adv Drug Deliv Rev* **54**, 631–51.
12. Reddy, G. R., Bhojani, M. S., McConville, P., Moody, J., Moffat, B. A., Hall, D. E., Kim, G., Koo, Y. E. L., Woolliscroft, M. J., Sugai, J. V., Johnson, T. D., Philbert, M. A., Kopelman, R., Rehemtulla, A., and Ross, B. D. (2006) Vascular targeted nanoparticles for imaging and treatment of brain tumors. *Clin Cancer Res* **12**, 6677–6686.
13. van Vlerken, L. E. and Amiji, M. M. (2006) Multi-functional polymeric nanoparticles for tumour-targeted drug delivery. *Expert Opin Drug Deliv* **3**, 205–216.
14. Bruchez, M., Moronne, M., Gin, P., Weiss, S., and Alivisatos, A. P. (1998) Semiconductor nanocrystals as fluorescent biological labels. *Science* **281**, 2013–2016.
15. Chan, W. C. W., Maxwell, D. J., Gao, X. H., Bailey, R. E., Han, M. Y., and Nie, S. M. (2002) Luminescent quantum dots for multiplexed biological detection and imaging. *Curr Opin Biotechnol* **13**, 40–46.
16. Gao, X. H., Yang, L. L., Petros, J. A., Marshal, F. F., Simons, J. W., and Nie, S. M. (2005) In vivo molecular and cellular imaging with quantum dots. *Curr Opin Biotechnol* **16**, 63–72.
17. Smith, A. M., Ruan, G., Rhyner, M. N., and Nie, S. M. (2006) Engineering luminescent quantum dots for in vivo molecular and cellular imaging. *Ann Biomed Eng* **34**, 3–14.
18. Wu, X. Y., Liu, H. J., Liu, J. Q., Haley, K. N., Treadway, J. A., Larson, J. P., Ge, N. F., Peale, F., and Bruchez, M. P. (2003) Immunofluorescent labeling of cancer marker Her2 and other cellular targets with semiconductor quantum dots. *Nat Biotechnol* **21**, 41–46.
19. Alivisatos, A. P., Gu, W. W., and Larabell, C. (2005) Quantum dots as cellular probes. *Annu Rev Biomed Eng* **7**, 55–76.
20. Medintz, I. L., Uyeda, H. T., Goldman, E. R., and Mattoussi, H. (2005) Quantum dot bioconjugates for imaging, labelling and sensing. *Nat Mater* **4**, 435–446.
21. Michalet, X., Pinaud, F. F., Bentolila, L. A., Tsay, J. M., Doose, S., Li, J. J., Sundaresan, G., Wu, A. M., Gambhir, S. S., and Weiss, S. (2005) Quantum dots for live cells, in vivo imaging, and diagnostics. *Science* **307**, 538–544.
22. Stroh, M., Zimmer, J. P., Duda, D. G., Levchenko, T. S., Cohen, K. S., Brown, E.

B., Scadden, D. T., Torchilin, V. P., Bawendi, M. G., Fukumura, D., and Jain, R. K. (2005) Quantum dots spectrally distinguish multiple species within the tumor milieu in vivo. *Nat Med* **11,** 678–682.
23. Wang, L., Yang, C. Y., and Tan, W. H. (2005) Dual-luminophore-doped silica nanoparticles for multiplexed signaling. *Nano Lett* **5,** 37–43.
24. Wang, L., Zhao, W., and Tan, W. (2008) Bioconjugated silica nanoparticles: development and applications. *Nano Res* **1,** 99–115.
25. Santra, S., Wang, K. M., Tapec, R., and Tan, W. H. (2001) Development of novel dye-doped silica nanoparticles for biomarker application. *J Biomed Opt* **6,** 160–166.
26. Jin, Y. H., Kannan, S., Wu, M., and Zhao, J. X. J. (2007) Toxicity of luminescent silica nanoparticles to living cells. *Chem Res Toxicol* **20,** 1126–1133.
27. Xue, Z. G., Liang, D. S., Li, Y. M., Long, Z. G., Pan, D. A., Liu, X. H., Wu, L. Q., Zhu, S. H., Cai, F., Dai, H. P., Tang, B. S., Xia, K., and Xia, J. H. (2005) Silica nanoparticle is a possible safe carrier for gene therapy. *Chin Sci Bull* **50,** 2323–2327.
28. Charreyre, M. T., Yekta, A., Winnik, M. A., Delair, T., and Pichot, C. (1995) Fluorescence energy-transfer from fluorescein to tetramethylrhodamine covalently bound to the surface of polystyrene latex-particles. *Langmuir* **11,** 2423–2428.
29. Charreyre, M. T., Zhang, P., Winnik, M. A., Pichot, C., and Graillat, C. (1995) Adsorption of rhodamine-60 onto polystyrene latex-particles with sulfate groups at the surface. *J Colloid Interface Sci* **170,** 374–382.
30. Gao, H. F., Zhao, Y. Q., Fu, S. K., Li, B., and Li, M. Q. (2002) Preparation of a novel polymeric fluorescent nanoparticle. *Colloid Polym Sci* **280,** 653–660.
31. Harma, H., Soukka, T., and Lovgren, T. (2001) Europium nanoparticles and time-resolved fluorescence for ultrasensitive detection of prostate-specific antigen. *Clin Chem* **47,** 561–568.
32. Makarova, O. V., Ostafin, A. E., Miyoshi, H., Norris, J. R., and Meisel, D. (1999) Adsorption and encapsulation of fluorescent probes in nanoparticles. *J Phys Chem B* **103,** 9080–9084.
33. Schlupen, J., Haegel, F. H., Kuhlmann, J., Geisler, H., and Schwuger, M. J. (1999) Sorption hysteresis of pyrene on zeolite. *Colloids Surf A Physicochem Eng Asp* **156,** 335–347.
34. Bagwe, R. P., Yang, C. Y., Hilliard, L. R., and Tan, W. H. (2004) Optimization of dye-doped silica nanoparticles prepared using a reverse microemulsion method. *Langmuir* **20,** 8336–8342.
35. Zhao, X. J., Bagwe, R. P., and Tan, W. H. (2004) Development of organic-dye-doped silica nanoparticles in a reverse microemulsion. *Adv Mater* **16,** 173–176.
36. Tapec, R., Zhao, X. J. J., and Tan, W. H. (2002) Development of organic dye-doped silica nanoparticles for bioanalysis and biosensors. *J Nanosci Nanotechnol* **2,** 405–409.
37. Wang, S. and Low, P. S. (1998) Folate-mediated targeting of antineoplastic drags, imaging agents, and nucleic acids to cancer cells. *J Control Release* **53,** 39–48.
38. Zhao, X. J., Hilliard, L. R., Mechery, S. J., Wang, Y. P., Bagwe, R. P., Jin, S. G., and Tan, W. H. (2004) A rapid bioassay for single bacterial cell quantitation using bioconjugated nanoparticles. *Proc Natl Acad Sci U S A* **101,** 15027–15032.
39. Ross, J. F., Chaudhuri, P. K., and Ratnam, M. (1994) Differential regulation of folate receptor isoforms in normal and malignant-tissues in-vivo and in established cell-lines – physiological and clinical implications. *Cancer* **73,** 2432–2443.
40. Franklin, W. A., Waintrub, M., Edwards, D., Christensen, K., Prendegrast, P., Woods, J., Bunn, P. A., and Kolhouse, J. F. (1994) New anti-lung-cancer antibody cluster-12 reacts with human folate receptors present on adenocarcinoma. *Int J Cancer* 89–95.
41. Lee, J. W., Lu, J. Y., Low, P. S., and Fuchs, P. L. (2002) Synthesis and evaluation of taxol-folic acid conjugates as targeted antineoplastics *Bioorg Med Chem* **10,** 2397–2414.
42. Evans, C. O., Reddy, P., Brat, D. J., O'Neill, E. B., Craige, B., Stevens, V. L., and Oyesiku, N. M. (2003) Differential expression of folate receptor in pituitary adenomas. *Cancer Res* **63,** 4218–4224.
43. Ke, C. Y., Mathias, C. J., and Green, M. A. (2003) The folate receptor as a molecular target for tumor-selective radionuclide delivery. *Nucl Med Biol* **30,** 811–817.
44. Santra, S., Dutta, D., and Moudgil, B. M. (2005) Functional dye-doped silica nanoparticles for bioimaging, diagnostics and therapeutics. *Food Bioprod Process* **83,** 136–140.
45. Santra, S., Yang, H., Dutta, D., Stanley, J. T., Holloway, P. H., Tan, W. H., Moudgil, B. M., and Mericle, R. A. (2004) TAT conjugated, FITC doped silica nanoparticles for bioimaging applications. *Chem Commun* 2810–2811.
46. Ellington, A. D. and Szostak, J. W. (1990) Invitro selection of RNA molecules that bind specific ligands. *Nature* **346,** 818–822.

Chapter 11

Polymeric Nanoparticles for Drug Delivery

Juliana M. Chan, Pedro M. Valencia, Liangfang Zhang, Robert Langer, and Omid C. Farokhzad

Abstract

The use of biodegradable polymeric nanoparticles (NPs) for controlled drug delivery has shown significant therapeutic potential. Concurrently, targeted delivery technologies are becoming increasingly important as a scientific area of investigation. In cancer, targeted polymeric NPs can be used to deliver chemotherapies to tumor cells with greater efficacy and reduced cytotoxicity on peripheral healthy tissues. In this chapter, we describe the methods of (1) preparation and characterization of drug-encapsulated polymeric NPs formulated with biocompatible and biodegradable poly(D,L-lactic-co-glycolic acid)-poly(ethylene glycol) (PLGA-b-PEG) copolymers; (2) surface functionalization of the polymeric NPs with the A10 2′-fluoropyrimidine ribonucleic acid (RNA) aptamers that recognize the prostate-specific membrane antigen (PSMA) on prostate cancer cells; and (3) evaluation of the binding properties of these targeted polymeric NPs to PSMA-expressing prostate cancer cells in vitro and in vivo. These methods may contribute to the development of other useful polymeric NPs to deliver a spectrum of chemotherapeutic, diagnostic, and imaging agents for various applications.

Key words: Polymeric nanoparticles, polymer conjugation chemistry, targeted drug delivery, surface functionalization, aptamers, chemotherapy, microfluidics.

1. Introduction

Biodegradable polymers such as poly(D,L-lactic acid) (PLA), poly(D,L-lactic-co-glycolic acid) (PLGA), and poly(ε-caprolactone) (PCL) and their copolymers diblocked or multiblocked with poly(ethylene glycol) (PEG) have been commonly used to form polymeric nanoparticles (NPs) to encapsulate a variety of therapeutic compounds. These include polymeric micelles, capsules, colloids, dendrimers, etc. One such polymeric NP is Genexol-PM™, a PLGA-*b*-methoxyPEG NP encapsulating paclitaxel, which has received regulatory approval in South Korea for clinical use and is currently undergoing phase II clinical trials for a number of cancer indications in the United States. Polymeric NPs can be formulated by self-assembly of block copolymers consisting of two or more polymer chains with different hydrophobicity. These copolymers spontaneously assemble into a core-shell structure in an aqueous environment to minimize the system's free energy. Specifically, the hydrophobic blocks form the core to minimize their exposure to aqueous surroundings, whereas the hydrophilic blocks form the corona-like shell to stabilize the core through direct contact with water. Drug release rates from the polymeric NPs can be controlled by modifying polymer chemical and physical properties.

In this chapter, we describe the preparation and characterization of prostate cancer-targeted PLGA-*b*-PEG NPs as a model controlled-release drug delivery platform. We functionalized the NPs using the A10 2′-fluoropyrimidine ribonucleic acid (RNA) aptamers as a model targeting moiety, which binds to the prostate-specific membrane antigen (PSMA), a well-known prostate tumor marker, and characterized these targeted polymeric NPs for targeting to human prostate cancer cell lines in vitro and tumors in xenograft mouse models of prostate cancer in vivo.

2. Materials

2.1. PLGA-b-PEG Polymer Conjugation

1. Heterobifunctional PEG (amine-PEG-carboxylate) at molecular weight of 3,400 g/mol (NOF Corporation, Tokyo, Japan) is stored in dark at −20°C.
2. Poly(D,L-lactide-*co*-glycolide) (PLGA) with terminal carboxylate groups (PLGA-carboxylate) is stored at −20°C (Lactel Absorbable Polymers, Cupertino, CA).
3. Conjugation crosslinkers: 1-ethyl-3-(3-dimethylaminopropyl)carbodiimide hydrochloride (EDC) is stored in dark at −20°C; *N*-hydroxysuccinimide (NHS) is stored at 4°C (both from Pierce, Rockford, IL).
4. *N*,*N*-diisopropylethylamine (DIEA) is stored in dark at room temperature.
5. Solvents: dichloromethane (DCM), ethyl ether, acetonitrile, methanol are molecular biology grade (> 99% in purity).
6. Washing solution: anhydrous ethyl ether and methanol (50/50).

2.2. PLGA-b-PEG NP Preparation

1. Solvents: acetonitrile (> 99% in purity), ultrapure water.
2. Docetaxel (> 97% in purity, Fluka).
3. Doxorubicin (> 98% in purity, Sigma).
4. Poly(vinyl alcohol) (PVA) (88% hydrolyzed, ~22 kDa, Fisher).
5. Amicon ultracentrifugation tubes with molecular weight cut-off (MWCO) of 10,000 Da (Millipore).
6. PDMS T-shaped microchannel (20 × 60 μm) mounted on a glass slide. Channels are made using PDMS Sylgard 184 (Dow Corning, Midland, MI).
7. Standard microfluidics equipment: syringe pumps, syringes, plastic tubing, and bright-field microscope for visualization.

2.3. Polymer and NP Characterization

2.3.1. Polymer Characterization

1. Bruker AVANCE 400 nuclear magnetic resonance (NMR, 400 MHz) (Bruker, Billerica, USA). Solvent: CDCl$_3$.
2. Gas permeation chromatography (GPC) (Waters Corporation). Solvent: tetrahydrofuran. Standards: polystyrene.

2.3.2. NP Characterization

1. Brookhaven 90 Plus particle sizer (676 nm laser) and ZetaPALS (Brookhaven Instruments Corporation). Standard-size disposable cuvettes.
2. Transmission electron microscope (TEM). Formvar-carbon-coated grids. Negative stain: 3% uranyl acetate solution stored at 4°C in dark (both from Electron Microscopy Sciences, Hatfield, PA).
3. Slide-A-Lyzer MINI dialysis unit, 10 K MWCO and floats (Pierce, Rockford, IL).
4. Phenomenex Curosil-PFP column (250 × 4.6 mm; 5 μm) (Phenomenex, Torrance, CA).
5. High-performance liquid chromatography (HPLC, Agilent 1100 series, Palo Alto, CA).

2.4. Targeted NP Preparation

1. Targeting aptamer: PSMA A10 2′-fluoropyrimidine RNA aptamer (sequence: 5′-NH$_2$-spacer GGG/AGG/ACG/AUG/CGG/AUC/AGC/CAU/GUU/UAC/GUC/ACU/CCU/U GU/CAA/UCC/UCA/UCG/GCiT-3′ with 2′-fluoropyrimidines, a 5′-amino group attached by a hexaethyleneglycol spacer, and a 3′-inverted T cap) custom synthesized by Integrated DNA Technologies (IDT, Leuven, Belgium). Aptamers are stored as lyophilized powder at −80°C.
2. DNase- and RNase-free water (Invitrogen, Carlsbad, CA).

3. Dimethylsulfoxide (DMSO) (> 99% for molecular biology, Sigma).
4. 10% TBE-urea polyacrylamide gel (Invitrogen).

2.5. Reagents for In Vitro Cell Culture and Immunohistochemistry

1. LNCaP prostate epithelial cell line (Cat #: CRL-1740) cultured in RPMI-1640 medium and PC3 prostate epithelial cell line (Cat #: CRL-1435) cultured in F-12 K medium. All materials are from ATCC (Manassas, VA).
2. Both LNCaP and PC3 culture media are supplemented with 10% fetal bovine serum (FBS) and 1× (100 units/mL penicillin, 100 μg/mL streptomycin) of 100× penicillin–streptomycin (Invitrogen).
3. Opti-MEM I Reduced-Serum Media (Invitrogen).
4. CellBIND 75 cm^2 flask with rectangular, canted neck, vented cap; CellBIND 48-well plates (Corning, Lowell, MA) (*see* **Note 1**).
5. NBD cholesterol (22-(N-(7-nitrobenz-2-oxa-1,3-diazol-4-yl)amino)-23,24-bisnor-5-cholen-3β-ol) (Molecular Probes, Invitrogen).
6. NBD-encapsulated targeted NPs (preparation described in **Section 3.4**) (*see* **Note 2**).
7. Freshly prepared 4% paraformaldehyde in PBS.
8. 0.1% Triton X-100 (Sigma) in PBS buffer.
9. Mouse monoclonal EEA-1 antibodies, mouse monoclonal mannose-6-phosphate receptor antibodies, Cy5 goat anti-mouse antibodies (Abcam, Cambridge, MA).
10. Vectashield mounting medium with DAPI (Vector Laboratories, Burlingame, CA).
11. Glass cover slips (Size: No. 1) (VWR, Batavia, IL).
12. Delta Vision Deconvolution Microscope (Applied Precision, Issaquah, DC).
13. Cell Proliferation Assay kit (ATCC).

2.6. Reagents for In Vivo Experiments

1. Male, 8-week-old, BALB/c nude mice (Charles River Laboratories, Wilmington, MA) (*see* **Note 3**).
2. 3×10^6 LNCaP cells/mouse in 200 μL RPMI-1640 medium with 10% FBS and 1× penicillin–streptomycin.
3. BD Matrigel matrix phenol-red free (BD Biosciences, San Jose, CA) (*see* **Note 4**).
4. 2.5% Avertin. To make 100% Avertin, mix 10 g of 2,2,2-tribromoethanol (99%) with 10 mL of tertiary amyl alcohol (Sigma). To make 2.5% Avertin, add 100% Avertin dropwise with constant stirring into PBS at 37°C (*see* **Note 5**).

5. ^{14}C-paclitaxel (Sigma)-encapsulated targeted NPs (preparation described in **Section 3.4**).
6. Solvable tissue solubilizer (Perkin-Elmer, Waltham, MA).
7. Hionic-Fluor scintillation cocktail (Perkin-Elmer).
8. 0.5 M EDTA, pH 8.0 (Invitrogen).
9. 30% H_2O_2.
10. Packard TriCarb Scintillation Analyser (Downers Grove, IL).

3. Methods

3.1. Synthesis of PLGA-b-PEG Polymer

Two of the most common methods to synthesize PLGA-*b*-PEG diblock copolymers are (i) conjugation of PLGA homopolymer with a carboxylate end group to a heterobifunctional amine-PEG-carboxylate using EDC and NHS as conjugation crosslinkers (1), and (ii) melt or solution copolymerization of lactide and glycolide in the presence of monomethoxy-PEG using stannous octoate as a catalyst (2). Here, we describe polymer conjugation using EDC/NHS chemistry (*see* **Note 6**).

1. Dissolve 250 mg of PLGA-carboxylate (0.005 mmol) in 1–2 mL DCM (*see* **Note 7**).
2. Dissolve NHS (3.0 mg, 0.025 mmol) and EDC (4.8 mg, 0.025 mmol) in 1 mL DCM (*see* **Note 8**).
3. PLGA-carboxylate is converted into PLGA-NHS by adding the EDC/NHS solution to PLGA-carboxylate solution with gentle stirring.
4. PLGA-NHS is precipitated with 20 mL ethyl ether/methanol washing solvent by centrifugation at 2,700×*g* for 10 min to remove residual EDC/NHS.
5. Repeat washing and centrifugation two times (*see* **Note 9**).
6. The PLGA-NHS pellet is dried under vacuum for 30 min to remove residual ether and methanol.
7. After drying under vacuum, PLGA-NHS (200 mg, 0.004 mmol) is dissolved in DCM (4 mL) followed by addition of amine-PEG-carboxylate (20.4 mg, 0.006 mmol) and DIEA (7.5 mg, 0.06 mmol). The mixture solution is incubated for 24 h at room temperature under gentle stirring.
8. Precipitate the resulting PLGA-*b*-PEG block copolymer with ether/methanol washing solvent and centrifuge to remove unreacted PEG.
9. Dry the purified PLGA-*b*-PEG polymer under vacuum (*see* **Note 10**).

3.2. PLGA-b-PEG NP Preparation

There are several methods available to prepare PLGA-b-PEG NPs including the (i) emulsification-solvent evaporation method (this method itself includes single emulsion and double emulsion) (3); (ii) nanoprecipitation (also known as solvent displacement method) (4); and the (iii) salting-out method (5). The choice of method depends on the nature of the drug to be entrapped within the NPs. For the encapsulation of hydrophilic drugs, double emulsion is preferred. For hydrophobic drugs, nanoprecipitation, single emulsion, and salting-out methods can be used. Concomitantly, recent interest exists in the use of microfluidic devices for the formation of polymeric particles because of the fast mixing and homogeneous reaction conditions in the microscale (6). Our group prepared homogeneous NPs through nanoprecipitation using microfluidics devices (7). Here, we describe in detail the preparation of NPs that encapsulate hydrophobic compounds using nanoprecipitation "in bulk" and in microfluidic channels, and the preparation of NPs that encapsulate hydrophilic compounds using double emulsion.

3.2.1. Nanoprecipitation for Encapsulating Hydrophobic Compounds

3.2.1.1. "Bulk" Nanoprecipitation

1. Dissolve PLGA-b-PEG (10 mg/mL) and docetaxel (0.1 mg/mL) in acetonitrile.
2. Add the polymer/drug mixture dropwise to 3–5 volumes of stirring water giving a final polymer concentration of 3.3 mg/mL (*see* **Note 11**).
3. Stir NPs for 2 h, and remove remaining organic solvent in a rotary evaporator at reduced pressure.
4. The NPs are concentrated by centrifugation at $2,700 \times g$ for 15 min using an Amicon filter, washed with deionized water and reconstituted in PBS.

3.2.1.2. Microfluidic-Based Nanoprecipitation

1. Dissolve PLGA-b-PEG (20 mg/mL) and docetaxel (0.2 mg/mL) in acetonitrile (*see* **Fig. 11.1**).
2. Fill one syringe with water and place it in a syringe pump. Fill the other syringe with polymer/drug solution and place it in another syringe pump.
3. Set water and acetonitrile flow rate at 10 μL/min and 1 μL/min, respectively (*see* **Note 12**).
4. NPs are collected at the outlet stream (*see* **Note 13**).
5. NPs are washed and recovered as described in Step 4 of **Section 3.2.1.1**.

3.2.2. Double Emulsion (w/o/w) for Encapsulating Hydrophilic Compounds

1. An aqueous solution of doxorubicin (2.5 mg/mL, 0.4 mL) is emulsified in 2 mL PLGA-b-PEG dissolved in DCM (50 mg/mL) using a probe sonicator (Fisher Scientific) at 20 W for 45 s.

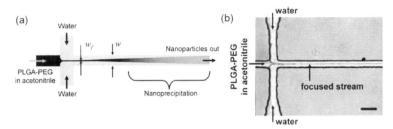

Fig. 11.1. (a) Schematic of synthesis of NPs by nanoprecipitation in microfluidic channels. The polymer stream is focused into a thin stream between two faster flowing water streams, in a process commonly called hydrodynamic flow focusing. In the channel, rapid mixing and solvent displacement occur by the diffusion of the organic solvent out of the focused stream and diffusion of water into the focused stream. (b) Micrograph of T-shaped device in operation. Scale bar = 50 μm. Reproduced with permission from *Nano Lett* 2008, 8, 2906–2912 (8). Copyright 2008 American Chemical Society.

2. Transfer the emulsion to a PVA aqueous solution (0.1% w/v, 50 mL) and sonicate at 20 W for 1 min.

3. Gently stir the w/o/w emulsion formed at room temperature for 2 h.

4. NPs are washed and recovered as described in Step 4 of **Section 3.2.1.1**.

3.3. Characterization of PLGA-b-PEG Polymer and NPs

3.3.1. Characterization of PLGA-b-PEG Block Copolymer

The composition of PLGA-*b*-PEG is characterized using a 400 MHz ^{1}H nuclear magnetic resonance (NMR). Prepare samples by dissolving 5 mg of the PLGA-*b*-PEG diblock copolymer in 1 mL of deuterated chloroform ($CDCl_3$). An example of a PLGA-*b*-PEG NMR spectrum is shown in **Fig. 11.2**. Conjugation of PLGA-PEG is confirmed using GPC. Compare the PLGA-*b*-PEG molecular weight distribution curve and elution time to PLGA and PEG alone. The GPC sample is prepared by dissolving 4–6 mg of diblock copolymer in 1 mL of tetrahydrofuran.

3.3.2. Characterization of PLGA-PEG NPs

The particle size and size distribution are measured by dynamic light scattering at 25°C, scattering angle of 90°C, using a NP concentration of approximately 1 mg/mL (*see* **Note 14**). The NP surface zeta potential is measured by ZetaPALS and is recorded as the average of three measurements. Transition electron microscopy (TEM) is used to confirm the size and structure of the NPs. A solution of NPs in distilled water (0.5–2 mg/mL) is absorbed on grids and negatively stained for 1 min. For each sample, 5–6 grids are prepared and viewed with a JEOL 200 CX TEM equipped with an AMT 2 k CCD camera. Image at 27–41,000× magnification (*see* **Note 15**).

3.3.2.1. NP Drug Release Kinetics

1. Prepare drug-encapsulated NPs at 5–20% wt of the polymer (*see* **Note 2**).

2. Wash away free drug three times using an Amicon filter.

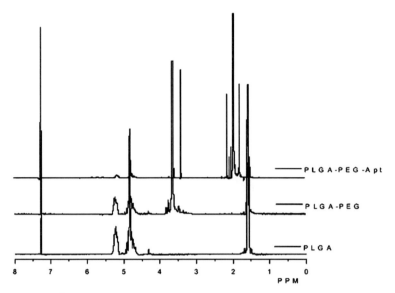

Fig. 11.2. ^{1}HNMR characterization of PLGA-*b*-PEG and PLGA-*b*-PEG-*b*-APT. PLGA: δ 5.2 (m, ((OC$\underline{H}$(CH$_3$)C(O)OCH$_2$ C(O))$_n$)); δ 4.8 (m, ((OCH(CH$_3$)C(O)OC$\underline{H}_2$C(O))$_n$)); δ 1.6 (d, ((OCH(C$\underline{H}_3$)C(O)OCH$_2$C(O))$_n$). PEG: δ 3.7 (s, (C$\underline{H}_2$C$\underline{H}_2$O)$_m$). APT: peaks between δ 1.8 and 2.2 ppm. Reproduced with permission from *Proc Natl Acad Sci USA* 2008, 105, 2586–2591 (2). Copyright 2008 National Academy of Sciences, USA.

3. Resuspend NPs in PBS buffer and split them equally into 30 Slide-A-Lyzer MINI Dialysis units (100 µL of sample per tube).
4. Dialyze these microtubes in 4 L of PBS buffer with gentle stirring at 37°C.
5. Change the PBS buffer every 24 h during the whole dialysis process.
6. Collect samples ($n = 3$) at specific time points, such as at 3, 6 or 12 h intervals.
7. Mix samples with an appropriate volume of organic solvent (as required for the mobile phase in Steps 9 and 10) and vortex overnight to dissolve the NPs.
8. Assay free drug content in each sample by measuring drug absorbance using a UV–Vis detector at the appropriate wavelength and mobile phase, against a standard curve of known drug content.
9. Measure docetaxel absorbance at a wavelength of 227 nm and a retention time of 12 min in 1 mL/min nongradient (50/50) acetonitrile/water mobile phase.
10. Measure doxorubicin absorbance at a wavelength of 490 nm and a retention time of 3 min in 1 mL/min nongradient (40/60) acetonitrile/water mobile phase.

3.4. Synthesis of Targeted NPs

3.4.1. Surface Functionalization of Polymeric NPs

1. Suspend 10 mg/mL PLGA-*b*-PEG NPs prepared as described in **Sections 3.1** and **3.2** in DNase- and RNase-free water, and incubate them with EDC (400 mM) and NHS (200 mM) for 20 min with gentle stirring.
2. Wash NPs three times in DNase- and RNase-free water using an Amicon filter.
3. Aptamers are dissolved in water and denatured for 5 min at 90°C followed by snap-cooling on ice, to allow the aptamers to assume binding conformation.
4. The resulting NHS-activated NPs are then reacted with aptamers (1 mg/mL) for 2 h at room temperature with gentle stirring.
5. Wash NP-Apt conjugates three times using an Amicon filter.
6. Keep the NP suspensions at 4°C until use.

3.4.2. Characterization of Targeted PLGA-b-PEG NPs

To verify the presence of the aptamer in the NPs, incubate PLGA-PEG NPs with (+EDC) and without (−EDC) the crosslinker to confirm covalent conjugation. Wash the targeted NPs and separate by polyacrylamide gel electrophoresis (PAGE) and visualize with ethidium bromide (8).

3.5. In Vitro Cell Culture Experiments

3.5.1. In Situ Hybridization to Visualize Endocytosis on Targeted NPs

1. LNCaP and PC3 cells were grown in 8-well microscope chamber slides at concentrations that allow 70% confluence in 24 h (i.e., LNCaP: 40,000 cells/cm^2).
2. On the day of the experiments, wash cells with pre-warmed PBS and incubate with pre-warmed Opti-MEM I Reduced Serum Media for 30 min at 37°C.
3. Incubate cells with ~50 μg of targeted NPs (with a final dye concentration of 1 μg/mL) for 30 min at 37°C in the Opti-MEM media.
4. Wash cells twice with pre-warmed PBS and fix them with 4% formaldehyde for 20 min.
5. Wash cells three times with PBS and permeabilize the cell membrane in PBS containing 0.1% Triton X-100 and 1% BSA and rinse again twice with PBS.
6. Incubate early endosomal marker (mouse monoclonal EEA-1) and late endosomal marker (mouse monoclonal mannose-6-phosphate receptor) antibodies with cells for 1 h at room temperature.
7. Wash cells twice with PBS.
8. Incubate cells with Cy5 goat anti-mouse antibodies for 1 h at room temperature and wash cells twice with PBS.
9. Mount the microscope chamber slides with Vectashield mounting medium with DAPI and glass coverslips. Observe slides by fluorescence microscopy (*see* **Note 16**).

3.5.2. In Vitro Cytotoxicity Assays with Drug-Encapsulated Targeted NP

1. LNCaP and PC3 cells were grown in CellBIND 48-well plates at concentrations that allow 70% confluence in 24 h (i.e., LNCaP: 40,000 cells/cm^2).
2. On the day of the experiments, wash cells with pre-warmed PBS.
3. Incubate cells with targeted NPs (final drug concentration of 1 μg/mL) for 1 h at 37°C.
4. Wash cells twice with pre-warmed PBS. Incubate in fresh complete media for 72 h at 37°C.
5. Assess cell viability colorimetrically with the MTT reagent following the standard protocol provided by ATCC.

3.6. In Vivo Experiments (see Note 17)

3.6.1. In Vivo Biodistribution Experiments

1. LNCaP cells were cultured as described in **Section 2.5**. They were grown to 90% confluency, counted, and resuspended to give 15 million cells/mL (*see* **Note 18**).
2. Weigh the mice and anesthesize intraperitoneally with 2.5% Avertin (200 mg/kg body weight) (*see* **Note 5**).
3. Resuspend 3×10^6 LNCaP cells in 200 μL media/Matrigel mixture suspensions with a media/Matrigel volume ratio of 1:1. Subcutaneously inject the suspensions into the left flank of each mouse. Between injections, gently invert the vials to mix suspensions for more regular-sized tumors. Allow LNCaP tumors to develop for ~3 weeks (*see* **Note 19**).
4. When tumors are sufficiently large (~250–300 mm^3), prepare NPs for administration. Tumor length and width can be measured by digital calipers using the formula: (width^2 × length)/2. Divide mice randomly into different groups to minimize tumor size variations between groups ($n = 4$–7).
5. Suspend ^{14}C paclitaxel-NP formulations in 200 μL PBS before administration sterile filter.
6. Anesthetize mice with 2.5% Avertin and dose with NPs via tail-vein intravenous injection.
7. After dosing, euthanize different groups at different time points such as ~3, 6, 12, or 24 h. Draw 200 μL of blood by cardiac puncture from each mouse. Harvest the tumor, heart, lungs, liver, spleen, and kidneys from each animal, weigh them, and place them directly in scintillation vials. The liver from each mouse has to be homogenized due to its large size and only ~100 mg of tissue is analyzed.
8. Solubilize each organ in 2 mL Solvable for ~12 h at 60°C. For the blood sample, add only 400 μL Solvable.

9. Add 200 μL of 0.5 M EDTA to each vial to help reduce foaming that occurs upon the addition of H_2O_2.
10. Add 200 μL of 30% H_2O_2 to each vial for 1 h at 60°C to decolorize the sample.
11. Cool samples and add Hionic-Fluor scintillation cocktail to the top of the vial (Perkin-Elmer).
12. The ^{14}C content of tissues were counted using a scintillation counter. To determine the 100% dose, count vials of the formulated NPs with tissue samples. Data are presented as percent injected dose per gram of tissue (% i.d./g).

4. Notes

1. LNCaP cells are an adherent cell line that originated from human prostate carcinomas. They demonstrate slow growth and poor attachment to tissue culture plates. The use of CellBIND plates (Corning) increased cell attachment.
2. Dye-encapsulated NPs are prepared similar to drug-free and drug-encapsulated NPs by mixing the dye or drug with the polymer in the organic phase.
3. Since this was a prostate cancer study, only male mice were used.
4. Phenol-red free media should be used for experiments that require fluorescence microscopy to reduce background auto-fluorescence.
5. When making 2.5% Avertin, dropwise addition with constant stirring at 37°C avoids crystals in the final solution that will cause death in mice via intestinal necrosis. The 2.5% stock solution should be sterile filtered, aliquoted into a series of sterile microcentrifuge tubes, capped tightly, and stored wrapped in foil at 4°C (stable for at least 1 year).
6. The reagent amounts included in this protocol is adequate for in vitro experiments.
7. PLGA viscosity can influence the rate of PLGA-*b*-PEG conjugation. For high-viscosity PLGA, dilute PLGA in DCM to 0.1–0.25 g/mL before adding EDC/NHS.
8. For maximum conjugation efficiency, dissolve EDC/NHS in DCM immediately before adding to PLGA-carboxylate.
9. Supernatant from the washing steps should be clear, especially after the second wash.
10. To achieve a more efficient polymer conjugation, use a high-power vacuum pump to rapidly evaporate residual solvents. The reaction yield should be between 90 and 95%.

11. In order to avoid NP aggregation, the acetonitrile/water volume should be larger than 1:2.

12. The ratio of aqueous stream to organic stream is important. It has been found that as this ratio increases, mixing time decreases as well as particle size (7). As the ratio of water to organic solvent increases, the focused stream becomes thinner and mixing by diffusion occurs faster. A range of 10–30 yields more homogeneous particles and narrower size distributions.

13. The amount of NPs collected at the current flow rates (10 μL/min) is relatively low compared to the "bulk" method. Flow rates can be increased but always maintaining the flow ratio of aqueous to organic stream constant.

14. To maintain NP colloidal stability, always formulate NPs in pure water before reconstituting in PBS or other desired media.

15. For better results, try to use freshly made NPs and avoid waiting longer than 1 h between the time the stain is applied and imaging by TEM.

16. To preserve imaging quality, NPs should be freshly encapsulated with fluorescent dyes and slides should be imaged immediately. Slides can be stored at −20°C in the dark.

17. Animals care and experimental procedures were performed in accordance with the regulations of the Massachusetts Institute of Technology Division of Comparative Medicine and the Principles of Laboratory Animal Care of the National Institutes of Health.

18. To obtain fast-growing tumors, reconstitute LNCaP cells in complete growth medium before mixing with Matrigel.

19. Carefully monitor health status and blood vessel growth around the tumor in the mice. If tumors are too big, the central region would have necrosed and will not be accessible by blood vessels; conversely, smaller tumors would have insufficient neovasculature. Observe for blood vessels around the tumor area.

References

1. Farokhzad, O. C., Cheng, J., Teply, B. A., et al. (2006) Targeted nanoparticle–aptamer bioconjugates for cancer chemotherapy in vivo. *Proc Natl Acad Sci USA* **103**, 6315–6320.
2. Avgoustakis, K. (2004) Pegylated poly(lactide) and poly(lactide-*co*-glycolide) nanoparticles: preparation, properties and possible applications in drug delivery. *Curr Drug Deliv* **1**, 321–333.
3. Gref, R., Domb, A., Quellec, P., et al. (1995) The controlled intravenous delivery of drugs using peg-coated sterically stabilized nanospheres. *Adv Drug Deliver Rev* **16**, 215–233.
4. Fessi, H., Puisieux, F., Devissaguet, J. P., Ammoury, N., and Benita, S. (1989) Nanocapsule formation by interfacial polymer deposition following solvent displacement. *Int J Pharm* **55**, R1–R4.

5. Allemann, E., Gurny, R., and Doelker, E. (1992) Preparation of aqueous polymeric nanodispersions by a reversible salting-out process – influence of process parameters on particle-size. *Int J Pharm* **87**, 247–253.
6. DeMello, J. and DeMello, A. (2004) Microscale reactors: nanoscale products. *Lab Chip* **4**, 11n–15n.
7. Karnik, R., Gu, F., Basto, P., et al. (2008) Microfluidic platform for controlled synthesis of polymeric nanoparticles. *Nano Lett* **8**, 2906–2912.
8. Cheng, J., Teply, B. A., Sherifi, I., et al. (2007) Formulation of functionalized PLGA-PEG nanoparticles for in vivo targeted drug delivery. *Biomaterials* **28**, 869–876.

Chapter 12

Synthesis, Characterization, and Functionalization of Gold Nanoparticles for Cancer Imaging

Gary A. Craig, Peter J. Allen, and Michael D. Mason

Abstract

This chapter describes the methodology by which mAb-F19-conjugated gold nanoparticles were prepared and used to label human pancreatic adenocarcinoma. Specifically, gold nanoparticles were coated with dithiol bearing hetero-bifunctional PEG (polyethylene glycol), and cancer-specific mAb F19 was attached by means of NHS-EDC coupling chemistry taking advantage of a carboxylic acid group on the heterobifunctional PEG. These conjugates were completely stable and were characterized by a variety of methods, including UV–Vis absorbance spectrometry, darkfield microscopy, DLS (dynamic light scattering), TEM (transmission electron microscopy), SEC (size-exclusion chromatography), and confocal microscopy. Nanoparticle bioconjugates were used to label sections of healthy and cancerous human pancreatic tissue. Labeled tissue sections were examined by darkfield microscopy and indicate that these nanoparticle bioconjugates may selectively bind to cancerous tissue and provide a means of optical contrast.

Key words: mAb-F19, pancreatic adenocarcinoma, gold nanoparticle, cancer targeting, heterobifunctional PEG, bioconjugate.

1. Introduction

The optical properties of small metallic particles have led to their use as pigments in paints and glasses for centuries (1). As the physical dimension of these particles is reduced to the nanoscale, their optical and electronic properties deviate dramatically from those of the bulk material. The interaction between light and small particles was first generalized by Gustav Mie over a century ago, but until recently detailed studies leading to practical applications have been severely limited by a general inability to grow and analyze nanoparticles of controlled size and geometry.

Driven largely by the needs of the computer industry to understand the optical and electronic properties of semiconductor materials at decreasing length scales, new solution phase chemistries have been developed providing effective size and geometry control over the growth of nanocrystals (2). These same synthetic strategies have been translated into vastly improved growth mechanisms for metallic particles. As such, metal nanoparticles are once again attracting strong interest in the fundamental sciences and are being widely investigated for their potential use in a range of technological and biological applications. Potential uses include sub-wavelength optical devices (3), solar cells (4), flexible electronics, conducting inks and adhesives (5–7), surface-enhanced spectroscopies (such as Raman) (8), chemical catalysis (9, 10), and for biological labeling and detection (11, 12).

1.1. Visualization of Metallic Nanoparticles

A broad range of instrumental geometries, using visible radiation, has been explored for imaging nanoparticles. Individual nanoparticles can be readily viewed at video rates on substrates, in live cells, or in thin tissue sections using conventional darkfield microscopy (**Fig. 12.1**). Thick or opaque samples, however, mandate the use of reflectance geometries where optical images are generated from either emission (fluorescence) or back-scattering (reflectance). When imaged in a back-scattering geometry metal nanoparticles have several potential advantages over commercial organic molecular and semiconductor quantum dot fluorophores (8, 13). Because photons are being scattered and not absorbed in this arrangement, these nanoprobes do not exhibit power-dependent excitation limitations such as photo-bleaching or intermittency, making it possible to image over extended periods of

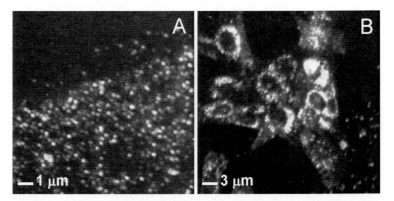

Fig. 12.1. Darkfield transmission images of gold nanoparticles (**a**) dispersed on glass and (**b**) in live cells. Bright circular features indicate the presence of nanoparticles. The gray scale of these features indicates the particle size (color). Here a broad size distribution centered around 20 nm (diameter) was observed.

time improving signal to noise. They can be engineered for peak optical activity at longer wavelengths, allowing for the use of red to near-infrared (NIR) light sources capable of improved optical penetration into biological samples while simultaneously reducing background autofluorescence. When compared to semiconductor materials (Cd, Se), or organic dyes, noble metals are relatively nontoxic making them well suited for in vivo studies (14).

While noble metal nanoparticles show great promise, there are a number of parameters that must be evaluated before they can be used effectively and quantitatively as probes in biological systems. When selecting the desired nanoparticle geometry, one must first carefully consider the final application (i.e., in vivo, ex vivo), the type of signal to be collected (i.e., mono- or polychromatic), and the instrumental geometry to be employed (reflection or transmission). Understanding these constraints allows for appropriate selection of nanoparticle geometry based on predicted photophysical properties.

The total extinction coefficient (σ_{ext}), the extent to which light is attenuated when a particle is placed in its path, is a sum of the absorption and scattering cross-sections, $\sigma_{ext} = \sigma_{abs} + \sigma_{sca}$. For spherical particles with radius smaller than the incident light wavelength ($R < \lambda/10$), the so-called Rayleigh criterion yields the following:

$$\sigma_{abs} = \frac{8\pi^2}{\lambda} R^3 \, Im\left[\frac{\varepsilon_p - \varepsilon_m}{\varepsilon_p - 2\varepsilon_m}\right]^2 \qquad [1]$$

$$\sigma_{sca} = \frac{128\pi^5}{\lambda^4} R^6 \left[\frac{\varepsilon_p - \varepsilon_m}{\varepsilon_p - 2\varepsilon_m}\right]^2 \qquad [2]$$

where ε_p and ε_m are the complex dielectric constants of the particle and the surrounding medium, respectively. The term in brackets is referred to as the polarizability (often denoted as $\alpha(\lambda)$), is itself wavelength dependent, and is a measure of the ability of the incident light to polarize electrons within the particle. The fact that scales as R^6, while σ_{abs} scales as R^3 implies that for very small gold particles ($R < 10$ nm) absorption is the dominant optical process. For gold nanoparticle sizes around 50 nm, equations [1] and [2] suggest that for visible wavelengths absorption and scattering are of the same approximate magnitude, and for larger particles scattering begins to dominate. For metal nanoparticles an additional process, arising from the interaction of the electric field of the incident light and conduction electrons in the metal surface, gives rise to a resonance condition which occurs when $\varepsilon_p \approx -2\varepsilon_m$. This process yields a peak in both the scattering and absorption spectra at a nanoparticle size and

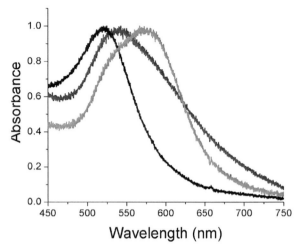

Fig. 12.2. Extinction spectra (absorption plus scattering) for a series of spherical gold nanoparticles with increasing mean diameters.

material-dependent resonance wavelength (plasmon resonance) as shown in **Fig. 12.2** (15). In general terms, the strong wavelength dependence of equation [2] suggests that smaller nanoparticles preferentially scatter shorter wavelengths, and larger nanoparticles scatter longer wavelengths, which is proven out in experiments as demonstrated in **Figs. 12.1–12.3**.

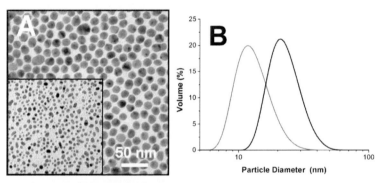

Fig. 12.3. (**a**) TEM images of Au spherical cores. (**b**) DLS size distributions for two nanoparticle preparations similar to those in (**a**).

Generally, for biological labeling schemes, larger nanoprobes increase the risk of biological sample perturbation or may show limited circulation or mobility. Unfortunately, as nanoparticle sizes decrease, the optical cross-section (σ_{ext}) also decreases dramatically. For free particles in solution, this effect scales approximately with the nanoparticle volume, and for the smallest nanoprobes results in dramatically reduced signal to noise. As such, spherical nanoparticles for use as optical contrasting agents are typically selected to be larger than 35 nm. It has now been demonstrated, however, that measurable scattering signals in biological systems can be observed for metallic nanoparticles, with diameters less than 10 nm, when incident light, typically laser radiation, matching the nanoparticle resonance energy is used (15).

1.2. Nanoparticle Characterization

As with core selection, one must keep in mind the detection geometry and desired signal type when selecting a characterization method and while interpreting nanoparticle data. For example, transmission electron microscopy (TEM) is often used to confirm the synthesis of a desired geometry. While the images provided by this method can be reassuring, they are often not representative of the entire sample, and say nothing regarding the measurable optical properties. Similarly, due to its widespread availability and ease-of-use solution phase UV–Vis absorption spectroscopy is often used to determine the wavelength for peak optical activity (position of the resonance peak). In fact, this technique measures the extent to which light is transmitted, with contributions arising from both absorption and scattering processes. If the proposed contrast mechanism is based on scattering (i.e., reflectance or darkfield imaging), then the measured "absorbance" spectrum must be considered informative but nonquantitative. This is especially true in the case of larger (>50 nm) particles where scattering and absorption are of the same approximate magnitude. Although somewhat less common, scattering spectroscopy can be used in addition to absorption spectroscopy. In its most simple form, this method combines darkfield microscopy with UV–Vis spectroscopy where only those photons which are scattered are measured (16).

Absorption data have also been used to determine nanoparticle size and geometry based on equation [1]. While this can be useful for comparing synthetic schemes, the polydispersity of as-prepared samples restricts one to using only the peak intensity values (plasmon resonance positions), characterizing only those particles which dominate the optical response. A somewhat more complete picture of the entire distribution of nanoparticle sizes can be obtained using dynamic light scattering (DLS) as shown in **Fig. 12.3B**. This method, based on Stoke's law, essentially determines nanoparticle size based on the average time required to diffuse through a fixed focal volume. Unfortunately, DLS too has its limitations. A general assumption is made that all particles are spherical. For nonspherical particles only an effective size (comparable to volume) is determined and no shape information is obtained. Furthermore, one must carefully select the statistical method used to calculate the final distribution (i.e., number, intensity, volume) to emphasize sensitivity for the desired property (i.e., polydispersity, optical activity, surface area).

Simply put, no single analytical technique is adequate for proper nanoparticle characterization. In order to obtain a complete picture of the geometry and optical response of the as-prepared nanoparticles, a combination of TEM, UV–Vis absorption (extinction), scattering spectroscopy, and dynamic light scattering (DLS) should be employed. With this complete set of data, synthetic parameters can be systematically fine-tuned and components specific to the final imaging or analytical instrument (such as bandpass filters or laser sources) can be properly selected for optimal signal detection.

2. Materials

2.1. Gold Nanoparticle Cores

1. 500 mL round-bottom flask and Teflon stir bar, rinsed with aqua regia and then rinsed with 18 MΩ distilled water.
2. 132 mg of sodium citrate dissolved in 15 mL of 18 MΩ water. 50 mg of $HAuCl_4 \cdot 3H_2O$ in 150 mL of 18 MΩ water.

2.2. Nanoparticle Surface Modification

1. Colloidal gold dispersion.
2. Heterobifunctional PEG ligand, for every 500 μL of gold colloid, 2 mg of heterobifunctional PEG ligand is required.
3. Eppendorf tubes and centrifuge for concentration/purification.
4. 1× MES buffer (100 mM 2-(N-morpholino)ethanesulfonic acid, pH=5).

2.3. Nanoparticle–Antibody Conjugation

1. 1× MES buffer.
2. 10 mg of NHS (N-hydroxysuccinimide) and 10 mg of EDC (1-ethyl-3-(3-dimethylaminopropyl) carbodiimide) first dissolved into 100 μL of MES buffer. Centrifuge filters (Millipore Ultrafree 0.5, 30 kDa cut-off).
3. 1× PBS.
4. Size-exclusion chromatography (SEC) was performed using a Waters 650E chromatography system with a 10 mm × 100 mm Superose 6 column, followed by a Waters model 440 280 nm detector.

2.4. Tissue Labeling

1. Prepared gold nanoparticle–antibody conjugates
2. PBS 1×
3. Materials for mounting incubated sections on slide glass and sealing coverslips.

2.5. Optical Imaging of Nanoparticle-Labeled Tissue

1. Microscope equipped with a darkfield condenser
2. A dichroic filter (550 ± 20 nm).
3. A digital camera (Moticam 1,280×1,024 pixels).

3. Methods

Spherical gold nanoparticles of various sizes are now commercially available, however, their clinical utility is limited by indeterminate geometry, unwanted surface species (stabilizers), and poor size distribution. Because of this, we strongly recommend in-house synthesis as this provides an inexpensive source of nanoparticles and allows one to fine-tune the chemistry for varying desired geometries. Furthermore, this makes it feasible to work with volumes much larger than the typical (micro-scale), allowing for more rigorous purification and size separation while still yielding sufficient particles for biofunctionalization.

The synthesis of spherical gold nanoparticle cores with well-defined size, shape, and surface properties has been accomplished based upon documented methods involving the reduction of aqueous metal ions (17, 18). For spherical nanoparticles, the synthesis is relatively straightforward and typically makes use of a soluble metal salt (hydrogen tetrachloroaurate), a reducing agent (sodium citrate), and a stabilizing agent (excess sodium citrate). The stabilizing agent caps the particle and prevents further growth or aggregation after the reduced metal ions are consumed during the reaction. The ratio of the reducing agent to the metal salt, as well as the reaction conditions (temperature, relative concentrations), dictates the resulting distribution of sizes of the spherical nanoparticles. With careful control it is possible to synthesize a broad range of spherical nanoparticle sizes (2.5–62 nm) with relatively narrow size distributions (**Fig. 12.3A**). While the smallest and largest sizes in this range tend to be challenging, a number of standard recipes exist allowing for simple reproducible synthesis of particles with dimensions between 15 and 25 nm (19).

3.1. Synthesis of Gold Nanoparticle Cores

1. Initially, ~15 nm gold nanoparticles are prepared from hydrogen tetrachloroaurate by reduction with sodium citrate. To obtain this average diameter, 132 mg of sodium citrate dissolved in 15 mL water was added to a boiling solution of 50 mg of $HAuCl_4 \cdot 3H_2O$ in 150 mL of water (*see* **Note 1**).

2. For spherical nanoparticle cores, the long-term stability of the colloid depends largely upon the extent with which the excess citrate molecules remain physisorbed on the surface. While one is often tempted to remove unreacted reducing agent or surfactant by centrifugation and washing or by dialysis, which is not recommended. In either case, reducing the concentration of unbound surfactant from the solution shifts the adsorption equilibrium, reducing the number of

surface species and destabilizing the colloid. This can result in rapid aggregation rendering the sample useless. Using mass selective techniques, such as size-exclusion chromatography (SEC), one might hope to eliminate undesired particle geometries and simultaneously remove unbound surfactant. This too leads to thermodynamic instability and ultimately aggregation. For best results, sample purification and size selection should only be performed after irreversible attachment of surface stabilizers (surfactants) such as polyethylene glycol dithiol (**Section 3.2**).

3.2. Nanoparticle Surface Modification

1. When considering a nanoparticle system for use as a probe in biology one must carefully consider stability, biocompatibility, and specificity. While organic stains and fluorophores are typically soluble in biologically relevant solutions (aqueous) as-prepared nanoparticles are generally unstable owing to their high-energy surfaces. As such, a critical aspect of nanoprobe development involves surface stabilization of the nanoparticle system to promote biocompatibility, avoid aggregation, and reduce nonspecific protein adsorption. This has been particularly challenging for semiconductor-based quantum dots, where cytotoxicity of the elements used and surface charge require complicated chemistries to ensure biocompatibility and results in larger than desired nanoparticle diameters (14, 20). For nanoparticles targeted to a specific biochemical species (i.e., antigen–antibody), a balance between inertness and biostability and bioreactivity (selectivity) must be achieved.

   Recently, gold nanoparticles have been stabilized with a novel carboxy terminal heterobifunctional polyethylene glycol dithiol (PEG dithiol) of monodisperse chain length according to the structural scheme shown in **Fig. 12.4**. In this scheme the dithiol group on the end of the PEG chain firmly anchors the polymer on the particle surface, and the terminal carboxy groups on the outer end allow coupling of biologically directing molecules such as antibodies via amide bonds. Similar approaches are based on monothiol attachment, polydisperse PEG chain lengths, or hydrazide-antibody attachment (21). In all cases, the PEG coating makes the nanoparticles resistant against protein adsorption, enhances their biocompatibility, and stabilizes them against agglomeration in biological environments (22–31). By this approach PEGylated nanoparticles, with diameters below 100 nm, become long-circulating in the bloodstream of live animals and have been called "stealth" particles (29, 32) since they can evade recognition by T cells and macrophages in vivo and avoid rapid clearance by the immune system. This unique PEG ligand system thus permits preparation of

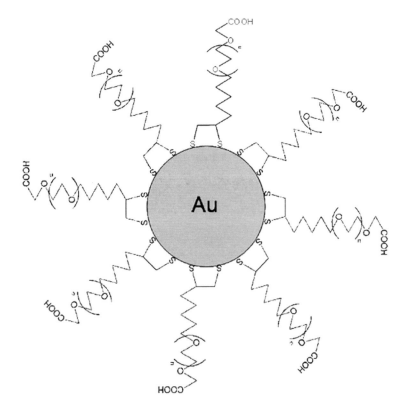

Fig. 12.4. Nanoparticle carboxy-pegylation scheme.

nanoparticles that are both stable in biological environment and highly bioselective.

Gold nanoparticles coated with the heterobifunctional PEG dithiol (or monothiol) ligand can be readily prepared from citrate-stabilized spherical gold nanoparticles by ligand exchange in water. Antibodies are easily attached to the PEGylated particles by activation of the terminal carboxy groups by standard NHS/EDC chemistry and formation of amide bonds (21).

One important factor to be considered is the PEG packing density on the particle surface. The packing density of PEG on the nanoparticles as well as the PEG molecular weight will determine properties such as protein repulsion, colloidal stability and ultimately adhesion strength to tissues, recognition by macrophages, and circulation times in living organisms. Ideally, the PEGylated particles will not adsorb any protein when the carboxy groups of the ligand are not chemically activated. On the other hand, we found that even NHS-activated PEGylated gold nanoparticles do not covalently bind any antibody when the packing density or molecular weight of the PEG chains is comparatively high. Therefore, an intermediate PEG packing density is necessary in order to combine high protein repulsion of the particles with efficient covalent binding of targeting antibodies. Since optimum PEG lengths and packing densities will vary with particle size and shape, care must be taken to accurately determine the appropriate relative concentrations of PEG to be used.

2. Pegylation is performed by adding 500 μL of the room temperature citrate-stabilized gold nanoparticle dispersion to 2 mg of the dry PEG dithiol ligand and mixed well. At this relative concentration of the PEG dithiol ligand in water coating occurs rapidly (*see* **Note 1**), and after several minutes, an increase of the hydrodynamic radius can be confirmed by dynamic light scattering. The mixture is allowed to stand for ~2 h at room temperature to ensure complete reaction. The nanoparticle dispersion is transferred into a 1.5 mL Eppendorf tube and centrifuged at $16,000 \times g$ for 30 min, forming a pellet. The supernatant is removed and 1 mL of 18 MΩ water was added. This process was repeated three times to remove any unreacted PEG ligand.

3. After the final washing and decanting, the particles are resuspended into 100 μL of salt containing medium (0.1 M MES buffer, pH 5), after which their size distribution remains completely stable (>1 year under exclusion of air and storage in a dark refrigerator), allowing for later functionalization with antibodies. The absence of free PEG dithiol ligand in solution is confirmed by size-exclusion chromatography using a refractive index detector and the particle size, compared to the citrate-stabilized particles, is determined by dynamic light scattering.

3.3. Nanoparticle–Antibody Conjugation

1. A variety of small molecules and monoclonal antibodies (mAb) have been recently developed and applied to the diagnosis, staging, and treatment of malignancy. Many of the therapeutic approaches have involved the blockade of cell surface or extra-cellular receptors with antibody, and we feel that application of the antibody–nanoparticle chemistry described above has great potential in the further application of these targeted strategies.

We have recently evaluated a monoclonal antibody (F19) that is specific to tumor stroma. The F-19 antigen is a cell surface glycoprotein (fibroblast activation protein, FAP-α) that is highly expressed by the stromal tissue of various cancer types such as breast, liver, lung, colon, pancreas, head, and neck cancer (33, 34). Our preliminary investigations of F19-conjugated gold nanoparticles focused on pancreatic adenocarcinoma because of the significant amount of tumor stroma arising in this malignancy.

The specificity of this antibody for stroma was initially confirmed by immunohistochemical (IHC) staining with F-19 mAb of ex vivo primary and metastatic human pancreatic cancer specimens. These studies demonstrated consistent and intense staining of the tumor stroma, which is nearly absent in adjacent normal tissue (see **Fig. 12.5**).

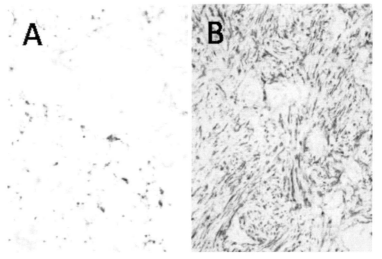

Fig. 12.5. Immunohistochemical staining with F-19 of (**a**) healthy and (**b**) cancer tissue. Cancer stroms are indicated as dark regions in both images.

2. Attachment of the F19 mAb to the PEGylated nanoparticles is performed using standard N-hydroxysuccinimide/1-ethyl-3-(3-dimethylaminopropyl) carbodiimide (NHS/EDC) coupling chemistry (35, 36). In this method, the carboxy groups on the particle surface are first activated by reaction with EDC hydrochloride and NHS in 0.1 molar MES buffer (pH 5). Ten milligrams of NHS and 10 mg of EDC are first dissolved into 100 μL of MES buffer. A measure of 25 μL of this solution is added to 100 μL of the PEGylated particle dispersion and allowed to stand for 30 min at room temperature.

3. Excess activation agents are removed by repeated washing (4 times) with 300 μL of MES (pH 5) at 0°C in centrifuge

filters (Millipore Ultrafree 0.5, 30 kDa cut-off), spinning down at 11,500×g to no more than 25 µL each time.

4. Antibody attachment is then performed by adding the concentrated activated nanoparticles to a dilute solution containing the antibody (see **Note 2**). First 15 µg (~100 pmol) of the F19 antibody was diluted to a volume of 300 µL with cold PBS buffer (0°C) at pH 7.4. This solution is added to the centrifuge filter containing the 25 µL solution of activated gold particles and mixed well. The mixture is then spun down to 25 µL and rinsed once more with 300 µL PBS (all at 0°C). Finally, enough PBS buffer to obtain a final volume of 25–50 µL was added. The solution is mixed well and transferred into an Eppendorf tube and shaken gently overnight at room temperature. After this time, all NHS-activated carboxy groups have reacted or been hydrolyzed, so no additional quenching was necessary.

5. The gold nanoparticle-F19 and nonspecific murine IgG conjugates (GNP-F19 and GNP-mIgG) are fractionated and analyzed by size-exclusion chromatography (SEC) using a Waters 650E chromatography system with a 10 mm × 100 mm Superose 6 column, followed by a Waters model 440 280 nm detector (**Fig. 12.6**). The mobile phase is phosphate-buffered saline (0.05 M sodium phosphate,

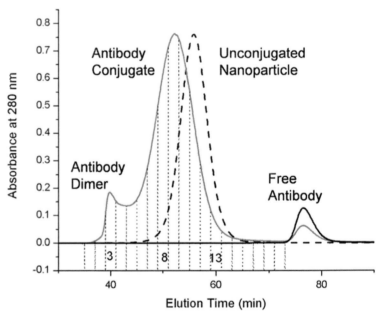

Fig. 12.6. SEC elution profile of as-prepared gold nanoparticle F-19 bioconjugate (*solid gray line*) as compared to the PEGylated nanoparticle core (*dashed line*). Collected fractions are indicated by the vertical dashed gray lines. Fractions 3, 8, and 13 were retained for further analysis.

0.15 M NaCl, pH 7.0, 0.02% sodium azide) at a flow rate of 0.2 mL/min.

6. Data are collected and analyzed using a Beckman 406 A/D converter and a Beckman System Gold system. The SEC eluates are fractionated into 400 μL aliquots that are selectively analyzed by dynamic light scattering and TEM (**Fig. 12.7**), as well as darkfield scattering spectroscopy (not shown).

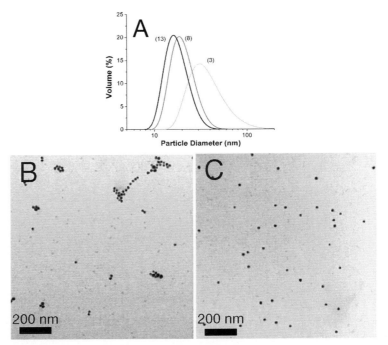

Fig. 12.7. DLS size distributions for individual fractions collected during SEC purification. Fraction 8 corresponds to the desired nanoparticle conjugate, while fractions 3 and 13 likely contain unwanted aggregates or un-conjugated particles, respectively. TEM of earlier fractions (**b**), clearly indicate aggregation while that of later fractions (**c**) show discrete particles.

7. Dynamic light scattering is performed with a Malvern Zetasizer Nano ZS using a 45 μL quartz cell either in water or in standard 1× PBS buffer with 1.02 cP as the viscosity and 1.335 as the refractive index of PBS at 25°C. Transmission electron microscopy is done on a JEOL JEM-1230 device at 80 kV. Samples are prepared by dilution of the nanoparticles in water, placement of a drop (2–3 μL) on a copper grid carrying a 20-nm thick carbon and drying overnight.

3.4. Pancreatic Tissue Labeling

1. Tissue samples of both cancerous and healthy human pancreas are obtained from patients undergoing pancreatic resection. Tissue sections are prepared by microtome to a thickness of approximately 5 μm. These sections were fixed on glass slides using cold acetone (0°C) for 10 min.

2. After washing in PBS, the sections are incubated individually in a 1:10 dilution of the nanoparticle conjugates, GNP-F19 and GNP-mIgG (~50 g/mL of bioconjugate to PBS buffer), for 3, 6, and 12 h (*see* **Note 4**). After incubation, the labeled samples are rinsed in PBS buffer multiple times to remove any unbound nanoparticle conjugate. The samples are then dried with a stream of N_2 and sealed under cover glass by standard methods. Control samples are similarly prepared using tissue sections of healthy pancreas labeled with GNP-F19 and cancer tissue labeled with a nonspecific mouse IgG monoclonal antibody.

3.5. Optical Imaging of Nanoparticle-Labeled Tissue

1. The F19-nanoparticle-labeled tissue sections are imaged by darkfield microscopy, with wavelength selection near the GNP-F19 resonance scattering maximum using a dichroic filter (550 ± 20 nm), onto a digital camera (Moticam 1280×1024 pixels). The resulting optical measurements are shown in **Fig. 12.8**. For comparison, an image area labeled by immunohistochemical (IH) secondary antibody staining of the F-19 mAb is shown (**Fig. 12.8A**). The forward scattering image (**Fig. 12.8B**) exhibits the same underlying stroma structure indicated by the IH-stained sample, whereas the healthy tissue sample (**Fig. 12.8C**) demonstrates minimal image contrast with only a few individual nanoparticles (small green spots) visible. This indicates

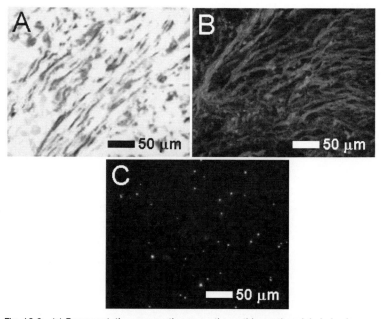

Fig. 12.8. (**a**) Representative pancreatic cancer tissue thin sections labeled using secondary antibody staining (darker regions), (**b**) darkfield transmission scattering images of GNP-F19-labeled pancreatic cancer tissue, (**c**) GNP-F19-labeled healthy tissue (25).

that the F19 mAb bioconjugates do selectively label tumor stroma. The wide-field optical contrast, shown in **Fig. 12.8**, proved to be sufficiently bright for visualization by eye and could be imaged routinely under only 5× (low NA) magnification, indicating the potential of this labeling technique for a number of clinical and surgical applications.

These antibody-functionalized PEGylated gold nanoparticles are one of the few examples of biologically targeted nanoparticles that have been used for specific labeling of human cancer tissue (**Fig. 12.8**). The PEG coating is especially important for this application as it ensures high redispersibility, biocompatibility, and bioselectivity of the particles. Non-PEGylated particles such as the ionically stabilized examples used for cancer cell labeling are generally not redispersible, may exhibit agglomeration upon contact to proteins, and can thus adhere nonspecifically to cells or neighboring tissues (37–40). Current directions include further optimization of antibody coupling, introducing methods for reproducibility, and defining the concentrations of gold and antibody necessary for targeted imaging of malignant lesions.

4. Notes

1. Consistent heating is important in making particles of uniform size.
2. Since gold nanoparticles stabilized by citrate agglomerate immediately upon transfer into salt containing buffer, the ligand exchange from citrate to PEG must be performed in pure water.
3. If the antibody storage solution contains sodium azide as a preservative, as is typical for many IgGs, it must first be removed by repeated washing with cold PBS buffer in centrifuge filters, as it competes for the activated carboxy groups on the particles.
4. No noticeable improvement in signal for the longer exposure times.

References

1. Bishop, P. T. (2002) The use of gold mercaptides for decorative precious metal applications. *Gold Bull* **35**(3), 89–98.
2. Alivisatos, P. A., Gu, W., and Larabell, C. (2005) Quantum dots as cellular probes. *Annu Rev Biomed Eng* **7**, 55–76.
3. Shiraishi, Y., et al. (2002) Frequency modulation response of a liquid-crystal electro-optic device doped with nanoparticles. *Appl Phys Lett* **81**(15), 2845–2847.
4. Law, M., et al. (2005) Nanowire dye-sensitized solar cells. *Nat Mater* **4**, 455–459.

5. Fuller, S. B., Wilhelm, E. J., and Jacobson, J. M. (2002) Ink-jet printed nanoparticle microelectromechanical systems. *J Microelectromech S* **11**(1), 54–60.
6. Carotenuto, G., Pepe, G. P., and Nicolais, L. (2000) Preparation and characterization of nano-sized Ag/PVP composites for optical applications. *Euro Phys J B* **16**, 11–17.
7. Lo, C. T., Chou, K. S., and Chin, W. K. (2001) Effects of mising procedures on the volume fraction of silver particles in conductive adhesives. *Adhes Sci Technol* **15**, 783–792.
8. Mulvaney, S. P., et al. (2003) Glass-coated, analyte-tagged nanoparticles: a new tagging system based on detection with surface-enhanced Raman scattering. *Langmuir* **19**, 4784–4790.
9. Hughes, M. D., et al. (2005) Tunable gold catalysts for selective hydrocarbon oxidation under mild conditions. *Nat Mater* **437**, 1132–1135.
10. Pradhan, N., Pal, A., and Pal, T. (2002) Silver nanoparticle catalyzed reduction of aromatic nitro compounds. *Coll Surf A* **196**(2), 247–257.
11. Maxwell, D. J., Taylor, J. R., and Nie, S. (2002) Self-assembled nanoparticle probes for recognition and detection of biomolecules. *J Am Chem Soc* **124**(32), 9606–9612.
12. Salata, O. (2004) Applications of nanoparticles in biology and medicine. *J Nanobiotech* **2**, 3–8.
13. Zheng, J., Zhang, C., and Dickson, R. M. (2004) Highly fluorescent, water-soluble, size-tunable gold quantum dots. *Phys Rev Lett* **93**, 077402(1)–077402(4).
14. Kirchner, C., et al., (2005) Cytotoxicity of colloidal CdSe and CdSe/ZnS nanoparticles. *Nano Lett* **5**, 331–338.
15. Daniel, M. C. and Astruc, D. (2004) Gold nanoparticles: assembly, supramolecular chemistry, quantum-size-related properties, and applications toward biology, catalysis, and nanotechnology. *Chem Rev* **104**(1), 293–346.
16. Mock, J. J., Smith, D. R., and Schultz, S. (2003) Local refractive index dependence of plasmon resonance spectra from individual nanoparticles. *Nano Lett* **3**(4), 485–491.
17. Turkevitch, J., Stevenson, P. C., and Hillier, J. (1951) Nucleation and growth process in the synthesis of colloidal gold. *Discuss Faraday Soc* **11**, 55–75.
18. Frens, G. (1973) Controlled nucleation for the regulation of the particle size in monodisperse gold suspensions. *Nature* **241**(105), 20–22.
19. Link, S. and El-Sayed, M. A. (2000) Shape and size dependence of radiative, non-radiative and photothermal properties of gold nanocrystals. *Int Rev Phys Chem* **19**(3), 409–453.
20. Chen, F. and Gerion, D. (2004) Fluorescent CdSe/ZnS nanocrystal-peptide conjugates for long-term, nontoxic imaging and nuclear targeting in living cells. *Nano Lett* **4**(10), 1827–1832.
21. Eck, W., et al. (2008) PEGylated gold nanoparticles conjugated to monoclonal F19 antibodies as targeted labeling agents for human pancreatic carcinoma tissue. *ACS Nano* **2**(11), 2263–2272.
22. Otsuka, H., et al. (2001) Quantitative and reversible lectin-induced association of gold nanoparticles modified with a-lactosyl-w-mercapto-poly(ethylene glycol). *J Am Chem Soc* **123**(34), 8226–8230.
23. Otsuka, H., Nagasaki, Y., and Kataoka, K. (2003) PEGylated nanoparticles for biological and pharmaceutical applications. *Adv Drug Deliv Rev* **55**(3), 403–419.
24. Kim, J., et al. (2006) Designed fabrication of multifunctional magnetic gold nanoshells and their application to magnetic resonance imaging and photothermal therapy. *Angew Chem Int Edit* **45**(46), 7754–7758.
25. Pierrat, S., et al. (2007) Self-assembly of small gold colloids with functionalized gold nanorods. *Nano Lett* **7**(2), 259–263.
26. Shenoy, D., et al. (2006) Surface functionalization of gold nanoparticles using heterobifunctional poly(ethylene glycol) spacer for intracellular tracking and delivery. *Int J Nanomed* **1**(1), 51–57.
27. Sperling, R. A., et al. (2006) Electrophoretic separation of nanoparticles with a discrete number of functional groups. *Adv Funct Mater* **16**(7), 943–948.
28. Liu, Y., et al. (2007) Synthesis, stability, and cellular internalization of gold nanoparticles containing mixed peptide-poly(ethylene glycol) monolayers. *Anal Chem* **79**(6), 2221–2229.
29. Gref, R. and Couvreur, P. (2004) Stealth and biomimetic core-corona nanoparticles. *Encyc Nanosci Nanotech* **10**, 83–94.
30. Dixit, V., et al. (2006) Synthesis and grafting of thioctic acid-PEG-folate conjugates onto Au nanoparticles for selective targeting of folate receptor-positive tumor cells. *Bioconj Chem* **17**(3), 603–609.
31. Liao, H. and Hafner, J. H. (2005) Gold nanorod bioconjugates. *Chem Mater* **17**(18), 4636–4641.
32. Owens, D. E. and Peppas, N. A. (2006) Opsonization, biodistribution, and

pharmacokinetics of polymeric nanoparticles. *Int J Pharm* **307**(1), 93–102.
33. Garin-Chesa, P., Old, L. J., and Rettig, W. J. (1990) Cell surface glycoprotein of reactive stromal fibroblasts as a potential antibody target in human epithelial cancers. *Proc Natl Acad Sci USA* **87**(18), 7235–7239.
34. Welt, S., et al. (1994) Antibody targeting in metastatic colon cancer: a phase I study of monoclonal antibody F19 against a cell-surface protein of reactive tumor stromal fibroblasts. *J Clin Oncol* **12**(6), 1193–1203.
35. Grabarek, Z. and Gergely, J. (1990) Zero-length crosslinking procedure with the use of active esters. *Anal Biochem* **185**(1), 131–135.
36. Hermanson, G. T. (ed) (1990) *Bioconjugate Techniques*. Academic Press, NY, 786.
37. Burda, F. C., et al. (2005) Chemistry and properties of nanocrystals of different shapes. *Chem Rev* **105**, 1025–1102.
38. El-Sayed, I. H., Huang, X., and El-Sayed, M. A. (2006) Selective laser photo-thermal therapy of epithelial carcinoma using anti-EGFR antibody conjugated gold nanoparticles. *Cancer Lett* **239**(1), 129–135.
39. Huang, X., et al. (2006) Cancer cell imaging and photothermal therapy in the near-infrared region by using gold nanorods. *J Am Chem Soc* **128**(6), 2115–2120.
40. Huang, X., et al. (2007) Cancer cells assemble and align gold nanorods conjugated to antibodies to produce highly enhanced, sharp, and polarized surface Raman spectra: a potential cancer diagnostic marker. *Nano Lett* **7**(6), 1591–1597.

Chapter 13

Identification of Pancreatic Cancer-Specific Cell-Surface Markers for Development of Targeting Ligands

David L. Morse, Galen Hostetter, Yoganand Balagurunathan, Robert J. Gillies, and Haiyong Han

Abstract

Pancreatic cancer is generally detected at later stages with a poor prognosis and a high-mortality rate. Development of theranostic imaging agents that noninvasively target pancreatic cancer by gene expression and deliver therapies directly to malignant cells could greatly improve therapeutic outcomes. Small-peptide ligands that bind cell-surface proteins and are conjugated to imaging moieties have demonstrated efficacy in cancer imaging. Identification of cancer-specific targets is a major bottleneck in the development of such agents. Herein, a method is presented that uses DNA microarray expression profiling of large sets of normal and cancer tissues to identify targets expressed in cancer but not expressed in relevant normal tissues. Identified targets are subsequently validated for protein expression using tissue microarray. Further validations are performed by quantifying expression in pancreatic cancer cells by quantitative real-time reverse-transcription polymerase chain reaction (qRT-PCR), by immunocytochemistry and immunohistochemistry, and by reviewing data and literature in public databases. Validated targets are selected for ligand development based on the existence of a known ligand or by known structure–activity relationships useful for development of novel ligands.

Key words: pancreatic adenocarcinoma, cancer target, cell surface, gene-expression profiling, DNA microarray, tissue microarray, imaging, ligand conjugate.

1. Introduction

The incidence of pancreatic cancer is increasing worldwide and is associated with a high-mortality rate. Since pancreatic adenocarcinoma (PanAdo) is typically diagnosed at later stages of disease, only a small fraction of patients have operable lesions at the time of diagnosis (1). Endoscopic ultrasound and other imaging modalities are currently used for detection of pancreatic cancer in suspect patients (2). Agents that noninvasively target pancreatic cancer by specificity of gene expression have great potential for theranostic use. Patient outcomes could be improved by noninvasively following tumor response to treatment through imaging; by selective delivery of therapy to tumor relative to normal tissue; by aiding in diagnosis through characterization of gene expression; and by providing treatment options for patients with inoperable or disseminated disease.

Development of imaging and therapeutic agents using antibody or small-peptide-based ligands has been moderately successful in targeting cancer. Effective treatment of non-Hodgkin's lymphoma was achieved using radiolabeled monoclonal antibodies targeting cell-surface epitopes (3). However, the use of large conjugated antibodies to deliver imaging or therapeutic compounds to solid tumors has not been ideal (4, 5). Several agents based on the relatively small RGD peptide have been developed to deliver therapeutic and imaging agents to solid tumor vasculature (6), e.g., an [^{18}F]galacto-RGD positron emission tomography (PET) agent was used to reliably image tumor $\alpha_v\beta_3$-integrin expression and has a favorable pharmacokinetic profile (7, 8). Hence, targeting of small-peptide conjugates to cell-surface proteins is a solid approach. Known structure–activity relationships (SAR) are routinely used to engineer specific binding ligands via computer modeling and high-throughput screening methodologies (9). These small-peptide ligands may be developed with binding constants in the nanomolar range and can subsequently be tethered to imaging or therapeutic moieties without significantly altering binding characteristics (10, 11).

Although such agents can be readily developed, there remains a critical need for agents that specifically target pancreatic cancer. The question might be asked, why aren't there a plethora of agents currently in development? Often, too little emphasis in study design has been made on target identification and validation. A target that has been reported in the literature as being "expressed in pancreatic cancer" may or may not be a good target. After further validation, such targets are often found to be commonly expressed in other vital tissues and are thus nonspecific. Both expression of a target in cancer and nonexpression in normal tissues must be considered. Often targets are identified using contrived cell lines that are grown in a medium that does not accurately reflect conditions found in human tissues and therefore may have an altered expression profile. Additionally, pancreatic cancers are heterogeneous in origin and a given validated target may be useful for only a subset of tumors (12). Hence, multiple targets may be required to cover all pancreatic cancers.

For target identification, it is necessary to quantify the differential expression of protein localized to the cell surface in cancer tissue relative to normal tissues. Unfortunately, the field of proteomics has not yet advanced to the degree that quantitative determinations can be made for the complete set of cell-surface proteins in tissue samples with high throughput (13). Alternatively, gene-expression profiling via DNA microarray determination of transcript levels is now routinely performed on tissue samples with robust and quantitative results. Although transcript levels are not necessarily linearly related to the level of translation and subcellular localization of gene product, transcript is required for translation and for a large percentage of gene products there is a linear relationship. When using mRNA levels to identify putative targets, further validation of protein expression and localization is required.

The following points are general guidelines for identification and validation of cancer targets. Determination and validation of protein expression in a panel of tumor tissues is a requirement for target identification. Furthermore, validation of nonexpression in a large panel of vital normal tissues (e.g., heart, lungs, liver, kidneys), and in normal tissues found associated with tumors (e.g., vascular tissues and monocytes), is also a requirement. Limiting a target identification search to cell-surface proteins is beneficial during agent development because strategies that enable the construct to cross the plasma membrane are not required. Also, knowledge of the biological function of the target protein may be of interest, but is not a requirement for agent development. For targeting, discovery of a small-peptide binding ligand with high affinity is sufficient.

2. Materials

All solutions were prepared using distilled and deionized H_2O and all chemicals were purchased from Sigma-Aldrich, St. Louis, MO, unless stated otherwise.

2.1. Tissue Samples and Cell Lines

1. For DNA microarray for expression profiling of pancreatic adenocarcinoma (PanAdo), 28 tissue samples were acquired (eight fresh-frozen from the Arizona Cancer Center Tissue Acquisition and Cellular/Molecular Analysis Shared Service, AZCC TACMASS, at the University of Arizona, Tucson, AZ, and 20 sets of array data from the Molecular Profiling Institute, Phoenix, AZ).

2. For DNA microarray of normal, unaffected tissue, four fresh-frozen normal pancreas tissue samples (AZCC TACMASS) and 103 RNA samples from normal tissues

representing 28 different organ sites (BioChain, Hayward, CA and Stratagene, La Jolla, CA) were acquired.

3. For tissue microarray (TMA), paraffin-embedded pancreatic tissues were obtained from the Biospecimen Repository Core of the Pancreatic Cancer P01 project (CA109552) at the Translational Genomics Research Institute (TGen), Phoenix, AZ.

4. All tissue samples were de-identified and an institutional review board exemption obtained for their use.

5. For DNA microarray, qRT-PCR, and immunocytochemistry, 17 PanAdo cell lines were obtained from American Type Culture Collection (ATCC).

2.2. Cell Culture

1. Cells were grown using RPMI medium with 10% fetal bovine serum (FBS), 1% penicillin, and 1% streptomycin added.

2.3. RNA Extraction and DNA Microarray

1. RNeasy kit (Qiagen, Valencia, CA).
2. Agilent low-input RNA fluorescent linear amplification kit (Agilent Technologies, Santa Clara, CA).
3. Human 1A Microarray Chips (Agilent Technologies, Santa Clara, CA).
4. GenElute Mammalian Total RNA Miniprep Kit and Amplification Grade DNase I (Sigma-Aldrich, St. Louis, MO) for qRT-PCR of specific targets in pancreatic cancer cell lines.

2.4. Tissue Microarray (TMA)

1. A tissue microarray, designed and constructed by the TMA Core Facility at TGen, Phoenix, AZ, comprised of 42 unique PanAdo cases and triple punched using 1.0 mm cores. When available, a normal duct (by morphology) was arrayed alongside tumor counterparts. TMA slides for normal tissues (version CHTN2002N1) were provided by the Cooperative Human Tissue Network funded by the National Cancer Institute/NIH.

2. The TMA block was sectioned at 5 μm and transferred by water floatation to standard charged slides.

3. TMA slides containing a variety of tumor and normal tissues were used in the antibody optimization process.

2.5. Quantitative Real-Time Reverse-Transcription Polymerase Chain Reaction (qRT-PCR)

1. Primer sets were designed in-house (*see* **Note 1**) and purchased from Invitrogen, San Diego, CA.
2. QuantiTect SYBR Green RT-PCR Kit (Qiagen, Valencia, CA).

2.6. Immunocytochemistry (ICC)

1. The same primary antibodies used for TMA staining were used for ICC.
2. Secondary antibodies: Alexafluor 488 goat anti-rabbit and AlexaFluor488 goat anti-mouse (Invitrogen, San Diego, CA).
3. 10× PBS stock solution: 80 g NaCl, 2.0 g KCl, 14.4 g Na_2HPO_4, and 2.4 g KH_2PO_4 in 1 L, adjust pH to 7.4 with HCl.
4. Paraformaldehyde solution was made fresh on the day of use (see **Note 2**): 2% paraformaldehyde in 1× PBS. Heat water in a microwave, then slowly add the powder while stirring, add 10% final volume of 10× PBS. Clarify by adding one drop of 1 N NaOH. Filter through paper-lined funnel. Cool on ice until cold to touch.
5. 20× SSC stock solution: 3.0 M NaCl and 0.3 M Na_3-citrate, pH to 7.4 with 1 N NaOH.
6. Antibody conjugation buffer: 1× SSC, 2% goat serum, 1% BSA, 0.05% Triton X-100, and 0.02% NaN_3.
7. Antibody wash buffer: 1× SSC and 0.05% Triton X-100.
8. Glycine wash for quenching paraformaldehyde: 0.75% glycine, pH 7.4 with 1 N NaOH and store at 4°C.
9. Permeabilization buffer: 1× SSC, 0.1% Triton X-100. Invert flask several times to mix thoroughly.
10. Vectashield H-1000 mounting medium for fluorescence (Vector Laboratories, Burlingame, CA).

3. Methods

Figure 13.1 is a flow chart describing the identification and validation of cancer targets, and the subsequent discovery of binding ligands and development of targeting nanoagents. To

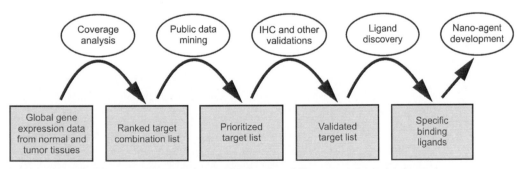

Fig. 13.1. Flow chart for target identification and validation, ligand discovery, and nanodevelopment.

identify potential pancreatic cancer targets, mRNA was obtained from multiple pancreatic tumor samples and multiple normal tissue samples from 28 organ sites including normal pancreas. DNA microarray data were generated and data for genes with products that are localized to the cell surface were parsed and analyzed for expression in tumor and normal tissues. To do this, a list of cell-surface genes was compiled and expression versus nonexpression threshold values determined for the array data (12). Genes determined to be expressed in tumor, but not expressed in normal tissues were prioritized based on percentage of expression among the tumor samples (tumor coverage). Targets intended for imaging were limited to nonexpression in normal pancreas and organs associated with drug toxicity and clearance. Targets intended for delivery of therapeutics were limited to nonexpression in all normal tissues (*see* **Note 3**). Putative targets were ranked and prioritized based on percent coverage among the tumor samples and potential for ligand development, i.e., known ligands or SAR. The highest ranked targets were verified by checking expression values reported in public databases, evaluated for availability of known ligands and structure–activity relationships (SAR), and selected for further validation. Protein expression was validated via tissue microarray (TMA) for the highest ranked targets that had commercially available antibodies (*see* **Notes 4 and 5**) (14–17). TMA-validated targets were further validated for expression in pancreatic cancer cell lines via quantitative real-time RT-PCR (qRT-PCR) (18) and immunocytochemistry (ICC) (*see* **Note 6**) (19). The most promising fully validated targets were selected for ligand development for future incorporation into targeted agents.

3.1. RNA Extraction

1. For DNA array, total RNA was isolated from fresh-frozen tissue samples and from pancreatic cancer cells grown to ~80% confluence using the RNeasy kit (Qiagen, Valencia, CA).

2. For qRT-PCR, RNA was extracted from pancreatic cancer cells using the GenElute Mammalian Total RNA Miniprep Kit and traces of genomic DNA removed using Amplification Grade DNase I (Sigma-Aldrich, St. Louis, MO).

3.2. DNA Microarray and Gene-Expression Profiling

1. CY5-labeled cRNA targets were generated from normal tissue samples (103), pancreatic cancer tissues (28), or PaAdo cell lines using 1 μg total RNA and the Agilent low-input RNA fluorescent linear amplification kit. For use as a reference, CY3 cRNA were generated from normal pancreatic tissue.

2. The concentration and integrity of fluorescence-labeled cRNAs were determined using an Agilent 2100 Bioanalyzer.

3. For each sample, equal amounts of labeled cRNA targets from sample and reference were hybridized onto an Agilent Human 1A oligonucleotide array.

4. Hybridization signals were acquired and analyzed using Agilent's feature extraction software (version 7.1).

5. Feature intensity values were normalized by the array median intensity.

6. Internal stability of the data set was determined using data analysis techniques such as cluster analysis and multidimensional scaling analysis (MDS). Multidimensional scaling analysis (MDS) was used to view the entire array data projected onto three dimensions to verify the consistency of groupings based on phenotypes (*see* **Note 7**).

3.3. Compilation of Cell-Surface Protein List

1. The entire Gene Ontology hierarchical vocabulary was manually browsed through using the Cancer Genome Anatomy Project Gene Ontology browser. Each category was followed through to the lowest possible level in order to select lists of genes that may encode proteins containing cell-surface epitopes (6,389 genes combined).

2. Genes that were not represented on the microarray chips (Agilent Human 1A v1 & v2 arrays) used in our study were removed (4,407 remaining genes).

3. Each remaining gene was manually checked using existing databases (Genecard, Harvester, Entrez, Protein Database, and UniProt), retaining genes that encode or are predicted to encode cell-surface products (2,177 genes total).

3.4. Determination of Cutoff Values for Coverage Analysis (What Is Zero Expression?)

1. The maximum level of mRNA expression in normal tissues that corresponds to nonexpression of protein at the cell surface was estimated. This estimate was used to establish a threshold value for normalized DNA microarray data of normal tissues, below which the corresponding protein is considered to be not expressed at the cell surface (*see* **Note 8**).

2. The minimum level of mRNA expression in tumor samples that corresponds with protein expression at the cell surface was estimated (*see* **Note 8**).

3. The above estimates were used to set the most stringent coverage analysis threshold values possible (*see* **Section 3.5**) that still provided targets (*see* **Note 8**).

3.5. Target Identification by Coverage Analysis

1. An algorithm was prepared, where for a given cell-surface DNA array probe, an expression flag was assigned for each normal tissue and tumor sample (*see* **Notes 9** and **10**). Expression flag values for probes on each array were assigned as "0" if the median normalized value was $\leq$ the threshold

value; or as "1" if > the threshold value (*see* **Section 3.4** *for determining threshold values*).

2. For each probe, the normal and tumor expression flag values were summed.

3. The percent normal tissue coverage and pancreatic tumor coverage for each probe was calculated by dividing the summed value by the number of normal or tumor samples (*see* **Note 3**).

4. All probes that had 0% tumor coverage were removed from the analysis.

5. The remaining probes were sorted by ascending percent normal coverage and descending percent tumor coverage.

6. Genes with low or 0% normal tissue coverage, but with high tumor coverage were ranked highest.

3.6. Target Selection for Validation

1. Since targets were identified based on "expression" versus "nonexpression," tumor expression level was considered for the highest ranked targets. Targets with the highest expression in tumor tissues were preferred.

2. Targets with known small MW peptide binding ligands were given priority (*see* **Note 11**).

3. Targets with known biology or structure–activity relationships (SAR) were also preferred in order to enable a directed approach toward small ligand development.

4. Targets with available monoclonal antibodies that specifically target extracellular epitopes were considered desirable. In particular if the structure was known for the binding region of the antibody.

5. Published databases and current literature were consulted for agreement, e.g., a given target may be expressed in a specific tissue type that was not represented in the sample set.

6. Pancreatic tumors display heterogeneity of cell-surface gene expression (12). Thus, multiple targets are required to cover all pancreatic tumor types.

3.7. TMA Sectioning and (IHC) Staining/Scoring

1. The TMA block was sectioned at 5 μm and sections were transferred to standard glass slides by water floatation. Slides were baked for 20 min at 56°C.

2. IHC optimization included titration of antibodies against regular tissue sections and "tester" TMA slides containing a variety of tumor and normal tissues. TMA slides underwent antigen retrieval by heating at 100°C in citrate buffer (0.1 mol/L, pH 6.0) for 5–30 min depending on the antibody.

3. Slides were incubated with primary antibody at optimal dilutions for 30 min at room temperature with incubation (and washes) with biotinylated secondary antibody were followed by application of streptavidin–peroxidase complex (Vision BioSystems) and resolved with diaminobenzidine chromogen staining. Primary antibodies and dilutions used were anticholecystokinin A receptor (CCKAR; R&D Systems), 7 μg/mL; and antiprotein tyrosine phosphatase receptor, type C (PTPRC; R&D Systems), 2 μg/mL.

4. Slides were then counterstained with hematoxylin for 5 min and rinsed with water. After dehydration with serial concentrations of ethanol (70, 80, 90, and 100%), the slides were soaked with xylene. After draining the xylene, mounting media and coverslips were applied to the slides (*see* **Fig. 13.2** for representative immunostained and counterstained TMA cores).

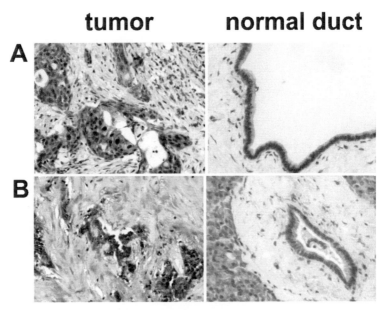

Fig. 13.2. Representative TMA cores immunostained for CCKAR (**a**) and PTPRC (**b**) from pancreatic adenocarcinoma cases (*left*) and pancreatic ducts with normal morphology (*right*).

5. Stained slides were evaluated using light microscopy and scored by a board-certified pathologist (G.H.) with 0 interpreted as negative to 3+ interpreted as strongly positive (*see* **Table 13.1**). When applicable, staining localization was listed as nuclear, cytoplasmic, or membranous.

Table 13.1.
Summarized results for TMA

Target	Sample classification	Score				% of cases with ≥2+
		0	1+	2+	3+	
CCKAR	Adjacent normal	8	5	3	0	23
	Tumor	5	4	10	2	57
PTPRC	Adjacent normal	10	5	1	0	7
	Tumor	5	6	7	1	42

3.8. Quantitative Real-Time Reverse-Transcription Polymerase Chain Reaction (qRT-PCR)

1. Pancreatic cancer cells were grown in 6-well plates to 80% confluence and RNA was extracted using the GenElute Mammalian Total RNA Miniprep Kit. Traces of genomic DNA were subsequently removed using Amplification Grade DNase I (Sigma-Aldrich, St. Louis, MO).

2. Primer sets were designed to generate cDNA and perform RT-PCR from transcripts of pancreatic cancer cell-surface targets of interest (*see* **Note 1**). Fragment lengths were approximately 100 bp long.

3. PCR conditions were optimized for maximum yield without spurious priming.

4. Real-time RT-PCR was performed using a Smart Cycler® (Cephid, Sunnyvale, CA) and the QuantiTect SYBR Green RT-PCR Kit (Qiagen).

5. A no-RT reaction and no-template reaction were included during each experiment as controls.

6. Melting curves yielded a single melt peak for all template reactions and a minimal melt peak for the no-template reaction.

7. A single reaction was performed per extract for each target template, three extracts per cell line. Overall reliability was high, Cronbach's $\alpha = 0.93$ (18).

8. Expression values were determined as 2^{-CT}, where CT is the second derivative of the fluorescence curve.

9. Raw expression values were normalized using ACTB transcript as an internal standard.

3.9. Immunocytochemistry (ICC)

1. Primary antibody dilutions (typically 1:50) were optimized individually to provide maximal staining without using excess antibody. The same primary antibodies were used for ICC as was used for TMA staining. Secondary

antibodies were conjugated with AlexaFluor488 fluorescent dye (Invitrogen) and dilutions (typically 1:200) were optimized to provide maximal staining without background.

2. Pancreatic cancer cells were grown to 80% confluence on round glass coverslips, 22 mm diameter, in 6-well tissue culture plates.

3. Paraformaldehyde solution was made fresh on the day of staining (see **Section 2.6**).

4. Primary antibodies prepared were diluted to the optimized concentration using antibody conjugation buffer (see **Section 2.6**).

5. Media were aspirated from the plates and paraformaldehyde solution (see **Section 2.6**) added until coverslips were submerged and incubated for 15 min.

6. Paraformaldehyde was quenched with an equal volume of warm 50 mM glycine buffer (see **Section 2.6** and **Note 12**). The resulting solution was removed using a disposable tip and discarded in a paraformaldehyde waste bottle.

7. Plates were washed twice for 5 min in glycine buffer. The first wash was discarded in a paraformaldehyde waste bottle.

8. The second glycine wash was discarded and the cell membranes permeabilized by incubating for 10–15 min in 0.1% Triton X-100 permeabilization buffer (**Section 2.6**).

9. The permeabilization buffer was discarded and primary antibody solution, 80 μL, dispensed on the top of each coverslip (see **Note 13**). Plates were covered and incubated at room temperature for 1 h (see **Note 14**).

10. Coverslips were washed three times, 5 min per wash, using antibody wash buffer (see **Section 2.6** and **Note 15**).

11. Secondary antibodies were prepared during the washes (Step 10) using the optimized dilution (Step 1) and antibody conjugation buffer (see **Section 2.6**). The tubes were wrapped in aluminum foil in order to prevent quenching of the fluorophore. Secondary antibody solution, 80 μL, was dispensed on the top of each coverslip (see **Note 13**). Plates were covered and incubated at room temperature in the dark for 45 min.

12. While keeping the plates in the dark as much as possible, coverslips were washed three times, 5 min per wash, using antibody wash buffer (see **Section 2.6** and **Note 15**).

13. Vectashield H-1000 mounting medium for fluorescence (Vector Laboratories), 10 μL, was dispensed onto the center of one microscope slide per coverslip.

14. Coverslips were removed from the antibody wash solution using forceps, gently dried on the back side with a kimwipe, and placed cell-side down onto the mounting media (*see* **Note 16**).
15. Excess mounting medium was removed from the coverslip and the outside edges sealed using clear fingernail polish.
16. Slides were air dried for 15 min at room temperature in the dark and moved to a −20°C freezer for long-term storage.
17. Duplicate slides were prepared for each cell line and target, and background was determined by staining only with secondary antibody as a control.
18. Relative staining intensities were compared to the no-primary antibody control and recorded as +++ = high, ++ = moderate, and + = low.

3.10. Verification Using Public Databases and Expression Signal Intensity Distributions

1. In order to further verify expression, or nonexpression in normal tissues, additional microarray gene-expression data sets were obtained from public databases such as the Gene-Expression Omnibus (GEO) and the GeneAtlas by the Genomics Institute of the Novartis Research Foundation (GNF).
2. Expression signal intensity distribution analyses were performed for each validated target using public data for a broad range of cancers and normal tissues. These analyses are useful to identify expression of a given target in normal tissues that were not included in the set used for DNA microarray identification and TMA validations. Also, these analyses can provide insight into the broader applicability of a given target among a range of cancer types.

4. Notes

1. When designing primer sets for real-time RT-PCR, the following should be considered: the optimal product length when using the QuantiTect SYBR Green RT-PCR Kit (Qiagen) is ~100 bp; it is best if primers span an intron so that amplified cDNA can be readily distinguished from genomic DNA; some primer sequences form secondary structures, e.g., stem loops, or can anneal to sequence from the reverse direction primer (primer-dimerization), these structures can be predicted by available computer algorithms or by eye and should be avoided; the annealing temperature for both primers in a set should be nearly identical; and NCBI-BLAST database searches should be performed for both primer sequences and no cDNA template other

than the intended sequence should be primed by both primers in a set. Optimize PCR conditions for each primer set by varying annealing temperature and Mg^{2+} concentration if necessary, so that maximum yield without spurious priming is achieved.

2. Paraformaldehyde is toxic. Wear mask while weighing and handling, and work in the fume hood. Dispose of liquid and dry waste appropriately.

3. A major hindrance to the development of targeted agents for imaging or therapy of cancer is the difficulty in identifying targets that are specifically expressed in cancer relative to normal unaffected tissue. In the case of targeted therapeutic agents and in order to avoid toxicity and serious side effects, it is best to identify targets that are not expressed in the broadest possible range of normal tissues, but are expressed in cancer. However, since imaging agents generally have significantly lower toxicities, the range of normal tissues surveyed can be decreased to include tissues involved in respiration, clearance, and the site of origin of the cancer (normal pancreas). Thus, increasing the likelihood of identifying targets suitable for early detection imaging.

4. If not available for a specific target of interest, antibodies can be commercially produced for a price.

5. TMA validations were largely in agreement with DNA microarray assessments, but not for 100% of the cases. Some differences are to be expected due to posttranslational regulation of the gene product. In addition to the determination of expression in tumor tissue, TMA provides useful detail, such as identification of specific cell types expressing the target within the tumor and determination of target expression in surrounding tissues of different pathologies among the sample, e.g., tumor versus adjacent normal pathology.

6. As a substitute for validation of protein expression in cell lines via ICC, Western analyses may be performed. To assure that cell-surface expression is determined both whole cell and plasma membrane extracts can be performed. Other alternatives include ligand-binding assay or functional assay, if these are available for the given target.

7. Multidimensional scaling analysis is a data analysis technique for mapping data of higher dimensionality (e.g., expression data with a number of genes across multiple samples) to a smaller dimension (typically 3 or lower) where distance between any two points corresponds to similarities or dissimilarities (20). It allows the visualization of

the entire data sets on lower dimensions and the identification of any discrepancies that may result from data acquisition and processing.

8. When analyzed by DNA microarray, nearly all transcripts exhibit some expression value, albeit values may be quite small for a large percentage of transcripts. For any given transcript, it is difficult to determine an expression value, or threshold, above which corresponds to gene product localized to the cell surface at quantities large enough to allow visualization by a targeted imaging modality. Or conversely, below which corresponds to nonexpression or detection at the cell surface. Also, since there is variation among individual transcripts in terms of posttranscriptional regulation, it is impossible to determine a universal threshold that will be ideal for all transcripts. However, a best estimate that will allow identification of expression in tumor versus nonexpression in normal tissues while limiting the number of false identifications is needed for this analysis. We used the following practical approaches with the intention of identifying errors during validation:
    a. Always allow for a gap between the lower normal tissue cutoff value and the higher tumor cutoff value, e.g., if the lower value is set at say 0.3 of the array median, then set the upper tumor cutoff value to 0.4 of the array median value.
    b. Perform the coverage analysis (see **Section 3.5**) at a range of lower normal tissue cutoff values, e.g., 0.2–0.6 of the array median. If set too low, a large and unmanageable number of targets will be identified, many of which may not be expressed in tumor. If set too high, few targets will be identified, and these targets may be expressed in normal tissues.
    c. Choose the lowest normal expression threshold value that provides a manageable number of targets, i.e., less than 100 rather than thousands. Further validation of select targets by TMA will provide feedback. For example, if many target proteins are found to be expressed in normal tissues, the normal threshold value may be set too high.
9. Rather than identifying targets that are differentially expressed in tumor relative to normal, for targeted agents it is vital that the target not be expressed in normal tissues. Hence, representing the data in binary form as "expressed" versus "not-expressed" is required.
10. Alternatively, in order to eliminate outliers in the normal tissue data set, all values for a given normal tissue type may

first be averaged prior to determining an expression flag value. Thus, determining an expression flag value for each normal tissue type rather than for each normal tissue sample.

11. Small-peptide ligands are optimal for attachment to nanoparticles, or attachment of linkers and imaging or therapeutic moieties. Small organic ligands are generally too small for attachment without disruption of binding or biological activity. Peptide ligands can be altered and developed via rational design and high-throughput synthesis and screening to improve the desired properties, e.g., reduced size, incorporation of peptidomimetic residues to decrease degradation, and to increase or decrease binding affinity and agonist or antagonist properties.

12. Stock glycine wash solution is stored at 4°C. It is important that the glycine solution is warm before quenching paraformaldehyde, so bring the solution to 37°C in a water bath before use.

13. Alternatively, in order to use less antibody 40–50 μL primary antibody solution per coverslip can be dispensed on parafilm in a petri dish. Coverslips are then removed from the 6-well plate, dabbed with a kimwipe to remove excess permeabilization or wash buffer, and placed cell-side down onto the primary antibody on parafilm making sure that there are no bubbles. Following incubation, carefully remove the coverslip from the parafilm and place them cell-side up in a 6-well culture plate for subsequent washes.

14. Primary antibody incubation time may vary depending on the cells and antibodies used. Another common procedure is to incubate overnight at 4°C. In this case, the incubation should be performed on parafilm in a covered petri dish.

15. To prevent washing cells off the coverslip, wash buffer should be added to the side of the well, not directly on the coverslip. To prevent antibody from being transferred among the different slips, use a new pipette tip to remove the antibody wash solution from each coverslip.

16. If there are bubbles in the mounting medium after placing the slide, move the coverslip to the edge of the slide, and gently peel up and replace.

Acknowledgments

We would like to thank Dr. Michael Bittner and Sonsoles Shack for microarray data acquisition, and Dr. Ronald Lynch for immunocytochemistry advice.

References

1. Dunphy, E. P. (2008) Pancreatic cancer: a review and update. *Clin J Oncol Nurs* **12**, 735–741.
2. Klapman, J. and Malafa, M. P. (2008) Early detection of pancreatic cancer: why, who, and how to screen. *Cancer Control* **15**, 280–287.
3. Goldenberg, D. M. and Sharkey, R. M. (2007) Novel radiolabeled antibody conjugates. *Oncogene* **26**, 3734–3744.
4. Jhanwar, Y. S. and Divgi, C. (2005) Current status of therapy of solid tumors. *J Nucl Med* **46 Suppl 1**, 141–150.
5. Goldenberg, D. M. and Sharkey, R. M. (2006) Advances in cancer therapy with radiolabeled monoclonal antibodies. *Q J Nucl Med Mol Imaging* **50**, 248–264.
6. Temming, K., Schiffelers, R. M., Molema, G., and Kok, R. J. (2005) RGD-based strategies for selective delivery of therapeutics and imaging agents to the tumour vasculature. *Drug Resist Updat* **8**, 381–402.
7. Haubner, R., Weber, W. A., Beer, A. J., et al. (2005) Noninvasive visualization of the activated avb3 integrin in cancer patients by positron emission tomography and [^{18}F]galacto-RGD. *PLoS Med* **2**, e70.
8. Beer, A. J., Haubner, R., Wolf, I., et al. (2006) PET-based human dosimetry of ^{18}F-galacto-RGD, a new radiotracer for imaging avb3 expression. *J Nucl Med* **47**, 763–769.
9. Fung, S. and Hruby, V. J. (2005) Design of cyclic and other templates for potent and selective peptide α-MSH analogues. *Curr Opin Chem Biol* **9**, 352–358.
10. Handl, H. L., Vagner, J., Yamamura, H. I., Hruby, V. J., and Gillies, R. J. (2005) Development of a lanthanide-based assay for detection of receptor–ligand interactions at the delta-opioid receptor. *Anal Biochem* **343**, 299–307.
11. Black, K. C., Kirkpatrick, N. D., Troutman, T. S., Xu, L., Vagner, J., Gillies, R. J., Barton, J. K., Utzinger, U., and Romanowski, M. (2008) Gold nanorods targeted to delta opioid receptor: plasmon-resonant contrast and photothermal agents. *Mol Imaging* **7**, 50–57.
12. Balagurunathan, Y., Morse, D. L., Hostetter, G., Shanmugam, V., Stafford, P., et al. (2008) Gene expression profiling-based identification of cell-surface targets for developing multimeric ligands in pancreatic cancer. *Mol Cancer Ther* **7**, 3071–3080.
13. Tangrea, M. A., Wallis, B. S., Gillespie, J. W., Gannot, G., Emmert-Buck, M. R., and Chuaqui, R. F. (2004) Novel proteomic approaches for tissue analysis. *Expert Rev Proteomics* **1**, 185–192.
14. Kononen, J., Bubendorf, L., Kallioniemi, A., et al. (1998) Tissue microarrays for high-throughput molecular profiling of tumor specimens. *Nat Med* **4**, 844–847.
15. Andersen, C. L., Hostetter, G., Grigoryan, A., Sauter, G., and Kallioniemi, A. (2001) Improved procedure for fluorescence in situ hybridization on tissue microarrays. *Cytometry* **45**, 83–86.
16. Mousses, S., Bubendorf, L., Wagner, U., et al. (2002) Clinical validation of candidate genes associated with prostate cancer progression in the CWR22 model system using tissue microarrays. *Cancer Res* **62**, 1256–1260.
17. Watanabe, A., Cornelison, R., and Hostetter, G. (2005) Tissue microarrays: applications in genomic research. *Expert Rev Mol Diagn* **5**, 171–181.
18. Morse, D. L., Carroll, D., Weberg, L., Borgstrom, M. C., Ranger-Moore, J., and Gillies, R. J. (2005) Determining suitable internal standards for mRNA quantification of increasing cancer progression in human breast cells by real-time reverse transcriptase polymerase chain reaction. *Anal Biochem* **342**, 69–77.
19. Lynch, R. M., Fogarty, K. E., and Fay, F. S. (1991) Modulation of hexokinase association with mitochondria analyzed with quantitative three-dimensional confocal microscopy. *J Cell Biol* **112**, 385–395.
20. Bittner, M., Meltzer, P., Chen, Y., Jiang, Y., Seftor, E., Hendrix, M., Radmacher, M., Simon, R., Yakhinik, Z., Ben-Dork, A., Sampask, N., Dougherty, E., Wang, E., Marincola, F., Gooden, C., Lueders, J., Glatfelter, A., Pollock, P., Carpten, J., Gillanders, E., Leja, D., Dietrich, K., Beaudry, C., Berens, M., Alberts, D., Sondak, V., Hayward, N., and Trent, J. (2000) Molecular classification of cutaneous malignant melanoma by gene expression profiling. *Nat Lett* **406**, 536–540.

Chapter 14

Preparation and Characterization of Doxorubicin Liposomes

Guoqin Niu, Brian Cogburn, and Jeffrey Hughes

Abstract

During nanoparticle system in drug delivery, liposomes were perhaps the best characterized and one of the first to be developed. Stealth liposomes (SLs), containing polyethylene glycol-conjugated lipid, which can form a hydro-layer around liposomes bilayer, have a long circulation time and hence result in enhanced drug efficiency. Doxorubicin (DOX), an effective anticancer drug, can be loaded into liposomes by transmembrane pH gradient method to get high encapsulation efficiency with high drug/lipid ratio. Liposomal doxorubicin is a successful clinical formulation, and also a perfect model drug system for cancer-therapy research. Here we described the preparation of SLs via extrusion, DOX loading by transmembrane pH gradient method, and characterization analysis, including phospholipid concentration, size, transmission electronic microscopy graph, encapsulation efficiency, and in vitro drug release.

Key words: Doxorubicin, liposome, stealth liposome, transmembrane pH gradient loading, size distribution, encapsulation efficiency, in vitro release.

1. Introduction

There are several methods for the incorporation of drugs into liposomes depending on the chemical characteristics of the drug and the liposome formulation. In some cases simple methods can be used to dramatically increase drug encapsulation. Transmembrane pH gradients drug loading (1, 2) is an active drug-loading process, which means drug is loaded into preformed vesicles with a chemical gradient. When doxorubicin ($pK_a = 8.6$) is incubated at neutral pH in the presence of liposomes exhibiting a ΔpH (interior acidic), the neutral (nonionized) form of the drug will diffuse down its concentration gradient into the liposome interior, where it will be subsequently protonated and precipitated.

To directly establish the trans-bilayer pH gradient, liposomes are prepared in an acidic buffer (300 mM citrate buffer), and the exterior buffer of the liposomes is then adjusted to a desired pH (7.0 – 8.0) using bases (sodium carbonate, sodium phosphate) or, alternatively, exchanging the outside buffer using column chromatography or dialysis. Protons (H^+) are permeable than any other cations, which result in a ΔpH between outside and inside liposome bilayer.

2. Materials

2.1. Preparation of Doxorubicin Liposomes

1. Distearoyl phosphatidylcholine (DSPC), cholesterol (CHOL), distearoyl phosphatidylethanolamine-*N*-monomethoxy polyethylene glycol (M_w 2,000) (mPEG-DSPE) were purchased from Avanti Polar Lipids Inc. Alabaster, AL. All lipids were stored at under –20°C. Prior to weighing, lipids should be brought to room temperature.

2. Doxorubicin was purchased from Sigma Chemical Co., St. Louis, MO. As with the handling of any cytotoxic agent, gloves and masks must be used when weighing doxorubicin.

3. Hydration buffer: pH 4.0, 0.3 mol/L citrate buffer, 39.35 g citric acid (M_w 210.1), and 33.15 g sodium citrate (M_w 294.1) dissolved in deionized water to make 1,000 mL. Store at room temperature.

4. Base for adjusting liposomes external pH: 0.5 mol/L sodium carbonate, 52.995 g sodium carbonate (M_w 105.99) dissolved in deionized water to make 1,000 mL. Store at room temperature.

5. 0.9% Sodium chloride (NaCl).

6. High-pressure homogenizers, EmulsiFlex-C5, Avestin, Inc., Ontario, Canada.

2.2. Phosphorus Assay

1. Dipotassium hydrogen phosphate trihydrate (M_w 228.24) standard solution: 18.418 mg dissolved in deionized water to make 25 mL. At this concentration, 10 µL standard solution contains 1 µg phosphorus. Store at room temperature.

2. Perchloric acid (70% w/w), hazardous, handle with caution, wearing gloves, in fume hood.

3. 2.5% Ammonium molybdate: 2.5 g ammonium molybdate dissolved in 100 mL diH_2O, freshly made

4. 10% Ascorbic acid: 10 g ascorbic acid dissolved in 100 mL diH_2O, freshly made, prevent from light.

5. UV–VIS Spectrophotometer, UV-2401, Shimadzu Scientific Instruments, Columbia, MD.

2.3. Transmission Electron Microscopy

1. 2% Phosphotungstic acid (PTA): 2 g phosphotungstic acid dissolved in 100 mL diH_2O, adjust pH to 7.0 with KOH. Store at 2–8°C.
2. Hitachi H-7600 Transmission Electron Microscope, Hitachi High Technologies America, Inc., Electron Microscope Division Headquarters, Pleasanton, CA. Performed in EM Core Facility, University of Florida.

2.4. Size Determination

Submicron Particle Sizer (Nicomp 380 ZLS, Particle Sizing Systems, Inc., Santa Barbara, CA).

2.5. Encapsulation Efficiency

1. Doxorubicin liposomes lysis solution: 90% isopropanol containing 10% 0.075 mol/L hydrochloride.
2. Sephadex G50 (medium), 4 g power added into 200 mL diH_2O or the external buffer used for the liposomes, boiled for 1 h, cooled down to room temperature.
3. Column, 1.5 cm × 15 cm, clean and intact with the nets, net fasteners, silicon tubes.

2.6. In Vitro Release

1. Drug release buffer: pH 7.4, 10 mM PBS, 150 mM NaCl, and/or containing 1% human serum.
2. Dialysis bag, cutoff size 8,000–12,000, immersed in boiled diH_2O for 30 min, rinse with PBS buffer.
3. F-3000 spectrofluorometer (Hitachi, Japan).

3. Methods

3.1. Preparation of Doxorubicin Liposomes

1. Weigh 160 mg DSPC, 39.2 mg cholesterol, 39.8 mg MPEG2000-DSPE (with mole ratio 2:1:0.14) using an analytical balance, dissolve in 10 mL chloroform in a 50-mL round-bottom flask.
2. The round-bottom flask was set in a rotary evaporator, the organic solvent was evaporated under reduced pressure, and the flask was seated in a 30–35°C water bath. And after a dried thin film formed on the wall of the flask, the flask was further dried under vacuum for 4–6 h to eliminate the residual solvent.
3. The dry film was hydrated with 10 mL, pH 4.0, 0.3 mol/L citric buffer, vortex 5 min, and then shaking 1 h at 65°C. Multi-layer vesicles (MLV) were formed.

4. The size of the formed MLV was reduced by five freeze–thaw cycles using liquid nitrogen and 65°C water bath. Wear eye protection goggles and cotton gloves.

5. Clean the homogenizer with phosphate-free soap water, hot tap water, ethanol, and distilled water and last the hydration buffer. Maintain the extruder at 65°C (**Note 1**).

6. The MLV, after the freeze–thaw cycles, was extruded through two stacked 0.4 μm and then through 0.1 μm pore-diameter polycarbonate filters using high-pressure extruder device (3, 4), each extrusion step was performed 8–11 times at 65°C. And large unilamellar vesicles (LUV) were formed.

7. The prepared liposomes (volume V0 with lipids concentration C0) pH was adjusted with that of the outer liposome pH value to pH 6.5–pH 7.0 with 0.5 mol/L sodium carbonate. Write down the volume of sodium carbonate used (V1) and the lipid concentration was estimated by the formula: $C1 = V0 \times C0/(V0+V1)$. The precise lipid concentration was determined by phosphorus assay, which was described in **Section 3.2.1** (**Note 2**).

8. Preheat proper volume DOX (10.0 mg/mL in 0.9% sodium chloride, Drug/Lipid = 1:5–10 mole ratio) to 65°C, mix with 5-mL liposome solution with outside pH 6.5–7.0, shaking 20 min at 65°C (**Note 3**).

9. DOX liposome was prepared.

3.2. Liposome Characterization Analysis

This section includes the following several parts:
- Phospholipids concentration determination by phosphorus assay
- Liposome morphology by transmission electron microscopy
- Liposome-size distribution
- Liposomal encapsulation efficiency
- In vitro release

3.2.1. Phospholipids Concentration Determination by Phosphorus Assay

1. Take 0, 10, 20, 30, 40, and 50 μL dipotassium hydrogen phosphate trihydrate standard solution into a 15-mL glass tube with glass stopper, triplicate, and add deionized water to each tube to make 50 μL in total (5).

2. Add 0.5 mL perchloric acid (70% w/w), mix, and heat in oil bath for 4.5 h at 130°C, manipulate in hood.

3. The tubes were cooled down to room temperature, and added the fresh cocktail containing 3.0 mL deionized water, 1 mL 2.5% ammonium molybdate, and 0.5 mL 10% ascorbic acid. Mix well immediately.

4. Incubate 1.5 h at 37°C, shaking. Then cool down to room temperature.

5. Reading the absorbance at 822 nm wavelength via UV–VIS spectrophotometer. A standard curve of absorbance versus phosphorus concentration is obtained.

6. Take 10–50 μL liposome sample and add deionized water to make 50 μL, and then follow the above Steps 2–5.

7. The lipid concentration was calculated according to the standard curve.

3.2.2. Liposome Morphology by Transmission Electron Microscopy (TEM)

1. Place one drop of liposome specimen onto a sheet of parafilm (4).

2. Place plastic/carbon-coated 400-mesh copper grid (film face down) on drop and let absorb for approximately 10 min.

3. Wick away excess fluid with filter paper.

4. Stain: Place grid (plastic-side down) on drop of filtered 2% PTA, pH 7.0, and let stain for 1–2 min.

5. Wick away excess fluid with filter paper, and place grids, specimen-side up, in specimen petri dish, and further dried in air for 30 min.

6. The specimens were observed using a Hitachi H-7600 Transmission Electron Microscope operating at 80 kV.

3.2.3. Size-Distribution Analysis

1. DOX liposome samples of 0.2 mL was diluted to 1.0 mL with 0.9% NaCl (filtered through 0.2 μm membrane), generally, phospholipid concentration was in the range of 2–10 mg/mL and analyzed by Submicron Particle Sizer (6).

2. Turn on the Submicron Particle Sizer (Nicomp 380 ZLS, Particle Sizing Systems, Inc., Santa Barbara, CA) and turn on the computer and then the ZW 380 software.

3. Click "setup" on the menu, choose "Fixed angel 90 Deg," click OK, and "Correlator is connected" shows up.

4. Click "Particle sizing" on the menu, and choose "Control menu," "Autoprint/save menu" to set the measuring parameters and the file path.

5. Transfer the diluted sample into the small glass tube by pipette, the intensity reading of the sample should be around 300.

6. Choose "Vesicle" style for liposome-size measuring from the icon tools.

7. Print the size and its distribution. Generally, if Chi-squared is under 3, Gaussian distribution is used, and when Chi-squared is larger than 3, Nicomp distribution is used. And the volume-weighting is often used for liposomes.

3.2.4. Liposomal Encapsulation Efficiency

1. Swell 4 g of Sephadex G50 medium with 200 mL deionized water in a boiled water bath for 1 h. Prepare a media slurry in a ratio of 70% settled gel to 30% buffer. Equilibrate to room temperature (7).

2. Prepare the column 1.5 cm × 15 cm, make sure that the nets, net fasteners, and glass tube are clean and intact. Mount the column vertically on a laboratory stand. Fill the column with a few milliliters of buffer using the syringe from the bottom, pour the media slurry into the column, down a glass rod against the wall of the column, in one continuous motion, and equilibrate the column with 100 mL buffer.

3. Add 1 mL liposome sample on the top of the column, let it run into the gel, and then add a few mL buffer to the column, elute with buffer, collect DOX liposomes, write down the volume (**Section 4**).

4. Dissolve 0.1 mL DOX liposome sample before and after the column with 0.9 mL of 90% isopropanol containing 10% 0.075 mol/L HCl, measure absorbance at 480 nm by UV–VIS spectrophotometer.

5. Liposomal DOX encapsulation efficiency (EE%) is
   EE% = [A1 × V1/A0] × 100%

   A1: The absorbance of the sample after the column

   A0: The absorbance of the sample before the column

   V1: The volume obtained from 1 mL sample running the column

3.2.5. In Vitro Drug Release

1. Prepare the standard curve of fluorescence versus DOX concentration in PBS. The DOX standard solution of 0, 0.1, 0.2, 0.4, 0.6, 0.8, 1.0, and 1.2 μg/mL in PBS, triplicate, fluorescence was measured at excitation wavelength $\lambda_{Ex} = 501$ nm and emission wavelength $\lambda_{Em} = 555$ nm. The standard curves of DOX in 1% human serum–PBS and 0.075 mol/L HCl–90% isopropanol were the same as in PBS, except DOX dissolving in the corresponding buffer (8).

2. Cut dialysis bag (cutoff size 8,000–12,000) with 5 cm length, hydrated with PBS buffer. Seal at one end, add 1 mL DOX liposomes into the bag, and seal the other end.

3. Put the bag into a 50-mL round-bottom flask, filled with 50 mL PBS, triplicate each sample. Shake the flasks at 37°C at 100 rpm.

4. At 0, 0.5, 1, 2, 3, 5, 7, and 10 h, take 1 mL sample from the flask, and add 1 mL PBS at the same temperature to the

flask. Measure fluorescence at excitation wavelength $\lambda_{Ex} = 501$ nm and emission wavelength $\lambda_{Em} = 555$ nm.

5. At the end point, cut the dialysis bag and release all samples to the flask, as total released concentration after calibration with DOX content taken out of each point.

6. Drug release curve can be obtained by release percentage versus time.

3.3. Results

3.3.1. The Morphology of the LUV

The morphology of the LUV was observed by transmission electron microscopy and was shown in **Fig. 14.1**. The LUVs were spherical particles with integrated bilayers. A fingerprint-like surface on the liposomes was distinct. The vesicle sizes were about 80–120 nm.

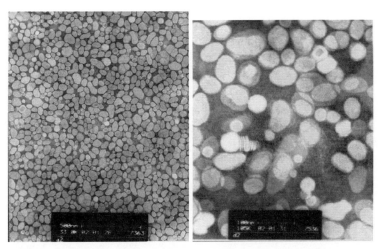

Fig. 14.1. TEM pictures of SLs prepared by high-pressure extrusion method. Samples for TEM were made by negative staining as described in Section 3. Scale: 500 nm (*left*) and 100 nm (*right*).

3.3.2. Particle Size of Prepared Liposomes and Doxorubicin Liposomes

According to results measured by dynamic light scattering method, the average diameters of stealth liposomes and doxorubicin liposomes were very similar. The volume-weighting size of LUVs was 134.85 nm ± 4.70 nm ($n = 4$), and that of DOX liposomes was 141.23 ± 4.83 nm ($n = 4$). The particle sizes of LUVs were slightly less than DOX liposomes. It may be due to the encapsulation of doxorubicin.

3.3.3. Liposomal DOX Encapsulation Efficiency

For the liposomes composed of DSPC: Cholesterol: MPEG2000-DSPE (with mole ratio 2:1:0.14), loaded DOX by transmembrane pH gradient method, the encapsulation efficiency was 96.27% ± 2.22% ($n = 3$), when DOX/Phospholipids = 1:5 (w/w).

3.3.4. In Vitro Drug Release Curve

In vitro drug release curve was shown in **Fig. 14.2**. At 10 h, DOX release percentage from Stealth liposomes in PBS at 37°C was about 13.5%, while from Immunoliposomes (DOX-SL-IgG) (9) it was about 20.8%. As in 1% human serum-PBS, DOX only released about 6.0% from Stealth liposomes and 8.7% from Immunoliposomes (DOX-SL-IgG) at the same condition. This may be due to the human serum preventing DOX's release and diffusion.

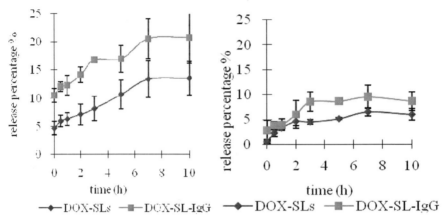

Fig. 14.2. In vitro DOX-SLs and DOX-SL-IgG drug release percentage versus time at 37°C. *Left*: DOX release curve in pH 7.4, 10 mM PBS. *Right*: DOX release curve in pH 7.4, 10 mM PBS, containing 1% human serum. *Diamond*: DOX-SLs, *square*: DOX-SLs-IgG.

4. Notes

1. The extrusion step may be performed by different extrusion device, such as Thermobarrel Extruder System (Northern Lipids Inc., Vancouver, BC, Canada). The key point is to maintain the whole sample extrusion circle at the temperature 5°C above the lipid's phase transition point (T_m).

2. Transmembrane pH gradient can be established directly or indirectly. For direct method, liposomes were hydrated with an acid buffer, then the eternal buffer was adjusted with base (illustrated in **Section 3**), or changed by column chromatography, or dialysis. For indirect method, ammonium sulfate (10) was often used another method to prepare DOX liposomes; and manganese sulfate and potassium sulfate were also used (11).

3. The success of getting a high encapsulation efficiency is to pre-incubate both DOX solution and liposomes at the temperature of 5°C above the lipid's phase transition point (T_m).

References

1. Mayer, L. D., Bally, M. B., and Cullis, P. R. (1986) Uptake of adriamycin into large unilamellar vesicles in response to a pH gradient. *Biochim Biophys Acta* **857**(1), 123–126.
2. Madden, T. D., Harrigan, P. R., Tai, L. C., Bally, M. B., Mayer, L. D., Redelmeier, T. E., Loughrey, H. C., Tilcock, C. P., Reinish, L. W., and Cullis, P. R. (1990) The accumulation of drugs within large unilamellar vesicles exhibiting a proton gradient: a survey. *Chem Phys Lipids* **53**(1), 37–46.
3. Schneider, T., Sachse, A., Rößling, G., and Brandl, M. (1994) Large-scale production of liposomes of defined size by a new continuous high pressure extrusion device. *Drug Dev Ind Pharm* **20**, 2787–2807.
4. Schneider, T., Sachse, A., Rößling, G., and Brandl, M. (1995) Generation of contrast-carrying liposomes of defined size with a new continuous high pressure extrusion method. *Int J Pharm* **117**(1), 1–12.
5. Mrsny, R. J., Volwerk, J. J., and Griffith, O. H. (1986) A simplified procedure for lipid phosphorus analysis shows that digestion rates vary with phospholipid structure. *Chem Phys Lipids* **39**, 185–191.
6. Berger, N., Sachse, A., Bender, J., Schubert, R., and Brandl, M. (2001) Filter extrusion of liposomes using different devices: comparison of liposome size, encapsulation efficiency, and process characteristics. *Int J Pharm* **223**(1–2), 55–68.
7. Mayer, L. D., Bally, M. B., and Cullis, P. R. (1986) Uptake of adriamycin into large unilamellar vesicles in response to a pH gradient. *Biochim Biophys Acta* **857**(1), 123–126.
8. Sivakumar, P. A. and Panduranga Rao, K. (2001) Polymerized (ethylene glycol) dimethacrylate-cholesteryl methacrylate liposomes: preparation and stability studies. *React Funct Polym* **49**, 179–187.
9. Allen, T. M., Brandeis, E., Hansen, C. B., Kao, G. Y., and Zalipsky, S. (1995) A new strategy for attachment of antibodies to sterically stabilized liposomes resulting in efficient targeting to cancer cells. *Biochim Biophys Acta* **1237**, 99–108.
10. Lasic, D. D., Frederik, P. M., Stuart, M. C., Barenholz, Y., and McIntosh, T. J. (1992) Gelation of liposome interior. A novel method for drug encapsulation. *FEBS Lett* **312**, 255–258.
11. Abraham, S. A., Waterhouse, D. N., Mayer, L. D., Cullis, P. R., Madden, T. D., and Bally, M. B. (2005) The liposomal formulation of doxorubicin. *Methods Enzymol* **391**, 71–97.

Chapter 15

PEGylated Nanocarriers for Systemic Delivery

N.K. Jain and Manoj Nahar

Abstract

In this chapter, we outline the protocols for PEGylation of some drug carriers, such as dendrimer, polymeric nanoparticles, liposomes, for systemic delivery. PEGylation simply refers to the modification of particle surface by covalently grafting, entrapping, or adsorbing PEG chains of vivid length. However, limitation of simple adsorption being easy displacement of the coating layer in vivo, covalent mode for PEGylation of nanoparticles is mostly preferred, and outlined herein. Derivatization and activation of polyethylene glycol is an important step during PEGylation and its chemistry chiefly relies on availability as well as type of functional groups on carrier periphery. A summarized set of protocols for PEGylation of widely explored nanocarriers for systemic delivery is presented.

Key words: PEGylation, dendrimer, nanoparticles, liposomes, covalent conjugation.

1. Introduction

The covalent coupling of poly(ethylene glycol) (PEG) to pharmaceutical drugs, to proteins, or to surfaces of carriers is commonly termed as PEGylation. PEG is a hydrophilic, nonionic polyether that has been shown to possess excellent biocompatibility. PEG is nontoxic and has been approved by the FDA for systemic use (1). It is a neutral polymer with hydroxyl end groups that are weak hydrogen bond acids, and weakly basic ether linkages in the backbone. Lower PEGs are viscous and colorless liquids, whereas higher molecular weight PEGs are waxy liquids. They are soluble in water, alcohol, acetone, and chloroform, miscible with glycols but practically insoluble in ether. PEG is linear polyether diol that possesses a number of outstanding physiochemical and biological properties, including hydrophilicity, solubility in water and organic solvent, absence of antigenicity and immunogenicity, and lack of toxicity. Terminal hydroxyl groups of PEG were activated, functionalized, and conjugated with nanoparticles. Higher molecular weight PEGs (2,000–5,000) suppress protein adsorption and are therefore preferred for steric stabilization. The steric stabilization conferred by PEG probably is due to its strongly hydrophilic nature, flexibility of PEG chains, and neutral charge at surface, which prevent interactions with biological components in vivo (2, 3). Various mechanisms have been established to explain the stealth behavior. Surface modification increases hydrophilicity, decreases interaction with serum components, provides flexibility, and thus disguises from being recognized by the opsonins thereby preventing its uptake by the macrophages resulting in steric stabilization of particles (4, 5).

Advantages of PEGylation include increased stability (against temperature, pH, solvent, etc.), enhanced drug solubility, lowered renal clearance, increased half-life, reduced toxicity, reduced immunogenicity, and antigenicity (6). PEGylation can be achieved by several methods such as physical or chemical adsorption, grafting and incorporation of PEG chain (7–11). However, the drawback of simple adsorption is an easy displacement of the coating layer in vivo and hence covalent mode for PEGylation of nanocarriers is preferred. The subject of chemical derivatization of the end groups of PEG, which is often an essential first step in the preparation of bioconjugates, was recently reviewed by our group (12). Derivatization and activation of polyethylene glycol is an important step in the synthesis of the PEGylated system. Schematic preparation of the PEGylated system with covalent modification is shown in **Fig. 15.1** (12).

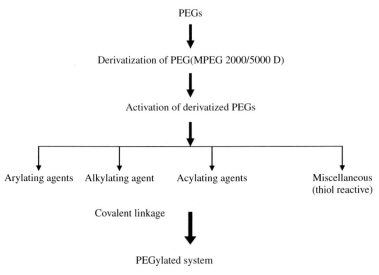

Fig. 15.1. Principle steps in the preparation of PEGylated systems.

Literature is replete with the reports on PEGylation of a variety of nanocarriers, namely dendrimer, liposomes and polymeric nanoparticles used for drug delivery. Chemistry of PEGylation of these carriers differs widely due to variance in availability of functional groups and their mode of preparation. For example, polymeric nanoparticles can be functionalized with PEG by (1) physical coating of preformed nanoparticles with PEG copolymer, (2) covalent conjugation of PEG with the preformed nanoparticles surface, and (3) use of block copolymer of PEG with polymer (7–11). On the other hand, PEGylated dendrimers can be developed on the basis of orientation of PEG chains required in the dendrimers. The first category includes preparation of simple PEGylated dendrimers having PEG chains conjugated to their periphery. The second category includes preparation of dendrimers having PEG as a core material. The inner PEG core increases the distance between branching units of the dendrimers and prevents the drug dumping into the dendritic core. Likewise preparation of dendrimers with PEG as branching monomer unit constitutes the third category of PEGylated dendrimers, whereas drug-conjugated PEGylated dendrimers constitute the fourth category having PEG chains in between the drug and the dendrimers. PEG increases steric hindrance over the dendrimer, which precludes entry of drug inside the dendrimer and causes controlled release (13). Moreover, PEGylated liposome is usually prepared by incorporation of PEG-conjugated lipid along with other lipids during liposome preparation.

2. Materials

1. Monomethoxy polyethylene glycol (PEG) with a molecular weight of 5,000 Da
2. Monomethoxy polyethylene glycol 2000 (MPEG-2000)
3. Polyethylene glycol 2000 (PEG-2000)
4. Lysine
5. Fluorenemethoxy carbonyl succinimide (FMOC-Su)
6. N,N'-Dicyclohexyl carbodiimide (DCC)
7. 1-Hydroxybenzotriazole (HOBT)
8. Dimethylamino pyridine (DMAP)
9. Sodium azide
10. 10% Pd catalyst adsorbed on charcoal
11. Ethylenediamine (EDA)
12. Methylmethacrylate (MAA)

13. Acrylonitrile
14. *N*-Hydroxysuccinimide (NHS)
15. Raney nickel (in 10% NaOH)
16. Miglyol 812®, a triglyceride formed from medium-chain fatty acids
17. The surfactant soybean L-α-lecithin and Poloxamer 188 (Pluronic F-68®)
18. Chitosan hydrochloride salt (Protasan® Cl110)
19. *N*-(3-Dimethylaminopropyl)-*N*′-ethylcarbodiimide hydrochloride (EDC)
20. Poly(D,L-lactide-*co*-glycolide) PLGA (50:50 molar ratio, with free end carboxyl groups, MW 45,500 Da), Resomer® RG 503
21. Stannous octoate, $Sn(Oct)_2$
22. Sodium cholate (99%)
23. Type-B gelatin (225 bloom strength) with 100–115 mmol of free carboxylic acid per 100 g of protein, an isoelectric point of 4.7–5.2, and an average molecular weight of 40,000–50,000 Da
24. *N*,*N*-dimethylformamide
25. Epichlorohydrin
26. Ethanol
27. Cellulose dialysis tubing of MWCO 12,000–14,000 and pore size of 2.4 nm
28. Specialized equipments (*see* text).

3. Methods

The following sections describe the outline for (1) the synthesis of PEGylated dendrimers (lysine, PPI, and PAMAM); (2) synthesis and preparation of PEGylated polymeric nanoparticles (chitosan, PLGA, and gelatin); and (3) preparation of PEGylated liposomes.

3.1. PEGylated Dendrimers

3.1.1. Synthesis of MPEG-Lysine Dendrimers

The MPEG-lysine-diFMOC dendrimers are synthesized using MPEG-amine 2,000 Da and 5,000 Da as core and protected diFMOC-lysine for progressive linking on terminal amino groups of prior generations consecutively by liquid-phase peptide synthesis (14). **Figure 15.2** represents the synthesis of MPEG-lysine dendrimers.

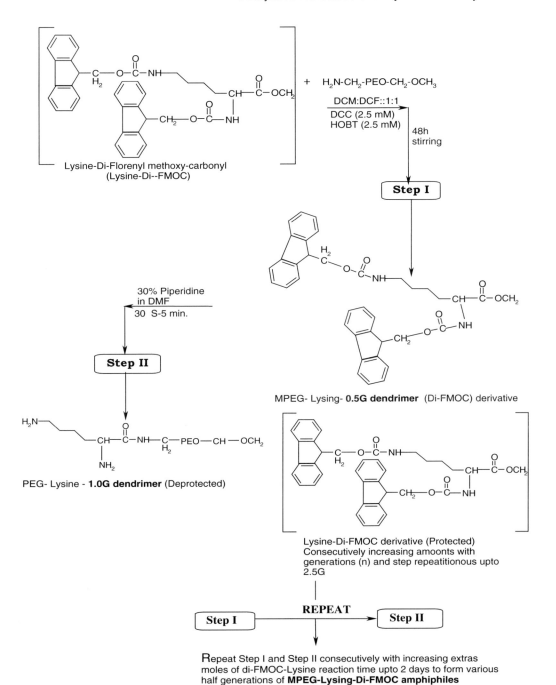

Fig. 15.2. Structural scheme for synthesis of PEGylated lysine dendrimer (adapted from 14 with copyright permission).

1. Synthesize MPEG-amine by stepwise synthesis scheme as suggested by Zalipsky et al. (15). Briefly, synthesis of MPEG-amine is carried out by first tosylation of PEG followed by reaction of the product with K-phthalimide and finally removal of the phthaloyl group by hydrazine.

2. Synthesize FMOC-protected lysine using FMOC-Su (fluorenylmethoxy carbonyl succinimide) to form diFMOC lysine by the method suggested by Lapatsanis et al. (16). (*see* **Note 1**).
3. Synthesize MPEG-terminated lysine-diFMOC micellar systems of various generations by the well-known DCC-HOBT coupling procedure in DCM:DMF (1:1) solvent system.
4. Deprotect diFMOC groups from the micelles by piperidine-based hydrolysis for synthesis of further higher generations.
5. Repeat protection and de-protection steps alternately with subsequent increase in reactants for every consecutive generations, up to 2.5G.
6. Separate products, dry, and store in a vacuum desiccator.
7. Characterize the products by FTIR, ^{1}H-NMR.

3.1.2. PEGylation of PAMAM Dendrimers

PEGylated PAMAM dendrimers are synthesized in two steps, i.e., synthesis of dendrimers followed by PEGylation at the periphery (17).

3.1.2.1. Synthesis of Poly(Amidoamine) (PAMAM) Dendrimers

The dendrimers are synthesized following two consecutive chain-forming reactions: the exhaustive Michael addition reaction and the exhaustive amidation reaction, repeated alternatively (18–20) (*see* **Note 2**).

1. React methanolic methyl methacrylate solution (5% molar excess) with methanolic solution of ethylenediamine in a light-resistant round-bottomed flask to form ester-terminated dendrimers. Evaporate excess methanol using a rotary vacuum evaporator.
2. Treat ester-terminated structure with methanolic ethylenediamine (10 molar times) and keep for 55 h in dark. Remove excess of ethylenediamine under high vacuum (5 mm of Hg) to yield 0.0G dendrimers.
3. Repeat this reaction sequence required number of times to produce PAMAM dendrimers up to generation four (4.0G PAMAM).
4. Confirm completion of every step in the synthesis by reacting with copper sulfate solution. The full generation yields a purple color while half-generation gives a deep-blue color due to copper chelation at the terminal groups of the dendrimers. The synthesized PAMAM dendrimers are characterized by FTIR and ^{1}H-NMR.

3.1.2.2. PEGylation of PAMAM Dendrimers

The end functional groups of MPEG-5000 are activated by first converting them into carboxylic acid derivatives and then into NHS ester as shown in **Fig. 15.3** (21), followed by PEGylation.

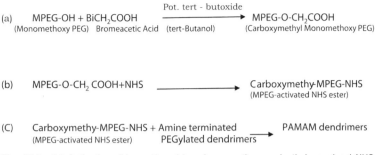

Fig. 15.3. (a) Activation, (b) reaction, (c) carboxy methoxy polyethylene glycol-NHS-activated ester with dendrimer.

1. Dissolve lyophilized 4.0G PAMAM dendrimers having 64 terminal amine groups of theoretical molecular weight 15.932 g (100 mg, 6.3 μM) in double-distilled water.
2. Add 16 molar times of MPEG-activated NHS ester (0.55 g) at basic pH (8–10) to dendrimers solution and stir vigorously for 2 h at room temperature (RT) in the dark.
3. Dialyze the final product to remove the by-products.
4. Concentrate the dialyzed product and lyophilize.
5. Dissolve the resultant product in dichloromethane and precipitate it from cold diethyl ether as oily viscid lump, separate and dry.

3.1.3. PEGylation of Poly(Propylene Imine) (PPI) Dendrimers

3.1.3.1. Synthesis of PPI Dendrimers

Poly(propylene imine) dendrimers are synthesized using repetition of double Michael addition of acrylonitrile to primary amines, followed by heterogeneously catalyzed hydrogenation of the nitriles, resulting in a doubling of the number of primary amines. In this sequence, ethylenediamine (EDA) has been used as dendrimer core, but a variety of molecules with primary or secondary amine groups such as 1,4-diaminobutane can also be used (22–24).

1. Add acrylonitrile (443 g, 8.35 mol), which is about 2.5 molar times per terminal NH_2 group of core amine moiety to a solution of ethylenediamine (100.34 g, 1.67 mol) in 1.176 kg water.
2. The exothermic reaction causes the temperature to rise to 38°C. After this exothermic effect of the reaction, heat the mixture at 80°C for 1 h to complete the addition reaction.
3. Remove the excess of acrylonitrile as a water azeotrope by vacuum distillation (16 mbar, bath temperature 40°C). The crystalline solid obtained is 0.5G PPI dendrimer. The general formula of half-generation can be represented as (EDA-dendr-$(CN)_{4n}$), where n is the generation of reaction or reaction cycle (*see* **Note 3**).

4. Dissolve EDA-dendr-(CN)$_4$ in methanol.

5. Add Raney nickel catalyst pretreated with hydroxide (900 g) and water to hydrogenation vessel. Hydrogenate EDA-dendr-(CN)$_4$ methanolic solution at 40 atm hydrogen pressure at 70°C for 1 h.

6. Cool and filter the reaction mixture and evaporate the solvent at reduced pressure. The residue contains 1.0G PPI dendrimer [EDA-dendr-(NH$_2$)$_4$].

7. Repeat all the above steps consecutively, with increasing quantity of acrylonitrile to prepare PPI dendrimer up to 5.0G. The general formula of half-generation can be represented as [EDA-dendr-(NH$_2$)$_{4n}$] where n is the generation of reaction or reaction cycle.

3.1.3.2. PEGylation of PPI Dendrimer

PEGylation of PPI dendrimer is reported by two schemes. In the first scheme, PEGylation is performed following the activation of end functional groups of PEG 2000 by converting them into dicarboxylic acid derivatives and subsequently into NHS ester according to Veronese et al. (21), with slight modification. This is the first report of PEGylation on dendrimer by dicarboxylic acid PEG 2000 as shown in **Fig. 15.4** (22). Chloroacetic acid is used to prepare dicarboxymethyl PEG 2000 diether (CM-PEG-CM). This generates two carboxylic acid functional groups on PEG 2000.

1. Dissolve PEG 2000(4 mM) in 50 mL of tertiary butanol at 50°C and add potassium tertbutanolate (32 mM) to it. The mixture is stirred at the same temperature overnight.

2. Solubilize chloroacetic acid (32 mM) in tertiary butanol and add slowly to the reaction mixture. Carry out the reaction under magnetic stirring for 24 h.

3. Evaporate the solvent and add 50 mL of dichloromethane to precipitate the product. Wash the product by stirring with 250 mL of water and separate the layers in a separating funnel. Remove the lower layer of dichloromethane and allow the mixture to stand for 1 h and concentrate to 10–15 mL.

4. Add cold ether (200 mL) to the mixture, keep in the refrigerator overnight with excess of ether.

5. Remove the precipitate and re-precipitate by dichloromethane and ether precipitation repeatedly to remove impurities.

6. Dry the precipitate of dicarboxylic acid PEG 2000 in a Petri dish.

7. Convert dicarboxylic acid PEG 2000 into NHS ester by DCC and NHS (*see* **Note 4**).

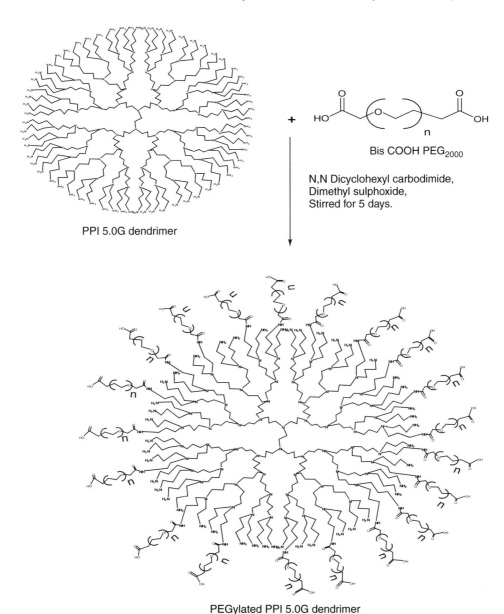

Fig. 15.4. Synthesis of PEGylated PPI dendrimers (adapted from 22 with copyright permission).

8. Mix solution of PPI 5.0G dendrimer (0.01 mM) in dimethyl sulfoxide (DMSO) (10 mL) and NHS ester of dicarboxylic acid PEG 2000 (0.32 mM) in DCM (10 mL) and stir the solution for 5 days at room temperature.

9. Precipitate the product from cold diethyl ether, filter, and dialyze through dialysis membrane (MWCO 12–14 kDa) to remove free bis carboxylic acid PEG 2000, DCC, and partially PEGylated dendrimers, followed by lyophilization.

While in the second scheme, MPEG is activated into MPEG carboxylic acid moiety and thereafter PEGylation is carried out with the amine terminal of dendrimers using DCC. Details of this scheme are given below (23).

1. Dissolve MPEG 2000 (8 g, 8 mmol), succinic anhydride (500 mg, 10 mmol), 4 dimethyl amino pyridine (488 mg, 8 mmol), and triethylamine (404 mg, 8 mmol) in dioxane and stir the resulting solution overnight at room temperature. Evaporate dioxane in vacuum and dissolve the residue in dichloromethane, filter, and concentrate the solution.

2. Precipitate MPEG-COOH 2000 with ether and dry in an oven to remove final traces of solvent.

3. Add MPEG-COOH 2000 (0.32 mmol) in DMSO (10 mL) and N,N' dicyclohexyl carbodiimide (DCC) (0.32 mmol) in DMSO (10 mL) to a solution of 4G EDA-PPI dendrimer (0.01 mmol) in dimethyl sulfoxide (DMSO) (10 mL), and stir the solution for 5 days at room temperature.

4. Precipitate the product by addition of water, filter, and dialyze (MWCO 12–14 kDa) against double-distilled water for 24 h to remove free MPEG-COOH 2000, DCC, and partially PEGylated dendrimers, followed by lyophilization.

3.2. PEGylated Nanoparticles

3.2.1. PEGylated Chitosan Nanocapsule

PEGylated chitosan nanocapsules are prepared by synthesizing PEGylated chitosan followed by coating of this synthesized conjugate over prepared plain chitosan nanocarriers (25).

3.2.1.1. Synthesis of PEGylated Chitosan

1. Dissolve chitosan hydrochloride (80 mg, 0.40 mmol) in water (11.5 mL) and add MeO-PEGCH$_2$COOH (14.2 mg, 2.79 μmol) and NHS (1.6 mg, 0.014 mmol) to the polymer solution.

2. Add EDC (21.7 mg, 0.113 mmol) in small portions (*see* **Note 3**).

3. Stir the resulting solution at room temperature for 22 h and ultrafilter (Amicon, YM30) and lyophilize.

3.2.1.2. Preparation of Chitosan–PEG Nanocapsules

Chitosan–PEG nanocapsules are prepared in two steps.

1. First, prepare a nanoemulsion by solvent displacement technique. Briefly, add an organic phase, composed of 125 μL de Miglyol, 40 mg of lecithin dissolved in 10 mL of acetone, to an aqueous phase containing Poloxamer 188 (0.25% w/v). The mixture turns milky immediately due to the formation of the nanoemulsion. Then, evaporate the solvents under vacuum.

2. Second, coat the colloidal carrier with chitosan–PEG separately with two degrees of PEGylation of chitosan, 0.5 and 1%, by simple incubation in polymer solutions. Briefly,

incubate 4 mL of the nanoemulsion for 1 h with 1 mL of chitosan–PEG aqueous solution (0.5% w/v) with different degrees of PEGylation of chitosan (0.5 and 1%), leading to the formation of chitosan–PEG 0.5% and chitosan–PEG 1% nanocapsules, respectively.

3.2.2. PEGylated PLGA Nanoparticles

3.2.2.1. Synthesis of PEGylated PLGA Diblock Copolymer

PLGA–mPEG diblock copolymers are synthesized by ring-opening polymerization of lactide and glycolide in the presence of mPEG as the initiator (10, 26).

1. Dissolve specified quantities of PLGA and mPEG in freshly distilled toluene.
2. Place the solution in a 250 mL three-necked flask equipped with a stirrer, a water-cooled condenser, and a nitrogen inlet.
3. Add stannous octoate (0.03% v/v) as a catalyst.
4. Carry out the reaction at 110°C for 6 h under continuous stirring at 250 rpm.
5. Evaporate the solvent under reduced pressure, dissolve the residue in DCM, filter, and recover a solid product against hot water.
6. Purify with excess of methanol and dry under vacuum at 40°C for 48 h.

3.2.2.2. Preparation of PEGylated PLGA Nanoparticles

1. Dissolve specified amounts of copolymer in 2 mL of DCM, vortex, and emulsify in 20 mL of a 0.1% sodium cholate solution in a sonicator at 20 W output for 1 min.
2. Evaporate organic solvent at room temperature for 4 h.
3. Recover nanoparticles by centrifugation ($33,900 \times g$, 20 min, 4°C), wash twice with water, and lyophilize.
4. Store dried nanoparticles in the refrigerator at 4°C.

3.2.3. PEGylated Gelatin Nanoparticles

3.2.3.1. Synthesis of PEGylated Gelatin

PEGylation of gelatin polymer is carried out according to the method described by Kaul and Amiji (27), using PEG-epoxide as activated derivative.

1. Dissolve poly(ethylene glycol) monomethyl ether in sufficient amount of dehydrated N,N-dimethyl formamide and 1% w/w triethanolamine mixture at 40°C.
2. Add 5 times molar excess of epichlorohydrin to the reaction mixture in a round-bottomed flask and reflux for 12 h.
3. Precipitate the PEG-epoxide in ice-cold diethyl ether and dry.
4. Add Type-A/B gelatin to a known quantity of PEG-epoxide. Proceed the reaction for 14 h at 40°C for grafting PEG-epoxide to primary amine groups of basic amino acids available at the gelatin surface.

5. Precipitate PEG-grafted gelatin derivative in acetone to remove unreacted PEG-epoxide, dialyze against deionized distilled water, and lyophilize.

3.2.3.2. Preparation of PEGylated Gelatin Nanoparticles

PEGylated gelatin nanoparticles are prepared by desolvation methods described by Balthasar et al. (28).

1. Dissolve a calculated amount of gelatin in a defined quantity of water at 50°C and add acetone to precipitate higher molecular weight gelatin.
2. Discard the supernatant and dissolve the precipitate in water at 50°C, adjust the pH to 2.5 (for gelatin A) or 12 (gelatin B) according to the type of gelatin used.
3. Add the acetone dropwise under vigorous stirring.
4. Crosslink nanoparticles with glutaraldehyde solution by keeping overnight.
5. Centrifuge the PEGylated gelatin nanoparticles at 15,000 rpm and lyophilize.

3.2.4. PEGylated Liposomes

Despite several methods used to conjugate PEG to lipids, most of the reported work utilizes PEG derivatives of the reactive primary amine of PE. Several materials such as PEG–DSPE containing a carbamate or urethane linkage are now available commercially. PEGylated liposomes are prepared by mixing commercially available PEG-conjugated lipids in mixture of lipids during the preparation of simple liposomes.

4. Notes

1. In the synthesis of lysine dendrimers, protected lysine is required for allowing uniform branching.
2. Maintain perfect nonaqueous condition in the synthesis of PAMAM dendrimer. Carry out the reaction using methanol as the medium. Use redistilled ethylenediamine whenever required. Cork the RBF tightly to avoid direct light and moisture and well cover with carbon black paper and silver foil.
3. Activate/store Raney nickel in 10% NaOH solution. Maintain the temperature below 80°C during refluxing of half-generation dendrimers. Maintain high pressure (about 40 atm) while hydrogenation.
4. Prepare EDC and NHS afresh and carry out EDC and NHS reactions in airtight containers.

References

1. Haris, J. (1992) Poly(ethylene glycol) Chemistry: Biotechnical and Biomedical Applications. Plenum Press, New York, 1.
2. Gref, R., Domp, A., Quellec, P., Blunk, T., Muller, R. H., Verbavatz, J. M., and Langer, R. (1995) The controlled intravenous delivery of drugs using PEG coated sterically stabilized nanospheres. *Adv Drug Deliv Rev* 16, 215–233.
3. Beletsi, A., Leotiadis, L., Klepetsanis, P., Ithakissios, D. S., and Avgoustakis, K. (1999) Effect of preparative variables on the properties of poly (DL-lactide-*co*-glycolide) methoxy poly (ethylene glycol) copolymers related to their application in controlled drug delivery. *Int J Pharm* 182, 187–197.
4. Strom, G., Beliot, S. O., Daemen, T., and Lasic, D. D. (1995) Surface modification of nanoparticles to oppose uptake by the mononuclear phagocyte system. *Adv Drug Deliv Rev* 17, 191–199.
5. Otsuka, H., Nagasaki, Y., and Kataoka, K. (2003) PEGylated nanoparticles for biological and pharmaceutical applications. *Adv Drug Deliv Rev* 55, 403–419.
6. Verones, F. M. and Pasut, G. (2005) PEGylation, successful approach to drug delivery. *Drug Deliv Tech* 10(21), 1451–1458.
7. Tobio, M., Sanchez, A., Vila, A., Soriano, I., Evora, C., Vila-Jato, J. L., and Alonso, M. J. (2000) The role of PEG on the stability in digestive fluids and in vivo fate of PEG–PLA nanoparticles following oral administration. *Coll Surf B Bioint* 18(3–4), 315–323.
8. Gref, R., Luck, M., Quellec, P., Marchand, M., Dellacherie, E., Harnishch, S., Blunk, T., and Muller, R. H. (2000) 'Stealth' corona-core nanoparticles surface modified by polyethylene glycol (PEG): influences of the corona (PEG chain length and surface density) and of the core composition on phagocytic uptake and plasma protein adsorption.. *Coll Surf B Bioint* 18(3–4), 301–313.
9. Calvo, P., Gouritin, B., Chacun, H., Desmaele, D., D'Angelo, J., Noel, J. P., Georgin, D., Fattal, E., Andreux, J. P., and Couvreur, P. (2001) Long circulating PEGylated polycyanoacrylate nanoparticles as new drug carrier for brain delivery. *Pharm Res* 18, 1157–1166.
10. Li, Y. P., Pei, Y. Y., Zhang, X. Y., Gu, Z. H., Zhou, Z. H., Yuan, W. F., Zhou, J. J., Zhu, J. H., and Gao, X. J. (2001) PEGylated PLGA nanoparticles as protein carrier; synthesis, preparation and bio distribution in rats. *J Control Rel* 71, 203–211.
11. Dong, Y. and Feng, S. S. (2004) Methoxy poly (ethylene glycol)-poly (lactide) (MPEG-PLA) nanoparticles for controlled delivery of anticancer drugs. *Biomaterials* 25, 2843–2849.
12. Bhadra, D., Bhadra, S., Jain, P., and Jain, N. K. (2002) Pegnology: a review of PEGylated systems. *Pharmazie* 57(1), 5–29.
13. Gajbhiye, V., Vijayarajkumar, P., Rakesh, T., and Jain, N. K. (2007) Pharmaceutical and biomedical potential of PEGylated dendrimers. *Cur Pharm Design* 13, 415–429.
14. Bhadra, D., Bhadra, S., and Jain, N. K. (2005) PEGylated lysine based copolymeric dendritic micelles for solubilization and delivery of artemether. *J Pharm Pharmaceut Sci* 8(3), 467–482.
15. Zalipsky, S., Gilon, C., and Zilkha, A. (1983) Attachment of drugs to polyethylene glycols. *Eur Polym J* 19(12), 1177–1183.
16. Lapatsanis, L., Milias, G., Froussios, K., and Kolovos, M. (1983) Synthesis of N-2,2,2-(trichloroethoxycarbonyl)-l-amino acids and N-(9-fluorenylmethoxy-carbonyl)-lamino acids involving succinimidoxy anion as a leaving group in amino acid protection. Synthesis, 8, 671–673.
17. Bhadra, D., Bhadra, S., Jain, S., and Jain, N. K. (2003) A PEGylated dendritic nanoparticulate carrier of fluorouracil. *Int J Pharm* 257, 111–124.
18. Tomalia, D. A., Naylor, A. M., and Goddard, W. A. (1990) Starburst, dendrimers, molecular level size, shape, surface, chemistry, topology and flexibility from atoms to macroscopic matter. *Angew Chem* 29, 138–175.
19. Peterson, J., Ebber, A., Allikmaa, V., and Lopp, M. (2001) Synthesis and CZE analysis of PAMAM dendrimers with an ethylenediamine core. *Proc Estonian Acad Sci Chem* 50(3), 156–166.
20. Tekade, R. K., Dutta, T., Gajbhiye, V., and Jain, N. K. (2008) Exploring dendrimers towards dual drug delivery. *J Microencap* 15, 1–10.
21. Veronese, F. M., Caliceti, P., Pastorino, A., Schiavon, O., and Sartore, L. (1989) Preparation, physicochemical and pharmacokinetic characterization of methoxy polyethylene glycol derivatized superoxide dismutase. *J Control Rel* 10, 145–154.
22. Virendra Gajbhiye, V., Vijayaraj Kumar, P., Tekade, R. K., and Jain, N. K. (2008) PEGylated PPI dendritic architectures for sustained delivery of H_2 receptor antagonist. *Eur J Med Chem* doi:10.1016/j.ejmech.2008.06.012.

23. Vijayaraj Kumar, P., Agashe, H., Dutta, T., and Jain, N. K. (2006) PEGylated dendritic architecture for development of a prolonged drug delivery system for an antitubercular drug. *Curr Drug Del* **3**(**4**), 11–19.
24. De Brabander-Van den Berg, E. M. M. and Meijer, E. W. (1993) *Angew Chem Int Ed Engl* **32**, 1308–1310.
25. Prego, C., Torres, D., Fernandez-Megia, E., Novoa-Carballal, R., Quiñoá, E., and Alonso, M. J. (2006) Chitosan – PEG nanocapsules as new carriers for oral peptide delivery effect of chitosan pegylation degree. *J Control Rel* **111**, 299–308.
26. Senthilkumar, M., Subramanian, G., Ranjitkumar, A., Nahar, M., Mishra, P., and Jain, N. K. (2007) PEGylated poly (lactide-*co*-lycolide) (PLGA) nanoparticulate delivery of Docetaxel: synthesis of diblock copolymers, optimization of preparation variables on formulation characteristics and in vitro release studies. *J Biomed Nanotech* **1**, 52–60.
27. Kaul, G. and Amiji, M. (2002) Long-circulating poly (ethyleneglycol)-modified gelatin nanoparticles for intracellular delivery. *Pharm Res* **19**(**7**), 1061–1067.
28. Balthasar, S., Michaelis, K., Dinauer, N., Briesen, H. V., Kreuter, J., and Langer, K. (2005) Preparation and characterization of antibody modified gelatin nanoparticles as drug carrier system for uptake in lymphocytes. *Biomaterials* **26**, 2723–2732.

Chapter 16

Nanoparticle–Aptamer Conjugates for Cancer Cell Targeting and Detection

M. Carmen Estévez, Yu-Fen Huang, Huaizhi Kang,
Meghan B. O'Donoghue, Suwussa Bamrungsap, Jilin Yan,
Xiaolan Chen, and Weihong Tan

Abstract

Aptamers are DNA or RNA oligonucleotide sequences that selectively bind to their target with high affinity and specificity. They are obtained using an iterative selection protocol called SELEX. Several small molecules and proteins have been used as targets. Recently, a variant of this methodology, known as cell-SELEX, has been developed for a new generation of aptamers, which are capable of recognizing whole living cells. We have used this methodology for the selection of aptamers, which show high affinity and specificity for several cancer cells. In this chapter, we describe (1) the process followed for the generation of aptamers capable of recognizing acute leukemia cells (CCRF–CEM cells) and (2) the method of enhancing the selectivity and sensitivity of these aptamers by conjugation with a dual-nanoparticle system, which combines magnetic nanoparticles (MNP) and fluorescent silica nanoparticles (FNP). Specifically, the selected aptamers, which showed dissociation constants in the nanomolar range, have been coupled to MNPs in order to selectively collect and enrich cells from complex matrices, including blood samples. The additional coupling of the aptamer to FNPs offers an excellent and highly sensitive method for detecting cancer cells. In order to prove the potential of this rapid and low-cost method for diagnostic purposes, confocal microscopy was used to confirm the specific collection and detection of target cells in concentrations as low as 250 cells. The final fluorescence of the cells labeled with the nanoparticles was quantified using a fluorescence microplate reader.

Key words: Fluorescent silica nanoparticle, magnetic nanoparticle, aptamer, cell-SELEX, cancer cells.

1. Introduction

Accurate and sensitive methods for cancer diagnosis are essential to track and monitor disease development and evolution. In the specific case of leukemia, current diagnostic methods involve the analysis of bone marrow or blood by karyotyping or immunophenotyping by flow cytometry or microarray (1–5), which are procedures usually requiring expensive instrumentation and time-consuming techniques. Nanobiotechnology, on the other hand, has opened a whole new area of development focused on using different types of nanoparticles (NP) both for diagnostic and therapeutic purposes. As a powerful alternative to conventional luminescent probes, the use of different types of highly fluorescent nanoparticles (FNP) has emerged with manifest advantages, including improved fluorescence signal and photostability. The success of FNPs can be attributed to the controllability of their size and shape and the versatility of their surface, which allows straightforward and simple bioconjugation. Among these FNPs, dye-doped silica NPs have been widely used in bioanalysis in combination with specific receptors, such as antibodies, peptides, and aptamers (6). Similarly, magnetic nanoparticles (MNP) with specific receptors immobilized on the surface have proven to be efficient probes for selective bioaffinity extraction and for the purification and separation of target substances in complex matrices (7). As a consequence of higher surface area, they usually offer improved capabilities compared with larger particles. Here, we describe an easy, fast, reproducible, and highly sensitive cell-detection assay based on the use of a dual-nanoparticle system, which combines MNPs and FNPs with aptamers as specific targeting molecules.

Briefly, the procedure involves the following steps. A panel of aptamers is first selected for the specific recognition of CCRF–CEM acute leukemia cells using the cell-SELEX process (8). The aptamer with the best capabilities in terms of affinity and specificity for the target cells is further selected to develop the detection methodology. In this study, we used the aptamer sgc8 which has a K_d of 0.8 nM. Both magnetic and fluorescent silica NPs are then prepared and conjugated to the specific aptamer using avidin–biotin interaction or covalent binding between amino and carboxylic groups, respectively. The magnetic NPs allow the specific extraction of the target cells and the subsequent enrichment, whereas the luminescent NPs allow fluorescent labeling for easy detection. This procedure allows high levels of cell-sample enrichment and achieves a limit of detection of ∼250 cells in buffer. This protocol has been further extrapolated to the measurement of more complex samples, such as spiked blood samples (9). The use of different spectrally resolvable fluorescent silica nanoparticles combined with the specificity provided for different aptamers selected for several cancer cell lines has also allowed the multiple detection of different cancer cells in the same sample (10). Overall, this simple method shows the potential of using specific aptamer and nanoparticles for the sensitive targeting and detection of cancer cells.

2. Materials

2.1. Aptamer Selection

2.1.1. Cell Culture

1. Target cell line against which to create aptamer: CEM, CCL-119 T-cell line, human acute lymphoblastic leukemia (ATCC, Manassas, VA).
2. Negative cell line to select against: Ramos, CRL-1596, B-cell line, human Burkitt's lymphoma (ATCC).
3. RPMI-1640 Medium (ATCC) supplemented with 10% heat-inactivated fetal bovine serum (FBS, GIBCO, Bethesda, MD) and 100 units/mL penicillin–streptomycin (Cellgro, Herdon, VA).

2.1.2. Cell-SELEX Process

1. Wash buffer: 4.5 g/L glucose and 5 mM $MgCl_2$ in Dulbecco's phosphate-buffered saline with $MgCl_2$ and $CaCl_2$ (Sigma, St. Louis, MO) stored at 4°C.
2. Binding buffer: 0.1 mg/mL yeast tRNA (Sigma) and 1 mg/mL bovine serum albumin (Fisher, Pittsburgh, PA) stored at 4°C.
3. HPLC-purified library containing a central randomized sequence of 52 nucleotides flanked by two 18-nt primer hybridization sites stored at –20°C (*see* **Note 1**).
4. Fluorescein isothiocyanate (FITC)-labeled 5′ forward primer and biotinylated 3′ reverse primer stored at –20°C under N_2 (*see* **Note 1**).
5. Sephadex G25, NAP 5 desalting column (GE Healthcare).
6. Streptavidin-coated Sepharose beads (Amersham Pharmacia Biosciences, Piscataway, NJ).
7. *Taq* polymerase, dNTPs, and 10× PCR buffer (Takara Bio, Inc.).
8. Electrophoresis grade agarose (Sigma).
9. Ethidium bromide (Sigma) to be handled with gloves, as this is a potent carcinogen.
10. Gel running buffer, 10× Tris–borate–EDTA (TBE) buffer (pH 8.3) (Fisher).
11. 1× Phosphate-buffered saline, PBS (Fisher).
12. Fetal bovine serum, FBS (Sigma)
13. 454 competant primers (IDT DNA)

2.2. NP Preparation

1. Tetraethoxyorthosilicate (TEOS), 3-aminopropyl triethoxysilane (APTS), and dye, Tris(2,2′-bipyridyl)-dichlororuthenium(II) hexahydrate (Rubpy), are stored at 4°C. Cyclohexane, *n*-hexanol, DMSO, and Triton X-100 used

for the preparation of the reverse microemulsion NPs are stored at room temperature (Sigma-Aldrich, St. Louis, MO).
2. Carboxylethylsilanetriol sodium salt (CTES) (Gelest, Inc., Morrisville, PA) is stored at 4°C.
3. Ammonium hydroxide 29% (Fisher, Inc.) is stored at 4°C.
4. Ferric chloride hexahydrate, ferrous chloride tetrahydrate from Aldrich, stored at room temperature.
5. Avidin (Molecular Probes).
6. 1 M Tris–HCl buffer
7. Washing buffer: 20 mM Tris–HCl, 5 mM $MgCl_2$, pH 8.0.
8. 10 mM MES buffer (pH 5.5).
9. 0.1 M Phosphate-buffered saline (PBS) (pH 7.4).
10. Glass reaction vessels and Teflon-coated magnetic stir rod.

2.3. Conjugation of NPs to Aptamers

1. MNPs: 0.1 mg/mL in 20 mM Tris–HCl, 5 mM $MgCl_2$, pH 8.0 buffer (see **Note 2**).
2. FNPs in 10 mM MES buffer (2-(N-morpholino) ethanesulfonic acid), pH 5.5 (Sigma).
3. N-Hydroxysulfosuccinimide (Sulfo-NHS) and 1-ethyl-3-(3-dimethylaminopropyl) carbodiimide hydrochloride (EDC) from Pierce Biotechnology, Inc. (Rockford, IL).
4. Washing buffer: 10 mM PBS at pH 7.4 for FNPs and 20 mM Tris–HCl, 5 mM $MgCl_2$, pH 8.0 for MNPs.
5. Aptamer selected for CCRF–CEM cells using the cell-SELEX process (sgc8) labeled with biotin at the 3′-end for coupling to MNPs and labeled with amino group in the 3′-end for coupling to FNPs.

2.4. Cancer Cell Targeting Using NP–Aptamer Conjugates

1. Glass-bottom culture dishes (35 mm Petri dish, 10 mm glass microwell, MatTek Corporation, Ashland, MA) are used to place the suspension of cells for imaging.
2. 384 microwell black plates for fluorescent measurements (Corning, Lowell, MA).

3. Methods

The cell-based SELEX process described here is developed for the selection of a panel of aptamers, which can specifically recognize the unique molecular features of target cancer cells. Briefly, after incubating the ssDNA pool with target cells, the unbound DNA is washed off the cells. By increasing the temperature to 95°C to elute the bound DNA, the eluent is then incubated with control cells for counterselection. After centrifugation, the supernatant is collected, and the selected DNA is amplified by PCR. The PCR products are then separated into ssDNA for the next-round selection. By several rounds of selection and PCR amplification, aptamer candidates exclusively binding to the target cells are enriched. The selected DNA is cloned and sequenced for aptamer identification in the last-round selection. Through this strategy, a panel of probes can be simultaneously generated to recognize unique features of the cancer cells with high affinity and specificity at the molecular level.

The aptamers selected through cell-based SELEX have been applied as the molecular recognition elements for the rapid collection and detection of leukemia cells using a novel dual-nanoparticle assay. The aptamer-modified MNPs enable the selective extraction and enrichment of the target cells from a cell mixture. The aptamer-modified FNPs are employed for sensitive cell detection. The enhanced fluorescent intensity achieved by the FNPs also allows significant signal amplification compared to that of individual dye-labeled probes. The combination of these two types of NPs allows rapid, selective, and sensitive detection not possible by using either particle alone. The use of this method has also been extended for the collection and detection of multiple cancer cells and applied to complex biological solutions, including whole blood and serum samples (9, 10).

3.1. Cell-SELEX Selection and Synthesis of Specific Aptamers for Cancer Cells

1. Before selection, 20 nmol ssDNA selection pool is dissolved in 500 µL of binding buffer.

2. For the first round of selection, the 500 µL ssDNA selection pool is incubated with 10×10^6 target CEM cells (*see* **Note 3**) at the temperature desired for selection (typically on ice) for 45 min, shaking on a platform at ~200 rpm. The cells are washed three times with 0.5 mL washing buffer and spun at 990 rpm for 4 min (*see* **Note 4**).

3. After washing, cells are reconstituted in 400 µL binding buffer. Bound DNA is eluted off the cells by heating the mixture at 95°C for 5 min. The mixture is then spun at either $4,000 \times g$ for 5 min or $14,000 \times g$ for 2 min.

4. The eluted ssDNA in the supernatant from the first round is collected and amplified with 8 cycles of PCR using the FITC- and biotin-labeled primers in a reaction that contains 80 µL dNTPs, 50 µL primer pool, ~500 µL of the sample, 3.0 µL *Taq* polymerase, and DNase water to 1,000 µL (*see* **Note 5**). This PCR product is then reamplified after optimizing the number of amplification cycles. For subsequent rounds of selection, the initial PCR of 500 µL of the pool is not done. Instead cycle optimization is performed and then only 10% of the pool is amplified.

5. The steps above result in a dsDNA pool of aptamers having one strand labeled with biotin and the other with FITC. In order to separate the two, streptavidin-coated beads are used. Follow these steps (1): Take a 5 mL syringe and insert it into the top of the empty DNA synthesis column on the side without the filter (2). Add 200 μL of streptavidin-coated bead solution into the syringe (3). Remove the streptavidin-coated bead solution by gently pressing the plunger (4). Wash the beads by adding 2.5 mL 1× PBS to the syringe (5). Load the PCR product onto the syringe and collect the flow-through. The dsDNA-enriched pool will stay bound to the beads (6). Wash the beads with 2–2.5 mL PBS to remove any forward FITC-labeled primer trapped on the beads. Since we want the enriched pool of ssDNA labeled with FITC, we need to unzip the biotin-labeled strand from the dsDNA. This is done by adding 500 μL of 200 mM NaOH to melt the DNA, taking care not to put too much pressure on the plunger. Let it drip slowly to collect the enriched FITC-labeled ssDNA.

6. The ssDNA pool now needs to be desalted to remove the NaOH. To do this, a NAP 5 desalting column is washed with 15 mL dH_2O. When the column is empty, the ssDNA pool is added, followed by 1 mL dH_2O. Once the sample is in the flow-through, the column is washed with 20 mL dH_2O and reused in the next round.

7. Absorbance of the sample is measured at 260 nm using a UV–Vis spectrophotometer. From this, the number of ssDNA moles in the sample is calculated.

8. The sample is dried using a speed-vac on low heat, and the ssDNA is resuspended in binding buffer to a concentration of 250 nM.

9. The enriched sense FITC-labeled ssDNA is used as the pool for binding in subsequent rounds of selection. Stringency of selection is gradually increased with each round. For example, the number of cells for selection is decreased (from 10×10^6 to 2×10^6 over several rounds); the number and amount of washing buffer used for each wash is increased (from 3× with 0.5 mL washes to 5× with 5 mL); and a counterselection step is introduced.

10. After 10–20 rounds of selection, or when the observed shift of the selected pool bound to cells seen with flow cytometry is both large enough and stable, the selected ssDNA pool is PCR-amplified using unmodified 454 DNA sequencing, competant primers, purified, and squenced on a 454 sequencer made by 454 Life Sciences.

11. The sequences are compared to determine the presence of any sequence homology or conserved regions.

12. The steps above should result in at least one good aptamer, which specifically recognizes and binds to the target cells (*see* **Note 6**).

3.2. NP Preparation

3.2.1. MNPs

1. Iron oxide core MNPs are synthesized by coprecipitating iron salts. $FeCl_3 \cdot 6H_2O$ (4.88 g) and $FeCl_2 \cdot 4H_2O$ (2.03 g) are weighed and placed in a glass beaker. HCl 37% (0.81 mL) is added and the solution is bubbled with N_2 for 5 min to remove the oxygen present in the solution.

2. At the same time, 155 mL of H_2O and 8.3 mL of NH_4OH are mixed in a glass beaker and stirred at 350 rpm with a mechanical stirrer. The solution is bubbled with N_2.

3. The ferrous/ferric chlorides/HCl solution is then added to the beaker, and the mixture is kept under mechanical stirrer at 350 rpm for 10 min. A brown suspension can be observed, which indicates the formation of the iron oxide NPs (Fe_3O_4). It is advisable to store the solution of F_3O_4 obtained in a brown bottle at room temperature. The solution is stable for several months. Particles of around 10–12 nm are usually obtained using these conditions.

4. To prepare the magnetic particles with the silica shell, 5 mL of the Fe_3O_4 NP solution are washed with H_2O (5 mL, twice) and with EtOH (5 mL, twice). The washes are performed by applying a magnet on the tube wall for 5 min. This allows the separation of the NPs from the media. The supernatant is then carefully removed with a plastic pipette. The magnet is removed, fresh EtOH is added, and the particles are resuspended.

5. In order to add a silica coating to the particles, the Fe_3O_4 NPs are resuspended in a solution of EtOH containing 1.2% of NH_4OH in a clean 20 mL glass tube (*see* **Note 7**). The volume of the ethanolic solution added should yield a final NP concentration of 7.5 mg/mL. TEOS (200 μL), a silica precursor, is then added to the suspension, which is sonicated for 90 min to allow hydrolysis to occur. A further postcoating can be performed by adding 10 μL more TEOS and sonicating the suspension again for 90 min.

6. The Fe_3O_4–SiO_2 NPs (magnetic core with silica shell) are washed as described above and resuspended in PBS buffer. The NPs protected with the silica shell are stable at room temperature for several months. Freezing of the NPs must be avoided. By following this protocol, particles of around 60 nm are obtained.

7. The aptamer is coupled to the MNPs through biotin–avidin linkage. First avidin is coated on the surface of the NP. Fe_3O_4–SiO_2 NPs (12 mL of a solution of 0.1 mg/mL in

PBS 10 mM) are mixed with 2 mL of a solution of avidin 5 mg/mL (in PBS) in a propylene tube. The mixture is vortexed for 5–10 min. The solution is placed in a shaker and left to react for 12 h at 4°C. The particles are washed again (H_2O, 5 mL; three times) to remove excess reagents by applying a magnet on the tube.

8. The NPs are resuspended in 1 mL of PBS 10 mM, and glutaraldehyde (1% in PBS) is added (29 mL) in order to stabilize the adsorption of the avidin by cross-linking on the surface of the NP.

9. The particles are washed under the same conditions described, but using 1 M Tris–HCl buffer (three times) and left in this buffer for 3 h at 4°C.

10. The particles are washed again with 20 mM Tris–HCl, 5 mM $MgCl_2$, pH 8.0 (5 mL, three times) and finally resuspended to a final concentration of 0.2 mg/mL. The NPs should be stored at 4°C when not in use. They can be stable for several months.

3.2.2. FNPs

1. A fresh solution of Rubpy is prepared (100 mM in water). The solution can take a few minutes to completely dissolve under continuous shaking. It is advisable to keep it protected from light.

2. Triton X-100 (1.77 g) is weighed in a clean tube glass (*see* **Note 7**) and dissolved with cyclohexane (7.5 mL) and *n*-hexanol (1.6 mL). The solution is kept under magnetic stirring at around 800 rpm.

3. Rubpy (80 µL) solution is then added, followed by 400 µL H_2O and 100 µL TEOS. The suspension is stirred for 30 min (*see* **Note 8**). A volume of 60 µL NH_4OH is then added to the microemulsion to initiate the silica polymerization, and it is left under stirring for around 15 h at room temperature, protected from light.

4. The NPs have now been formed, and a postcoating can be performed in order to introduce the desired functionalization on the surface, in this case, carboxy groups. TEOS (50 µL) and CTES (40 µL) are added, and the polymerization is left to react for another 15 h.

5. The microemulsion is broken by adding acetone to the suspension (4–5 mL). The solution is centrifuged at 14,000 rpm for 25 min and washed with EtOH (three times) and H_2O (three times). Usually, several minutes of sonication are required between the washes in order to completely resuspend the NPs.

6. The NPs can be resuspended in H$_2$O or buffer until further use. They are stable at room temperature, but it is advisable to keep them at 4°C (*see* **Note 9**).

3.3. Conjugation of Aptamer to NPs

3.3.1. Conjugation of FNPs to the Aptamer

1. Carboxyl functionalized Rubpy NPs (2 mg) are pipetted from the stock solution and resuspended in MES buffer, 0.5 mL. Sonication of a few seconds up to a couple of minutes is advisable in order to have a well-dispersed and homogenous NP solution.

2. EDC (1.2 mg dissolved in 0.5 mL of MES) and sulfo-NHS (3.2 mg dissolved in 0.5 mL of MES) are added to the NP solution, followed by 0.5 nmol of amino-labeled aptamer (from a stock solution of the aptamer of 100 μM in DNA-free H$_2$O). The reaction is allowed to proceed for 3 h at room temperature. Gentle shaking is advisable during the whole reaction. Both EDC and sulfo-NHS solutions must be prepared just before use.

3. The excess of reagents is removed, and the particles washed by centrifugation at 14,000 rpm for 20 min three times with PBS buffer (pH 7.2).

4. The NPs are dispersed in binding buffer to a concentration of 10 mg/mL. The NP–aptamer conjugates should be stored at 4°C and should remain stable for several weeks. The conjugates must not be frozen.

3.3.2. Conjugation of MNPs to Aptamers

1. Biotin-labeled aptamer with a concentration of 31 μM in Tris–HCl buffer is added to a suspension of avidin-coated MNPs in a concentration of 0.2 mg/mL in Tris–HCl buffer. The reaction is allowed to proceed for 12 h at 4°C. Gentle shaking of the suspension is recommended during the reaction.

2. Excess reagents are removed, and the particles are washed and collected by applying the magnet to the side of the sample container for 1 min. The unbound materials are then removed with a Pasteur pipette. Three washes are performed with Tris–HCl buffer (pH 8.0).

3. The NPs are dispersed in Tris–HCl buffer to a final concentration of 0.2 mg/mL. The particles should be stored at 4°C and never frozen.

3.4. Cancer Cell Enrichment and Detection Using NP–Aptamer Conjugates

1. For each experiment, CEM and RAMOS cells are used as target and control cells, respectively. The cells are counted in the hemocytometer, and the volume required is collected from the culture media considering the amount needed for the experiment (*see* **Note 10**).

2. The cells are centrifuged at 920 rpm for 5 min at 4°C and washed three times with washing buffer. The cells are resuspended in 200 μL of binding buffer and kept at 4°C.

3. The MNPs are then added (5 μL from the stock solution of 0.5 mg/mL). The suspension is gently stirred in order to mix the NPs with the cells and then left to incubate at 4°C for 15 min.

4. The cells are washed by magnetic extraction by placing the magnet on the side of the tube containing the cells. The magnet is left for 2–5 min, and the supernatant is decanted using a Pasteur pipette. The magnet is removed, and the samples are redispersed in 200 μL of washing buffer. The process is repeated three times, and the cells are finally resuspended in 200 μL binding buffer. Gentle shaking of the suspension is recommended between the washes to allow the resuspension of the MNPs. It is also recommended to keep the buffer at 4°C while performing the experiments.

5. FNPs are then added (2 μL from the stock solution of 10 mg/mL). The suspension is gently stirred and left incubating for 5 min. The cells are washed as described above.

6. The cells are reconstituted with 20 μL of binding buffer for confocal microscopy imaging, or 100 μL for microplate reader analysis.

7. A total of 20 μL of cell suspension is placed onto glass-bottom culture dishes and directly analyzed with confocal microscopy. Images of cells are taken with a 20×70 NA objective. Images are taken under confocal microscopy by exciting the FNPs with the 488 nm argon ion laser, and the emission is collected using a 610 nm long-pass filter. Software can be used to overlay the transmission image and the fluorescent image. Examples of the images observed after incubation of the MNPs and FNPs with target (CEM) and control (RAMOS) cells are shown in **Fig. 16.1**.

8. A total of 20 μL of the cell suspension is placed in different wells of the microplate, and the fluorescence is measured using a common fluorescent microplate reader, in this case, a Tecan Safire microplate reader. The excitation was set at 488 nm and the emission at 610 nm. **Figure 16.2** shows the calibration curve obtained after measuring the fluorescence from different samples with decreasing amounts of cells (from 10^5 to 10^3 cells).

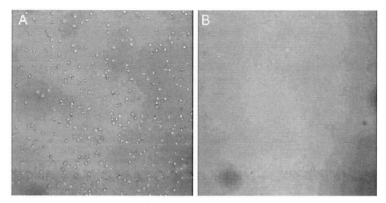

Fig. 16.1. Confocal microscopy images of extracted samples from (a) target CEM cells and (b) control RAMOS cells. (Reprinted with permission from (9). Copyright 2006 the American Chemical Society.)

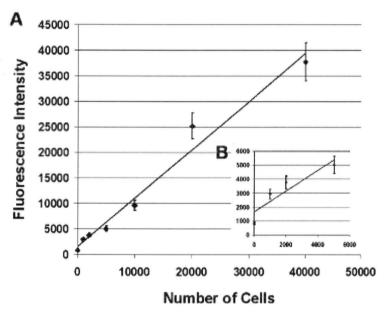

Fig. 16.2. Limit of detection for the stepwise addition of the MNPs and FNPs using the microplate reader for detection: (a) full calibration curve; (b) enlarged depiction of the lower concentration regime. A limit of detection of 250 cells can be achieved using this method (10). (Reprinted with permission from (10). Copyright 2007 the American Chemical Society.)

4. Notes

1. To minimize the possibility of nonspecific amplification of random library sequences in PCR, the primers and library sequences need to be carefully optimized. In particular, the ssDNA pool cannot be too stable, as it must easily

denature at 95°C. Furthermore, the 5′ end of the DNA pool should not be G, as it can quench the fluorescence of the fluorophore. The primers should be between 18 and 20 nts long and designed not to form self-dimers or heterodimers. Moreover, the primers must anneal to the library at a temperature between 55 and 60°C. To obtain such an annealing temperature, the primer must have a GC content of 50% or more. Since PCR machines have one annealing temperature, both primers must have the same annealing temperature (± 1°C). These design parameters can be easily optimized using free oligonucleotide prediction software such as Oligoanalyzer (Integrated DNA Technologies).

2. Unless indicated otherwise, all the noncommercial buffers used in these experiments should be prepared with DNA-free sterile water (Fisher Scientific, Pittsburgh, PA) and stored at 4°C.

3. The cells used for selection should be healthy, with >95% cells alive. Dead cells nonspecifically allow ssDNA from the pool into their membranes affecting the efficiency of the selection. A full 8-hour day for one technician should be planned to complete each round of selection.

4. For this selection, a suspension cell line is used as the target cell line. However, if an adherent cell line is desired, then the ssDNA pool can be incubated with a monolayer of the target cells in a T25 flask. After washing, the adhesive cells are gently scraped off on ice with a rubber policeman into a vial, and the eluted DNA is collected. Alternatively, a nonenzymatic cell-disassociation solution can be used to disassociate a monolayer of cells. Counterselection is done by simply incubating the DNA from the target cells onto a monolayer of the negative cell line in a 60-cm^2 dish for 1 h, followed by a collection of the unbound supernatant and proceeding with PCR amplification as above.

5. To perform PCR, it is first necessary to optimize the annealing temperature and number of cycles for the ssDNA selection pool. The annealing temperature with the number of cycles that produces the brightest band with the least nonspecific amplification for the initial ssDNA library should be chosen.

6. It has been the experience of our lab that, *if all goes well*, a complete selection takes from 4 to 6 months, from the first round until an aptamer is ready for screening.

7. The glass tubes used for the preparation of silica NPs should first be cleaned by adding a solution of NaOH for 15 min to inactivate the silanol groups on the glass surface

and avoid the silanization on the walls of the tube. The tubes are then washed thoroughly with H_2O and EtOH and are left to dry before use.

8. The addition of these reagents has to be performed while the solution is constantly kept under stirring at 800 rpm to allow the formation of the microemulsion.

9. The particles can be characterized in terms of size and brightness. Usually, the size obtained following this protocol and keeping the same ratio of reagents is about 50 nm. The brightness can be determined by comparing the fluorescent signal of the NP solution with a calibration curve of the pure dye under the same conditions. With Rubpy dye, the brightness obtained is usually equivalent to around 15,000 single dyes. Other methodologies for the preparation of fluorescent silica NPs can be used depending on the nature of the dye. The amount of NPs can vary from batch to batch, but usually around 50 mg can be obtained following this method.

10. For experiments involving pure cells and mixtures of cells, 10^5 cells are usually collected from the media. For the determination of the limit of detection of the procedure developed, a range of concentration of cells must be selected, in this case from 1000 to 10,000 cells.

Acknowledgments

This work was supported by NIH, NCI, and NIGMS grants and by State of Florida Center for NanoBiosensors. M.-C.E. acknowledges financial support from the Departament d'Universitats, Recerca i Societat de la Informació de la Generalitat de Catalunya, Spain.

References

1. Tchinda, J., Volpert, S., McNeil, N., Neumann, T., Kennerknecht, I., et al. (2003) Multicolor karyotyping in acute myeloid leukemia. *Leukemia Lymphoma* **44**, 1843–1853.
2. Kearney, L., Tosi, S., and Jaju, R. J. (2002) Detection of chromosome abnormalities in leukemia using fluorescence in situ hybridization. *Methods Mol Med* **68**, 7–27.
3. Faderl, S., Kantarjian, H. M., Talpaz, M., and Estrov, Z. (1998) Clinical significance of cytogenetic abnormalities in adult acute lymphoblastic leukemia. *Blood* **91**, 3995–4019.
4. Craig, F. E. and Foon, K. A. (2008) Flow cytometric immunophenotyping for hematologic neoplasms. *Blood* **111**, 3941–3967.
5. Belov, L., De la Vega, O., Dos Remedios, C. G., Mulliganm, S. P., and Christopherson, R. I. (2001) Immunophenotyping of leukemias using a cluster of differentiation antibody microarray. *Cancer Res* **61**, 4483–4489.
6. Wang, L., Wang, K., Santra, S., Zhao, X., Hilliard, L. R., et al. (2006) Watching silica nanoparticles glow in the biological world. *Anal Chem* **78**, 646A–654A.

7. Smith, J. E., Wang, L., and Tan, W. (2006) Bioconjugated silica-coated nanoparticles for bioseparation and bioanalysis. *Trends Anal Chem* **25**, 848–855.
8. Shangguan, D., Li, Y., Tang, Z., Cao, Z. C., Chen, H. W., et al. (2006) Aptamers evolved from live cells as effective molecular probes for cancer study. *Proc Natl Acad Sci* **103**, 11838–11843.
9. Herr, J. K., Smith, J. E., Medley, C. D., Shangguan, D., and Tan, W. (2006) Aptamer-conjugated nanoparticles for selective collection and detection of cancer cells. *Anal Chem* **78**, 2918–2924.
10. Smith, J. E., Medley, C. D., Tang, Z., Shangguan, D., Lofton, C., and Tan, W. (2007) Aptamer-conjugated nanoparticles for the collection and detection of multiple cancer cells. *Anal Chem* **79**, 3075–3082.

Chapter 17

Targeting of Nanoparticles: Folate Receptor

Sumith A. Kularatne and Philip S. Low

Abstract

Nanoparticulate medicines offer the advantage of allowing delivery of large quantities of unmodified drug within the same particle. Nanoparticle uptake by cancer cells can, however, be compromised due to the large size and hydrophilicity of the particle. To circumvent cell penetration problems and simultaneously improve tumor specificity, nanoparticulate medicines have been linked to targeting ligands that bind to malignant cell surfaces and enter cells by receptor-mediated endocytosis. In this chapter, we summarize multiple methods for delivering nanoparticles into cancer cells by folate receptor-mediated endocytosis, devoting special emphasis to folate-targeted liposomes. Folate receptor-mediated endocytosis has emerged as an attractive strategy for nanoparticle delivery due to both overexpression of the folate receptor on cancer cells and the rapid internalization of the receptor by receptor-mediated endocytosis.

Key words: Folate receptor-targeted drugs, cancer nanomedicines, ligand-targeted nanoparticles, folate-targeted imaging agents, folic acid coupling chemistries, pteroic acid synthesis, conjugation of amine, hydroxyl, thiol, or carboxyl functionalized nanoparticles to folate.

1. Introduction

Cancer is projected to become the leading cause of death in the United States by 2010, currently amounting to ~1.4 million new cases and ~565,000 fatalities per year (1). In 2008, cumulative expenditures for cancer therapies in the United States have been estimated at $219.2 billion. This enormous cost on lives and resources can be equally attributed to inadequacies in both early detection and treatment of the disease. Thus, current methods for diagnosis of cancer often reveal the malignant tissue only after it has already metastasized to other parts of the body (2). Further, treatment of metastasized disease is frequently limited to systemic chemotherapy, which can have marginal efficacy due to dose-limiting toxicities, inadequate potency, rapid clearance from the body, poor aqueous solubility, and compromised in vivo stability (3). In this opportunity-filled environment, nanoparticles have attracted considerable attention due to their ability to deliver large quantities of drug, remain in circulation for extended periods of time, passively accumulate in solid tumors, and release drug slowly at the site of action (4).

Biodegradable nanoparticles can be synthesized over a wide range of sizes; however, particles of 50–100 nm diameter are often preferred for optimal intracellular uptake and improved pharmacokinetics (5). While nanoparticles can be fabricated from a variety of polymeric building blocks, those containing hydrophilic polymers, such as polyethylene glycol (PEG), natural proteins, polysaccharides, polylactic acids, poloxamines, and poloxamers, often exhibit reduced plasma protein adsorption (and the consequent minimized clearance by the reticuloendothelial system), improved biocompatibility, increased water solubility, quicker biodegradation, and better pharmacokinetics (6–8). Further, when hydrophilic copolymers are assembled with a hydrophobic core, large quantities of drugs can be loaded into the composite nanoparticle, allowing delivery of significantly elevated payloads (9, 10).

Although nanoparticles will passively accumulate in tumor tissue as a consequence of the EPR effect (11, 12), internalization of such nanoparticles can be greatly improved by attachment of a high-affinity targeting ligand (13). Folic acid (FA) constitutes one of the most frequently employed targeting ligands, since its receptor [i.e., the folate receptor (FR)]: (1) is significantly overexpressed on cancer cells of the breast, lung, kidney, ovary, colon, brain, and myelogenous leukemias (14); (2) is present in low or nondetectable levels in most normal cells (15, 16); (3) binds folate-linked drugs and nanoparticles with nanomolar affinity (17); and most importantly, (4) undergoes internalization via receptor-mediated endocytosis, delivering its cargo into the cell interior (18). For these reasons, FA has been tethered to anticancer drugs (19), gene therapy vectors (20), immunotherapeutic agents (21), protein toxins (22), liposomes (23), dendrimers (24), polymeric micelles (25), imaging agents (26), and therapeutic siRNAs/miRNAs (27).

Delivery of imaging and therapeutic agents using folate-targeted nanoparticles can offer advantages over direct drug conjugation to FA. First, large quantities of drug can be internalized at each folate receptor, allowing treatment of cancers with lower potency drugs that may otherwise have desirable properties. Second, nanoparticle packaging can avoid the requirement for direct modification of the drug; i.e., a useful property when the drug contains no readily modifiable moiety. Third, intracellular trafficking can be directed to acidic compartments for facile drug release, since multivalent folate conjugates (e.g., nanoparticles derivatized with multiple folates) are trafficked to acidic endosomes (median pH∼5) (28), whereas monovalent folate conjugates are trafficked through endosomal compartments of median pH∼6.7 (29). And finally, drug release can be delayed until the nanoparticle has trafficked deep into the cell interior, thereby avoiding immediate efflux by multidrug-resistant pumps (30). Taken together, folate-targeted nanoparticles may possess properties that render them ideal drug delivery vehicles for a variety of applications. In the section that follows, we describe protocols for the preparation and preclinical analysis of FR-targeted nanoparticles for the subsequent diagnosis and treatment of cancer.

2. Materials

2.1. Synthesis of N^{10} (Trifluoroacetic)-Pteroic Acid

Chemicals: FA, tris(hydroxymethyl)aminomethane (tris–base), zinc chloride ($ZnCl_2$), carboxypeptidase G (CPG), hydrochloric acid (HCl), acetonitrile (ACN), phosphorous pentoxide (P_2O_5), trifluoroacetic anhydride (TFAA), trifluoroacetic acid (TFA), dimethyl sulfoxide (DMSO), ammonium acetate (NH_4OAc), sodium chloride (NaCl), ammonium bicarbonate (NH_4CO_3), sodium hydroxide (NaOH), diethylaminoethyl cellulose (DEAE), DMSO-d_6, and D_2O.

2.2. Synthesis of Folate Linkers

2.2.1. Synthesis of Folate-Cys and Folate-EDA

Chemicals: Fmoc-Cys(4-methoxytrityl)-Wang resin, 1,2-diaminoethane trityl resin, N10TFA-pteroic, Fmoc-Glu(O^{t}Bu)OH [where Fmoc = fluorenylmethyloxycarbonyl and ^{t}Bu = tertiarybutyl], diisopropylethylamine (DIPEA), TFA, benzotriazol-1-yl-oxytripyrrolidinophosphonium hexafluorophosphate (PyBOP), isopropanol (i-PrOH), piperidine, triisopropyl silane (TIPS), ethanedithiol (EDT), hydrazine, dichloromethane (DCM), dimethyl formamide (DMF), and diethyl ether.

2.2.2. Synthesis of Folate-PEG$_{2000}$-DSPE

Chemicals: chloroform ($CHCl_3$), triethylamine (TEA), distearoyl phosphatidylethanolamine (DSPE), N-hydroxysuccinimidyl-poly-ethyleneglycol-maleimide (NHS-PEG-MAL), folate-Cys, MeOH, $NaHCO_3$, diethyl ether, and sodium phosphate.

2.3. Preparation of Folate-Targeted Nanoparticles

Chemicals: dipalmitoyl phosphatidylcholine (DPPC), dimyristoyl phosphatidylglycerol (DMPG), DSPE, monomethoxy polyethylene glycol$_{2000}$-distearoyl phosphatidylethanolamine (mPEG$_{2000}$-DSPE), folate-PEG$_{2000}$-DSPE, imaging or therapeutic agents, methoxycarbonylsulfenyl chloride

[MeOC(O)SCl], 2-mercaptoethanol, 2,2′-dipyridyl disulfide, N-hydroxybenzotriazole (HOBT), folate-Cys, folate-EDA, triphosgene (should be handled by a trained personnel), DIPEA, DMSO, DCM, amine/hydroxyl/thiol/carboxyl functionalized nanoparticles, and $CHCl_3$.

2.4. In Vitro Studies of FA-Targeted Nanoparticles

Chemicals: FA, ^{3}H-FA, ^{3}H-thymidine, trichloroacetic acid (TCA), NaOH, Ecolume scintillation cocktail, and DMSO.

Cell culture/supplies: KB cells (FR positive), folate-free RPMI medium, heat-inactivated fetal bovine serum (HIFBS), penicillin–streptomycin (PS), and phosphate-buffered saline (PBS).

2.5. In Vivo Studies of FA-Targeted Imaging and Therapeutic Nanoparticles

Cells/animals: KB (FR^+) and A549 (FR^-) cells, folate-free RPMI medium, folate-free chow, female *nu/nu* mice, and 10% formalin in PBS.

3. Methods

3.1. Synthesis of N^{10}(Trifluoroacetyl)-Pteroic Acid

3.1.1. Preparation of Pteroic Acid (Ptc) by Enzymatic Hydrolysis of Folic Acid (FA)

1. Dissolve FA (20.0 g, 45.3 mmol) in 0.1 M tris–base (1.0 L). Add $ZnCl_2$ (50 mg, 0.367 mmol) and CPG (40 units) to the solution. Adjust the pH to 7.3 with 1 M HCl and heat to 30°C. Maintain the pH (assay daily) and the temperature throughout the reaction period. Wrap the flask in aluminum foil and stir for 7–10 days (**Fig. 17.1**; 31).

2. Monitor the reaction using analytical reverse-phase high-performance liquid chromatography (RP-HPLC) at wavelengths (λ) = 285 and 363 nm (1–50%B in 30 min, 80%B wash 35 min run: A = 10 mM NH_4OAc, pH 7; B = ACN;

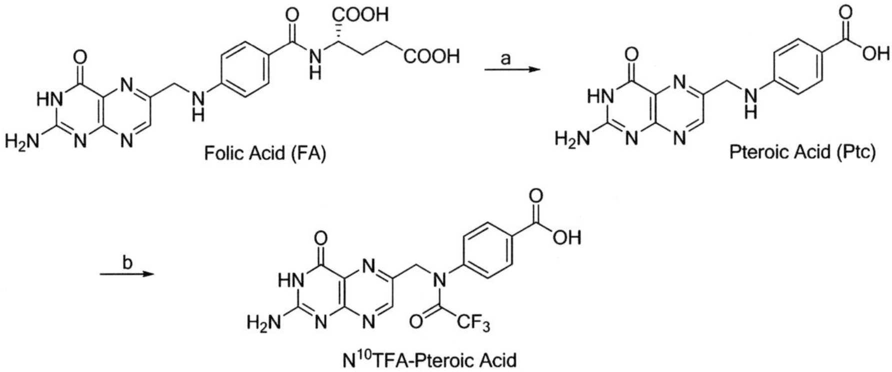

Fig. 17.1. Reagents and conditions: (**a**) $ZnCl_2$, CPG/tris–base, 30°C; (**b**) (i) TFAA, (ii) 3% TFA.

column: Waters, X-Bridge C$_{18}$ 5 μm, 3.0 × 50 mm, flow rate = 1 mL/min).

3. Precipitate the reaction mixture at pH 3.0 using 6 M HCl and transfer to centrifuge tubes. Centrifuge at 4,000 rpm for 10 min, decant, and discard the supernatant. Lyophilize the pellet for 48 h.

3.1.2. Purification of Pteroic Acid (Ptc)

1. Add HPLC-grade water (150 mL) to a flask containing crude Ptc (10 g) and adjust the pH to 11.5 using 1.0 M NaOH. Filter the solution through a Whatman type 1 filter paper. Load the sample onto a DEAE column and elute with 1.0 M NaCl/0.01 M NaOH (pH 11.5) at a flow rate of 17 mL/min. Collect the yellow fractions.

2. Analyze the fractions using analytical RP-HPLC followed by liquid chromatography/mass spectrometry (LC/MS) [m/z (M+H) = 313.28].

3. Combine the fractions containing pure Ptc and precipitate at pH 3.0 using 6 M HCl. Centrifuge at 3,000 rpm for 20 min, decant the supernatant, and wash the precipitate with HPLC-grade water (3×). Lyophilize for 48 h and dry in high vacuum in the presence of P$_2$O$_5$ for 2 days.

4. Characterize using proton nuclear magnetic resonance (^{1}H-NMR) spectroscopy in DMSO-d_6:D$_2$O (8:2 v/v) and electrospray ionization–high-resolution mass spectrometry (ESI-HRMS).

3.1.3. TFA Protection of Pteroic Acid

1. Add Ptc (10 g, 32.0 mmol) into a 500 mL round-bottom flask containing a magnetic stirring bar and evacuate under high vacuum overnight to remove all water.

2. Release the vacuum under argon (Ar), add TFAA (231.6 mL, 1.7 mol), and seal the flask with a rubber stopper. Wrap the flask in aluminum foil and stir the mixture at room temperature (r.t.) under argon for 4 days to protect N^{10} with TFA. Take 5 μL aliquot, dilute with HPLC-grade water (50 μL):DMSO (50 μL), and analyze using analytical RP-HPLC and LC/MS as above.

3. Remove TFAA using rotary evaporator. Add 3% TFA (250 mL) to the flask and stir for 2 days at r.t. Add HPLC-grade water (200 mL) to the reaction flask, transfer the resulting suspension to centrifuge bottles, and centrifuge at 3,000 rpm for 20 min. Decant the supernatant to a round-bottom flask, neutralize using NH$_4$OH$_{(aq)}$ while stirring inside a fume hood, and discard. Wash the pellet with HPLC-grade water (3×), centrifuge, discard the supernatant, and lyophilize for 48 h.

4. Transfer N^{10}TFA-pteroic acid to an amber bottle and dry in high vacuum in the presence of P_2O_5 for 2 days. Characterize using ^{1}H-NMR and ESI-HRMS.

3.2. Synthesis of Folate Linkers

3.2.1. Synthesis of Folate-γ-Cysteine (Folate-Cys)

1. Swell Fmoc-Cys(4-methoxytrityl)-Wang resin (1.0 equiv.) with DCM (3 mL) using a solid-phase peptide synthesis vessel (**Fig. 17.2**). After decanting, repeat swelling procedure with DMF (3 mL). After decanting DMF, add 3 mL of 20% piperidine in DMF to resin and bubble Ar to promote homogeneous mixing for 5 min. Repeat 3× and then wash the resin with DMF (3 × 3 mL) and i-PrOH (3 × 3 mL). Assess formation of free amine by the Kaiser test/ninhydrin test (*see* **Notes 1** and **2**).

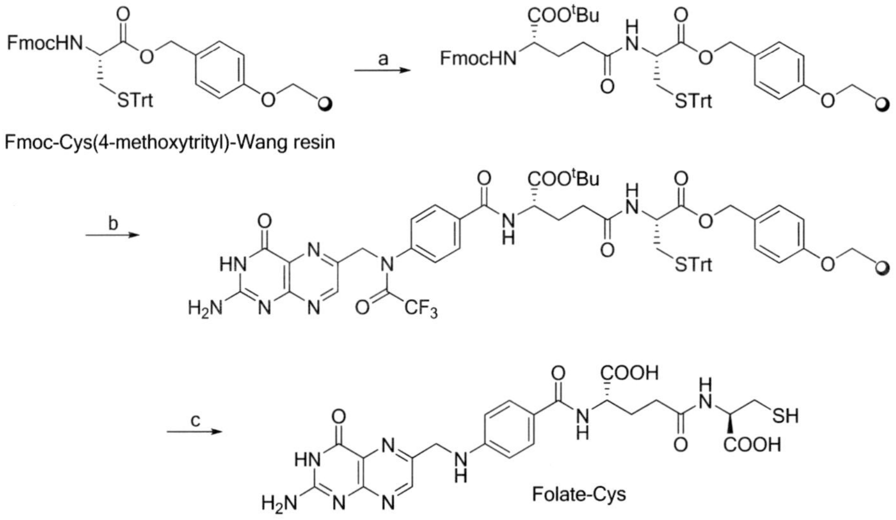

Fig. 17.2. Reagents and conditions: (**a**) (i) 20% piperidine/DMF, (ii) Fmoc-Glu(O^{t}Bu)-OH, PyBOP, DIPEA/DMF; (**b**) (i) 20% piperidine/DMF, (ii) N^{10}TFA-pteroic acid, PyBOP, DIPEA/DMF; (**c**) (i) 2% NH$_2$NH$_2$/DMF, (ii) TFA:TIPS:water:EDT (92.5:2.5:2.5:2.5).

2. Swell the resin again in DMF. Add solution of Fmoc-Glu(O^{t}Bu)-OH (2.5 equiv.), PyBOP (2.5 equiv.), and DIPEA (4.0 equiv.) in DMF. Bubble Ar for 2 h. Wash resin with DMF (3 × 3 mL) and i-PrOH (3 × 3 mL). Assess coupling efficiency using the Kaiser test. Swell the resin in DMF and decant DMF. Add 3 mL of 20% piperidine in DMF to resin and bubble Ar for 5 min. Repeat 3× and then wash the resin with DMF (3 × 3 mL) and i-PrOH (3 × 3 mL). Assess formation of free amine by the Kaiser test.

3. Swell the resin again in DMF. Add a solution of N^{10}TFA-pteroic acid (1.25 equiv.), PyBOP (2.5 equiv.), and DIPEA (4.0 equiv.) in DMF. Bubble Ar for 8 h and wash the resin with DMF (3 × 3 mL) and i-PrOH (3 × 3 mL). Assess

coupling efficiency using the Kaiser test and swell the resin in DMF.

4. Add 2% hydrazine in DMF (3 × 3 mL) (*see* **Note 2**) and bubble Ar for 5 min. Wash the resin with DMF (3 × 3 mL) and then i-PrOH (3 × 3 mL). Cleave the final compound from the resin using 3 mL TFA:H$_2$O:TIPS:EDT (92.5:2.5:2.5:2.5) cocktail (30 min × 3) (*see* **Note 2**) and concentrate under vacuum. Precipitate the concentrated product (folate-Cys) in diethyl ether and dry under vacuum.

5. Purify the crude product using preparative RP-HPLC at λ = 285 nm (1–50%B for 30 min, 80%B wash 5 min; A = 0.1% TFA, pH 2; B = ACN; column: Waters, xTerra C$_{18}$ 10 μm; 19 × 250 mm, flow rate = 26 mL/min). Analyze the fractions using analytical RP-HPLC and LC/MS. Combine the fractions containing pure folate-Cys, remove ACN, and lyophilize for 36 h to yield the final product as a yellow solid. Characterize folate-Cys using ^{1}H-NMR and ESI-HRMS.

3.2.2. Synthesis of Folate-γ-Ethylenediamine (Folate-EDA)

Swell 1,2-diaminoethane trityl resin (1.0 equiv.) with DCM (3 mL) using a solid-phase peptide synthesis vessel (**Fig. 17.3**). Follow Steps 2–5 in the synthesis of folate-Cys, except cleave the final compound from the resin using 3 mL TFA:H$_2$O:TIPS (95:2.5:2.5) cocktail (30 min × 3) and purify the crude product using preparative RP-HPLC (1–50%B for 30 min, 80%B 5 min; A = 10 mM NH$_4$OAc, pH 7; B = ACN).

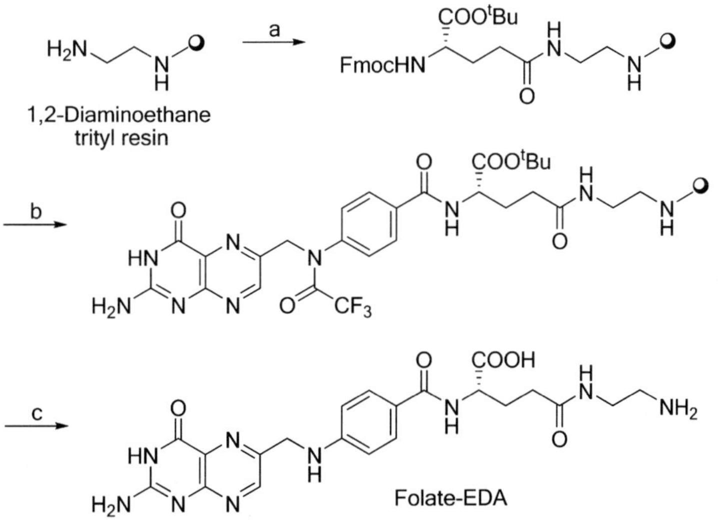

Fig. 17.3. Reagents and conditions: (**a**) Fmoc-Glu(O^{t}Bu)-OH, PyBOP, DIPEA/DMF; (**b**) (i) 20% piperidine/DMF, (ii) N^{10}TFA-pteroic acid, PyBOP, DIPEA/DMF; (**c**) (i) 2% NH$_2$NH$_2$/DMF, (ii) TFA:TIPS:water (95:2.5:2.5).

3.3. Synthesis of Folate-PEG$_{2000}$-DSPE (see Note 3)

1. Add a solution of DSPE (1.0 equiv.) and TEA (4.0 equiv.) in anhydrous CHCl$_3$ (1.0 mL) to a solution of NHS-PEG$_{2000}$-MAL (1.1 equiv.) in anhydrous CHCl$_3$ (1.0 mL) over 15 min under Ar with stirring. Stir the reaction overnight (15 h) at r.t. to yield DSPE-PEG$_{2000}$-MAL (32; see **Fig. 17.4**).

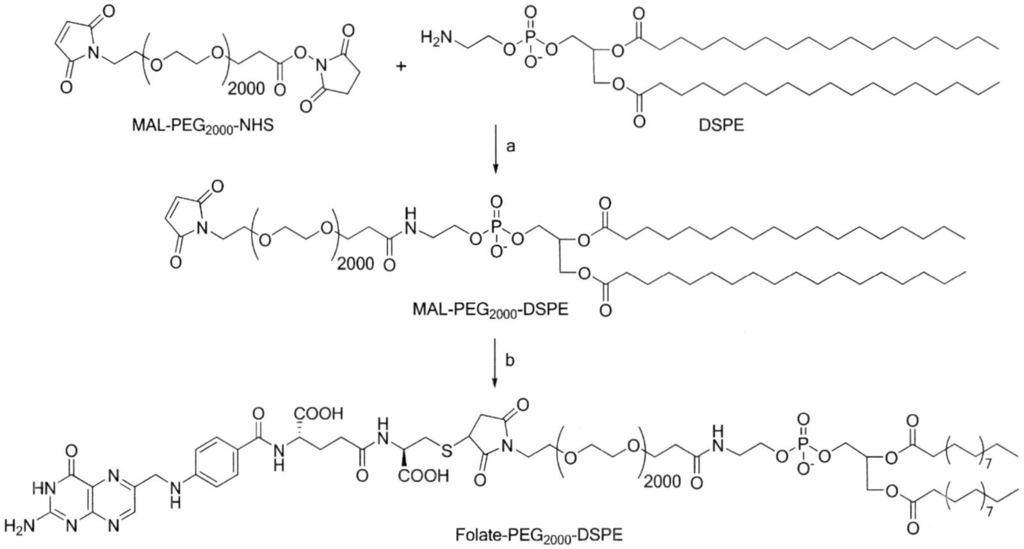

Fig. 17.4. Reagents and conditions: (**a**) NHS-PEG-MAL, TEA/CHCl$_3$; (**b**) folate-Cys/water, pH 7.2, bubble Ar, 40°C.

2. Dissolve folate-Cys (1.0 equiv.) in Ar-purged HPLC-grade water and adjust the pH to 7.2 with Ar-purged 1 M NaHCO$_3$ while continuing to bubble with Ar. Add a solution of DSPE-PEG$_{2000}$-MAL in CHCl$_3$ (reaction mixture from Step 1) and stir the reaction overnight at 40°C under Ar.

3. Concentrate the reaction mixture under vacuum and precipitate the product by adding it dropwise into diethyl ether over 10 min with constant stirring at 4°C, followed by centrifugation at 2,000×g for 10 min at 4°C. Wash the crude precipitate with ice-cold diethyl ether (2×).

4. Dissolve the crude product in HPLC-grade water to form micelles. Dialyze (3×) the micelles using a membrane (molecular weight cutoff = 14 kDa) with 8 h/cycle at r.t. Lyophilize the product for 36 h.

5. Determine the purity by analytical RP-HPLC at λ = 285 and 363 nm (isocratic mode, with MeOH:10 mM sodium phosphate pH 7.0 (92:8 v/v), column: Waters, X-Bridge C$_{18}$ 5 μm, 3.0 × 50 mm, flow rate = 1 mL/min) (see **Note 4**).

6. Determine folate-PEG$_{2000}$-DSPE concentration by measuring UV–vis absorbance of folate at $\lambda_{max} = 363$ nm (the molar extinction coefficient, $\varepsilon = 6{,}500$ per M/cm) or $\lambda_{max} = 285$ nm ($\varepsilon = 27{,}500$ per M/cm) in MeOH.

3.4. Preparation of Folate-Targeted Nanoparticles

3.4.1. Liposomal Nanoparticles

1. Dissolve lipids DPPC/DMPG/mPEG-DSPE/folate-PEG-DSPE (molar ratios 85:9.5:5:0.5) (see **Note 5**) or DPPC/DMPG/mPEG-DSPE (molar ratios of 85:10:5) in CHCl$_3$ to form folate-targeted and nontargeted nanoparticles, respectively (32, 33).

2. Evaporate the solvent at 40°C and dry under vacuum to form a thin film. Add the agent to be encapsulated and hydrate the lipid film in a buffer of choice at a drug-to-lipid molar ratio of 1:33 by vortexing (see **Note 6**). Subject the suspension to 10 cycles of freezing and thawing. Then sonicate for 2 min in a bath-type sonicator and extrude sonicated suspension 5× through 100 nm pore size polycarbonate membrane using an extruding device driven by high-pressure Ar.

3. Purify the liposomes from unencapsulated drug by size-exclusion chromatography on a Sepharose CL-4B column equilibrated in the above hydration buffer of choice. Sterilize the liposomal nanoparticles by passing through a 0.22 μm cellulose membrane.

4. Characterize physical properties of liposomes using photon correlation spectroscopy (liposome size), zeta (ζ)-potential using electrophoresis light-scattering method, amount of drug entrapped using analytical RP-HPLC, folate concentration using UV–vis absorbance, phospholipid content using phosphate assay (34), and stability at 4°C (storing conditions) and 37°C (human plasma), etc.

3.4.2. Derivatization of Hydroxyl/Amine Functionalized Nanoparticles with Folate (see Note 7)

1. Dissolve methoxycarbonylsulfenyl chloride (1 equiv.) in DCM and stir under Ar at 0°C for 10 min. Add a solution of 2-mercaptoethanol (1 equiv.)/DCM dropwise and stir at 0°C for 30 min. Add a solution of 2,2′-dipyridyl disulfide (1 equiv.)/DCM dropwise and stir at r.t. for 2.5 h. Evaporate the solvent under vacuum, crystallize using acetone, and characterize the product by ^{1}H-NMR in DMSO-d_6 and ESI-HRMS (35; see **Fig. 17.5**).

2. Add a solution of 2-(2-hydroxy-ethyldisulfanyl)-pyridine (1 equiv.) and TEA (1 equiv.) in DCM to triphosgene (0.33 equiv.) in DCM and stir under Ar at r.t. for 10 min. Add a solution of HOBT (1 equiv.) and TEA (1 equiv.) in DCM and stir under Ar at r.t. for 6 h. Evaporate the solvent under vacuum, crystallize using acetone, and characterize activated carbonate product by ^{1}H-NMR and ESI-HRMS (35).

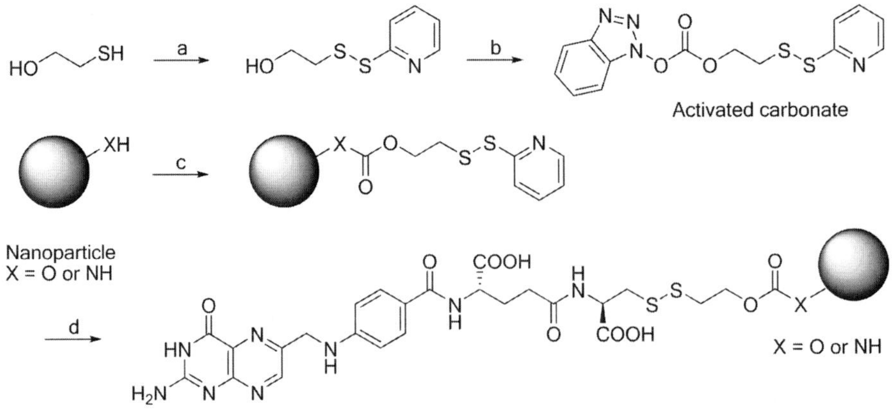

Fig. 17.5. Reagents and conditions: (**a**) (i) MeOC(O)SCl/DCM, 0°C, 30 min, (ii) 2-mercaptopyridine/DCM, 0°C, 2.5 h; (**b**) (i) triphosgene, TEA/DCM, r.t., 10 min, (ii) HOBT, TEA/DCM, r.t., 6 h; (**c**) activated carbonate, DIPEA/DCM, r.t.; (**d**) folate-Cys/water, pH = 7.2, bubble Ar, r.t., 30 min.

3. Dissolve the activated carbonate in $CHCl_3$ and add amine or hydroxyl functionalized nanoparticles and DIPEA dissolved in a solvent of choice. Stir the reaction mixture at r.t. for 2 h to form activated nanoparticles.

4. Dissolve folate-Cys in Ar-purged HPLC-grade water and adjust pH to 7.0 with Ar-purged 1 M $NaHCO_3$ while continuing to bubble with Ar. Add a solution of activated nanoparticles in solvent of choice and stir at r.t. under Ar for 30 min.

5. Lyophilize for 36 h or precipitate using diethyl ether to yield the final product.

3.4.3. Derivatization of Thiol Functionalized Nanoparticles with Folate

1. Dissolve the activated carbonate (1 equiv.) in DCM and add folate-EDA (1 equiv.) and DIPEA dissolved in DMSO (*see* **Fig. 17.6**). Wrap the flask in aluminum foil and stir the reaction mixture at r.t. for 2 h to form activated folate-EDA. Purify the product using preparative RP-HPLC (1–50%B for 30 min, 80%B 5 min; A = 1 mM phosphate, pH 7.2; B = ACN, column: Waters, xTerra C_{18} 10 μm; 19 × 250 mm, flow rate = 26 mL/min).

2. Dissolve thiol functionalized nanoparticles in a solvent of choice (e.g., DMSO). Add activated folate-EDA and 100-fold excess DIPEA to the reaction mixture. Wrap the flask in aluminum foil and stir the reaction at r.t. overnight. Follow Step 5 in **Section 3.4.2** to yield the final product. Follow Step 5 in **Section 3.4.3** to isolate the final product.

3.4.4. Derivatization of Carboxyl Functionalized Nanoparticles with Folate

Dissolve carboxyl functionalized nanoparticles in a solvent of choice and add NHS, TEA, and DCC sequentially (*see* **Fig. 17.7**). Stir the reaction mixture at r.t. for 1 h. Add folate-EDA dissolved

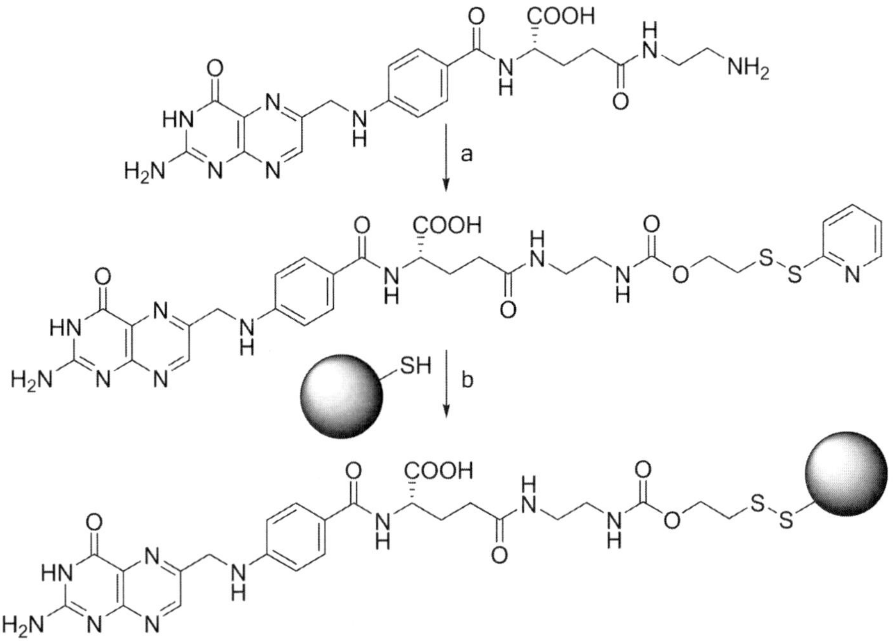

Fig. 17.6. Reagents and conditions: (a) activated carbonate, DIPEA/DMSO, r.t.; (b) nanoparticles/water, pH 7.2, bubble Ar, r.t.

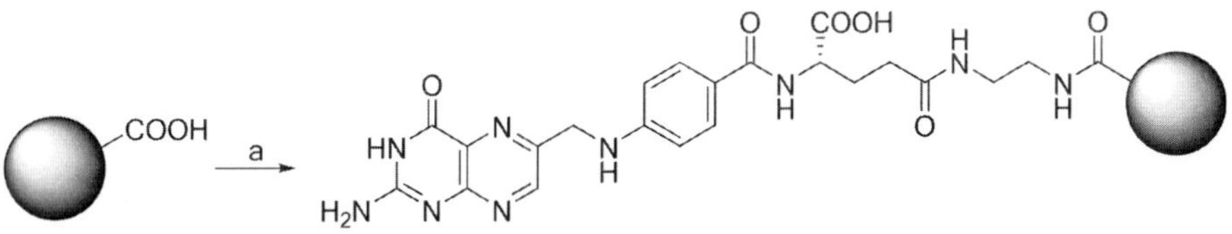

Fig. 17.7. Reagents and conditions: (a) (i) NHS, DCC, TEA/DMSO; (ii) folate-EDA, TEA/DMSO.

in DMSO to the reaction mixture, wrap the flask in aluminum foil, and stir overnight at r.t. Follow Step 5 in **Section 3.4.3** to isolate the final product.

3.5. Determination of In Vitro Efficacies FA-Targeted Nanoparticles

3.5.1. Determination of Affinity of FA-Targeted Nanoparticles Relative to Free FA (see **Note 8**)

1. Seed KB cells (50,000 cells/well in 500 μL) into a 48-well plate and allow to form monolayers overnight in folate-deficient RPMI medium (see **Note 9**) containing 10% heat-inactivated fetal bovine serum and 1% penicillin–streptomycin (culture medium). Replace spent medium with fresh culture medium containing a fixed amount of ^{3}H-FA (10 nM) plus increasing concentrations (0.01–1,000 nM) of either FA-targeted nanoparticle or free FA. Incubate cells at 37°C for 2 h and rinse gently with PBS (4 × 250 μL). Incubate rinsed cells with TCA (250 μL) at r.t. for 10 min and treat resulting white aggregate with 0.25 M NaOH solution (250 μL) for 30 min at r.t. Transfer resulting lysate (200 μL) into scintillation vial containing Ecolume (3 mL).

Count radioactivity using a liquid scintillation counter. Calculate relative affinity of the test article by plotting bound radioactivity versus log concentration of test article using GraphPad Prism 4.

3.5.2. Determination of Cell Labeling Efficiency and Extent of Internalization of FA-Targeted Fluorescence Nanoparticles

Flow cytometry for analysis of cell labeling efficiency: Seed KB cells into a T75 flask and allow cells to form a monolayer over 48 h. Digest cells with trypsin and transfer released cells to centrifuge tubes (10^6 cells/tube). Pellet cells by centrifuging at $1,000 \times g$ for 3 min and incubate pelleted cells with fresh culture medium containing fluorescent FA-nanoparticles (50 nM) in the presence or absence of 1,000-fold molar excess FA in a 5% CO_2:95% air-humidified atmosphere at 37°C for 2 h. Rinse cells with PBS (3×1.0 mL) and resuspend in PBS (1.0 mL) to analyze cell-bound fluorescence intensity (500,000 cells/sample) using a flow cytometer. Use untreated KB cells in PBS as a negative control (see **Note 10**).

Confocal microscopy to evaluate FA-nanoparticle internalization: Seed KB (100,000 cells/well in 1 mL) into micro-well petri dishes and allow to form monolayers overnight. Replace spent medium with fresh culture medium containing fluorescent FA-nanoparticles (50 nM) in the presence or lacking 1,000-fold excess FA. Incubate cells in 5% CO_2:95% air-humidified atmosphere at 37°C for 2 h. Rinse with PBS (3×1.0 mL) and evaluate abundance of liposomes in intracellular endosomes by confocal microscopy. Use untreated KB cells in PBS as a negative control.

3.5.3. Determination of In Vitro Potency of FA-Targeted Therapeutic Nanoparticles Using ^{3}H-thymidine Assay (see **Note 11**)

1. Seed KB cells (100,000 cells/well in 500 μL) in a 48-well plate and allow cells to form monolayers overnight. Replace spent medium with fresh culture medium containing increasing concentrations (0.01–1,000 nM) of drug-loaded nanoparticle in the presence or absence of 1,000-fold excess FA. Incubate cells in a 5% CO_2:95% air-humidified atmosphere at 37°C for 2 h.

2. Rinse cells with fresh culture medium (3×250 μL) and incubate in fresh medium (250 μL) in a 5% CO_2:95% air-humidified atmosphere at 37°C for 66 h.

3. Replace spent medium in each well with fresh medium containing [^{3}H]-thymidine (1 μCi/mL) and incubate cells in a 5% CO_2:95% air-humidified atmosphere at 37°C for 4 h.

4. Rinse cells with culture medium (3×250 μL) and incubate in 5% TCA (250 μL) for 10 min at r.t. Dissolve cells in 0.25 M $NaOH_{(aq)}$ (250 μL) for 30 min at r.t. and transfer into individual scintillation vials containing Ecolume (3.0 mL). Count radioactivity using a liquid scintillation counter. Calculate IC_{50} of test article using a plot

of %^{3}H-thymidine incorporation versus log concentration of test article using GraphPad Prism 4.

3.6. Determination of In Vivo Efficacy of FA-Targeted Imaging and Therapeutic Nanoparticles

3.6.1. Tumor Models

1. Maintain 6 weeks old female *nu/nu* mice on folate-free rodent chow for 2 weeks prior to tumor implantation and maintain mice on the same diet throughout the study (*see* **Note 12**).

2. Inoculate mice subcutaneously with KB or A549 cells (1.0×10^6 cell/mice in 100 μL of medium) on the right shoulder. Measure growth of tumors in two perpendicular directions every 2 days using a caliper and calculate tumor volume (V) as $0.5 \times L \times W^2$ (L = longest axis and W = axis perpendicular to L in mm). Monitor body weights on the same schedule.

3.6.2. Whole-Body Imaging and Biodistribution

1. Allow tumors on tumor-bearing mice to reach a volume of 400 mm^3. Inject mice with folate-targeted nanoparticulate imaging agent through the lateral tail vein (group 1).

2. Inject mice with nontargeted nanoparticulate imaging agent through the lateral tail vein (group 2; control).

3. Sacrifice animals by CO_2 asphyxiation 4 h after injection of radiolabeled nanoparticle. Acquire whole-body images by γ-scintigraphy.

4. Dissect animals after whole-body radioimaging and add tissues to pre-weighed γ-counter tubes. Count radioactivity of tissues and known amount of radioimaging agent in a γ-counter. Calculate results as % injected dose per gram of wet tissue and tumor-to-normal tissue ratios.

3.6.3. Determination of Chronic Maximum Tolerance Dose (MTD) and Site of Toxicity

1. Administer escalating doses of freshly prepared therapeutic agent dissolved in PBS (200 μL) to healthy *nu/nu* mice via lateral tail-vein injection (5 mice/group) on days 0, 2, 4, 6, 8, and 10.

2. Obtain body weights and clinical observations prior to dosing and daily thereafter from day 0 to 12. Prepare graph of %weight change versus days on therapy and euthanize any animals with a body weight loss of 20% or more over 2 consecutive days.

3. Collect blood via cardiac puncture from the left ventricle into tubes with or without heparin. Evaluate hematology (whole blood) and clinical chemistry (serum and/or plasma) parameters.

4. Dissect animals and collect selected tissues [e.g., brain, heart, lung, spleen, liver, kidneys, intestine, testes, and bone (tibia-fibula and sternum)]. Weigh tissues, fix in 10%

neutral-buffered formalin (in PBS), and submit for histopathology analysis.

3.6.4. In Vivo Potency

1. Treat *nu/nu* mice bearing tumor xenografts ($V = 100$ mm^3) with a dose of therapeutic nanoparticles equal to 25% of MTD (200 μL) via lateral tail-vein injection on days 0, 2, 4, 6, 8, and 10.

2. Monitor growth of subcutaneous tumor by measuring tumor volume 3× per week for 4 weeks. Monitor whole-body weight on the same schedule. Construct a graph of tumor volume (mm^3) versus days on therapy to evaluate in vivo efficacy of the drug. Construct a graph of % weight change versus days on therapy to evaluate in vivo toxicity of the drug.

4. Notes

1. Kaiser (AKA ninhydrin) test: Triketohydrindene hydrate reacts with primary or secondary amines to produce a purple/blue color. It is, therefore, a useful test to monitor formation of free amines and to evaluate the efficiency of amino acid coupling.

2. Piperidine (20%) deprotects Fmoc group, 2% deprotects TFA group, and TFA:H$_2$O:TIPS cocktail cleave the final product from the resin and deprotects ^{t}Bu group. EDT prevents the formation of disulfide bonds.

3. An alternative method for synthesis of folate-PEG$_{2000}$-DSPE involves dissolving FA in DMSO and adding NHS, DCC, and TEA sequentially. The addition of H$_2$N-PEG$_{2000}$-NH$_2$ dissolved in CHCl$_3$ then yields a mixture of γ- and α-folate derivatives (attachment at the γ-carboxyl is favored) of the H$_2$N-PEG$_{2000}$-NH$_2$ (along with some bis-folate derivative). In a separate flask, dissolve DSPE and TEA in CHCl$_3$ and add glutamic anhydride. Stir for 1 h and add the previously synthesized folate-PEG$_{2000}$-NH$_2$ dissolved in CHCl$_3$. Stir for an additional 12 h and purify as described in **Section 3**.

4. Purity can also be determined by thin-layer chromatography using the solvent system CDCl$_3$:MeOH:H$_2$O = 75:36:6 on a silica gel GF plates.

5. Lipid compositions and types of lipid can be varied.

6. Alternative method: Dissolve liposomal components and drug at requisite molar ratios in CHCl$_3$ and dry on a rotary evaporator. Rehydrate the lipid film with 10% sucrose or 5% dextrose/15 mM Hepes buffer (pH 7.4) (33).

7. Amine, hydroxyl, thiol, or carboxyl functionalized nanoparticles (e.g., liposomes, solid lipid nanoparticles, polymeric micelles, dendrimers, viral nanoparticles, nanotubes, and quantum dots) can be conjugated to either folate-Cys or folate-EDA using bi-functional linkers such as MAL-linker-NHS.

8. Relative affinity: the inverse molar ratio of the compound required to displace 50% of ^{3}H-folic acid bound to FR on cells; relative affinity of FA = 1; relative affinity <1 indicates weaker affinity; relative affinity >1 stronger affinity with respect to folic acid. Because folate-targeted nanoparticles cannot access as many folate receptors on a cell surface as ^{3}H-FA, only partial inhibition of ^{3}H-FA will be observed in the presence of FA-targeted nanoparticles whereas complete inhibition will be seen in the presence of excess free FA.

9. Fetal bovine serum (10%) contains sufficient FA to enable proliferation of KB cells and the resulting RPMI culture medium is physiologically more relevant than normal RPMI medium that contains 1,000-fold more FA than is present in the human body.

10. FR-mediated uptake (FR specificity) of a test article can be evaluated by quantitating uptake in the presence of excess FA, however, the use of nontargeted nanoparticles to determine the FR specificity is preferred. This is because monovalent folates (e.g., folic acid) do not compete well with multivalent folate-linked nanoparticles.

11. Alternative method: 3-(4,5-dimethylthiazol-2-yl)-2,5-diphenyltetrazolium (MTT) assay: Follow Steps 1 and 2 as described in the ^{3}H-thymidine assay. Add 20 µL of MTT stock solution (5 mg/mL) to each well and incubate cells in a 5% carbon dioxide:95% air-humidified atmosphere at 37°C for 4 h. Replace medium with DMSO (200 µL) to dissolve the blue formazan crystal generated during the MTT assay and assess cell viability by measuring absorbance at 570 nm.

12. Mice should be fed a folate-deficient diet to achieve a serum FA concentration closer to the range of normal human serum FA concentrations [normal rodent diet very high levels of FA (6 mg/kg chow)].

References

1. Jemal, A., Siegel, R., Ward, E., Hao, Y., Xu, J., Murray, J., and Thus, M. J. (2008) Cancer statistics, 2008. *CA Cancer J Clin* **58**, 71–96.

2. Menon, U. and Jacobs, I. J. (2000) Recent development in ovarian cancer screening. *Curr Opin Obstet Gynecol* **12**, 39–42.

3. Li, C. (2002) Poly(L-glutamic acid)-anticancer drug conjugates. *Adv Drug Deliv Rev* **54**, 695–713.
4. Gabizon, A. (1995) Liposome circulation time and tumor targeting: implications for cancer chemotherapy. *Adv Drug Deliv Rev* **16**, 285–294.
5. Nie, S., Xing, Y., Kim, G. J., and Simons, J. W. (2007) Nanotechnology applications in cancer. *Annu Rev Biomed Eng* **9**, 12.1–12.32.
6. Ringsdorf, H. (1975) Structure and properties of pharmacologically active polymers. *J Polm Sci Polym Symp* **51**, 135–153.
7. Moghimi, S. M. and Hunter, A. C. (2000) Poloxamers and poloxamines in nanoparticles engineering and experimental medicine. *Trends Biotechnol* **18**, 412–420.
8. Park, E. K., Lee, S. B., and Lee, Y. M. (2005) Preparation and characterization of methoxypoly(ethylene glycol)/poly(epsilon-caprolactone) amphiphilic block copolymeric nanospheres for tumor-specific folate-mediated targeting of anticancer drugs. *Biomaterials* **26**, 1053–1061.
9. Lichtenberg, D. (1988) Liposomes: preparation, characterization, and preservation. *Methods Biochem Anal* **33**, 337–468.
10. Litzinger, D. C. and Huang, L. (1992) Phosphatidylethanol amine liposomes: drug delivery, gene transfer, and immunodiagnostic applications. *Biochim Biophys Acta* **1113**, 201–227.
11. Matsumura, Y. and Maeda, H. (1986) A new concept for macromolecular therapeutics in cancer chemotherapy: mechanism of tumoritropic accumulation of proteins and the antitumor agent SMANCS. *Cancer Res* **46**, 6387–6392.
12. Meada, H. (2001) The enhanced permeability and retention (EPR) effect in tumor vasculature: the key role of tumor-selective macromolecular targeting. *Adv Enzyme Regul* **41**, 189–207.
13. Allen, T. M. (2002) Ligand-targeted therapeutics in anticancer therapy. *Nat Rev Cancer* **2**, 750–763.
14. Low, P. S. and Antony, A. C. (2004) Folate receptor-targeted drugs for cancer and inflammatory disease. *Adv Drug Deliv Rev* **56**, 1055–1231.
15. Ross, J. F., Chaudhuri, P. K., and Ratnam, M. (1994) Differential regulation of folate receptor isoforms in normal and malignant tissues in vivo and in established cell lines. Physiologic and clinical implications. *Cancer* **73**, 2432–2443.
16. Weitman, S. D., Lark, R. H., Coney, L. R., Fort, D. W., Frasca, V., Zurawski, V. R., and Kamen, B. A. (1992) Distribution of the folate receptor GP38 in normal and malignant cell lines and tissues. *Cancer Res* **52**, 3396–3401.
17. Reddy, J. A., Allagadda, V. M., and Leamon, C. P. (2005) Targeting therapeutic and imaging agents to folate receptor positive tumors. *Curr Pharm Biotech* **6**, 131–150.
18. Kamen, B. A. and Capdevila, A. (1986) Receptor-mediated folate accumulation is regulated by the cellular folate content. *Proc Natl Acad Sci USA* **83**, 5983–5987.
19. Henne, W. A., Doorneweerd, D. D., Hilgenbrink, A. R., Kularatne, S. A., and Low, P. S. (2006) Synthesis and activity of a folate peptide camptothecin prodrug. *Bioorg Med Chem Lett* **16**, 5350–5355.
20. Reddy, J. A. and Low, P. S. (2000) Enhanced folate receptor-mediated gene therapy using a novel pH-sensitive lipid formulation. *J Control Release* **64**, 27–37.
21. Lu, Y. and Low, P. S. (2002) Folate targeting of haptens to cancer cell surfaces mediates immunotherapy of syngeneic murine tumors. *Cancer Immunol Immunother* **51**, 153–162.
22. Leamon, C. P. and Low, P. S. (1992) Cytotoxicity of momordin-folate conjugates in cultured human cells. *J Biol Chem* **267**, 24966–24971.
23. Zhao, X., Li, H., and Lee, R. J. (2008) Target drug delivery via folate receptors. *Expert Opin Drug Deliv* **5**, 309–319.
24. Majoros, I. J., Thomas, T. P., Mehta, C. B., and Baker, J. R. (2005) Poly(amidoamine) dendrimer-base multifunctional engineered nanodevice for cancer therapy. *J Med Chem* **48**, 5892–5899.
25. Yoo, H. S. and Park, T. G. (2004) Folate-receptor-targeted delivery of doxorubicin nano-aggregates stabilized by doxorubicin-PEG-folate conjugate. *J Control Release* **100**, 247–256.
26. Leamon, C. P., Parker, M. A., Vlahov, I. R., Xu, L. C., Reddy, J. A., Vetzel, M., and Douglas, N. (2002) Synthesis and biological evaluation of EC20: a new folate-derived, ^{99m}Tc-based radiopharmaceutical. *Bioconjugate Chem* **13**, 1200–1210.
27. Yoshizawa, T., Hattori, Y., Hakoshima, M., Koga, K., and Maitani, Y. (2008) Folate-linked lipid-base nanoparticles for synthetic siRNA delivery in KB tumor xenografts. *Eur J Pharm Biopharm* **70**, 718–725.
28. Lee, R. J., Wang, S., Turk, M. J., and Low, P. S. (1998) The effects of pH and intraliposomal buffer strength on the rate of liposome content release and intracellular drug delivery. *Biosci Rep* **18**, 69–78.

29. Yang, J., Chen, H., Vlahov, I. R., Cheng, J., and Low, P. S. (2007) Characterization of the pH of folate receptor-containing endosomes and the rate of hydrolysis of internalized acid-labile folate-drug conjugates. *J Pharmacol Exp Ther* **321**, 462–468.
30. Larsen, A. K., Escargueil, A. K., and Skladanowski, A. (2000) Resistance mechanisms associated with altered intracellular distribution of anticancer agents. *Pharmacol Ther* **85**, 217–229.
31. Xu, L., Vlahov, I. R., Leamon, C. P., Santhapuram, H., and Li, C. (2006) Synthesis and purification of pteroic acid and conjugates thereof. *US Patent* WO2006101845.
32. Zhang, Y., Guo, L., Roeske, R. W., Antony, A. C., and Jayaram, H. N. (2004) Pteroyl-γ-glutamate-cysteine synthesis and its application in folate receptor-mediated cancer cell targeting using folate-tethered liposomes. *Anal Biochem* **332**, 168–177.
33. Wu, J., Liu, Q., and Lee, R. J. (2006) A folate receptor-targeted liposomal formulation for paclitaxel. *Int J Pharm* **316**, 148–153.
34. Rouser, G., Fleischer, J., and Yamamoto, A. (1970) Two dimensional thin layer chromatographic separation of polar lipids and determination of phospholipids by phosphorous analysis of spots. *Lipids* **5**, 494–496.
35. Vlahov, I. R., Santhapuram, H. R., Kleindl, P. J., Howard, S. J., Stanford, K. M., and Leamon, C. P. (2006) Design and regioselective synthesis of a new generation of targeted chemotherapeutics. Part 1: EC 145, a folic acid conjugate of desacetylvinblastine monohydrazide. *Bioorg Med Chem Lett* **16**, 5093–5096.

Chapter 18

Magnetic Aerosol Targeting of Nanoparticles to Cancer: Nanomagnetosols

Carsten Rudolph, Bernhard Gleich, and Andreas W. Flemmer

Abstract

Inhalation of aerosols represents the most frequently used drug delivery method for the treatment of lung diseases. To further improve drug efficacy in the lungs, it may be advantageous to control aerosol deposition and target aerosols to diseased or disease-causing lung tissue and cellular structures in order to maximize drug potency and minimize side effects in unaffected tissue. We have recently investigated a novel method which brings aerosol delivery to an advanced level of specificity by making use of magnetic gradient fields to direct magnetizable aerosol droplets containing superparamagnetic iron oxide nanoparticles (SPION) specifically to desired regions of the lungs in mice. In this chapter, we will present a detailed description of this procedure for application in mice.

Key words: Magnetic drug targeting, lung, aerosol, cancer.

1. Introduction

Although approximately 1.3 million patients are newly diagnosed with lung cancer every year, there is a lack of effective therapeutic options for a disease of such enormous dimension which is among one of the leading causes of death worldwide (1). There is currently no "gold standard" therapy for advanced lung cancer, although platinum-based therapies are the most widely used in the first-line setting for both non-small cell and small cell lung cancers. The median survival with the most commonly used chemotherapeutic regimens in advanced non-small cell lung cancer is only 8 months (1). The above facts illustrate the necessity of novel strategies to improve the therapeutic outcome for lung cancer treatment.

Among the major reasons of treatment failure are the devastating side effects caused by systemically applied chemotherapeutic agents (2). Indeed, pharmacologically effective drug concentrations have to be achieved in the diseased lung tissue to lead to tumor regression but simultaneously hazardous drug levels have to be avoided in non-diseased tissue. Although conventional chemotherapeutic agents are principally effective in killing cancer cells, one of their major limitations is the high dosage needed to achieve effective drug concentrations in the lung tissue when applied intravenously, which often results in unwanted dose-limiting side effects. One of the major unmet medical needs is therefore targeted delivery of the chemotherapeutic agents to only the diseased tissue as precisely as possible to minimize unwanted drug-related side effects and realize effective chemotherapy.

With respect to lung cancer, aerosol delivery of chemotherapeutic drugs by inhalation represents a straightforward strategy to target the lung tumor tissue. It allows delivery of a high dosage of the chemotherapeutic agent directly to the lung. Although only a few previous studies attempted to prove this attractive treatment option, these studies demonstrate that aerosol delivery of chemotherapeutics to the lungs by inhalation allows to reduce total drug dosage and drug-related side effects (2, 3).

We have recently attempted to bring this approach to an advanced level of specificity by making use of a magnetic gradient filed to direct magnetizable aerosol droplets, so-called *nanomagnetosols*, which comprise superparamagnetic iron oxide nanoparticles (SPIONs) packaged together into an aerosol droplet, to desired regions of the lungs (4). This novel approach overcomes the natural deposition mechanism of inhaled aerosol droplets in the lungs which is limited by targeting of aerosol deposition to the central airways or lung periphery but not to local regions in the lungs. Hence, this study opens up new perspectives to realize more specific treatment of lung tumors by increasing delivery of chemotherapeutic agents to the cancer cells and reducing unwanted drug-related side effects in non-diseased tissue.

2. Materials

2.1. Components for Electromagnet Construction

1. Magnetically soft material with high saturation flux density (up to 2.35 T, Vacuflux50) can be purchased from Vakuumschmelze Hanau, Germany (www.vacuumschmelze.de).

2. Magnetically soft material with medium saturation flux density (up to 2 T, Armco Telar 57 N) can be purchased from Remag AG, Germany.

3. Copper wire for coil windings with a diameter appropriate for the carrying current (www.pack-feindraehte.de).

2.2. Permanent Magnets

4. Cubic 4.8 mm × 4.8 mm × 4.5 mm (NE48) NeoDeltaMagnets made from neodymium–iron–boron (NdFeB, remanence 1,080–1,120 mT) can be purchased from IBS Magnet, Berlin, Germany (http://www.ibsmagnet.de/).

2.3. Intratracheal Aerosol Application

1. SAV FlexiVent system (Montreal, Quebec, Canada) for controlled ventilation of mice.

2. Aeroneb® Lab Micropump Nebulizer (Nektar Therapeutics, Mountain View, CA, USA; median mass aerodynamic diameter (MMAD) = 2.5–4 μm).

3. Blunt end 22-G gauge needle. A regularly clinically used 22-G gauge needle whose tip is made blunt end by using a file can be used. Just beneath the needle's blunt end, a fine chamfer should be added in order to exclude slipping of the fine cotton during fixation in the trachea.

4. Pentobarbital-Na (16 g/100 mL; Merial GmbH, Hallbergmoos, Germany) is used for anesthesia and diluted 1:10 with sterile, pyrogen-free saline from Braun Melsungen AG (Melsungen, Germany) before use.

2.4. Whole-Body Aerosol Application

1. Jet nebulizer (PARI BOY® LC plus; PARI GmbH, Starnberg, Germany).

2. The whole-body device comprises a sealed 9.8 cm × 13.2 cm × 21.5 cm plastic box which is connected directly to the nebulizer (5). At the opposite side of the plastic box, four small holes were inserted to allow aerosol flow through the plastic box (**Fig. 18.1a**). This device was further modified at one end with a 45 cm × 7.7 cm plastic cylinder (diameter of the connecting piece 2.1 cm) which in turn was connected to the jet nebulizer. The bottom of the connecting plastic cylinder was evenly covered with 150 g of silica gel (1–3 mm, #85330; Fluka, Switzerland) (*see* **Note 1**). Six small chambers of equal size were inserted into the box made from a fine non-magnetic mesh (**Fig. 18.1b**).

3. "UHU sekundenkleber blitzschnell" instant adhesive based on cyanoacrylates.

4. Gas cylinder containing synthetic air with 5% of carbon dioxide can be obtained custom-made from Westfalen AG (Münster, Germany).

A

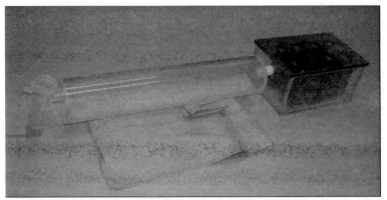

B

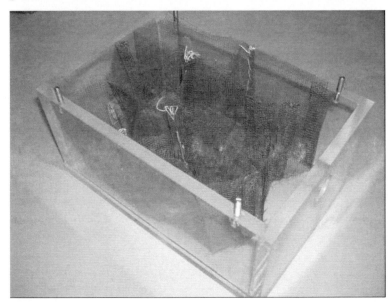

Fig. 18.1. Representation of the whole-body aerosol device. (**a**) A plastic box which houses the mice is connected to the nebulizer via an aerosol spacer placed in horizontal orientation. The detailed dimensions of the aerosol device are described in Rudolph et al. (5). (**b**) To avoid the mice from adhering together with their magnets, six small chambers of equal size are inserted into the box made from a fine non-magnetic mesh. The mesh size should allow unrestricted aerosol flow.

2.5. SPION and Polyethylenimine (PEI)–Plasmid DNA (pDNA) Solution

1. Custom-made superparamagnetic iron oxide nanoparticles coated with 25-kDa branched polyethylenimine are provided by Chemicell GmbH, Berlin, Germany (http://www.chemicell.com/home/index.html). The hydrodynamic particle diameter is 80 nm comprising a 50-nm multidomain core of 5-nm single-domain magnetite nanoparticles with a packaging density of 30% (*see* **Note 2**).

2. Branched PEI (average MW = 25 kDa, # 408727) is obtained from Sigma-Aldrich Chemie GmbH (Munich, Germany).

3. Plasmid DNA pCMV-Luc containing firefly luciferase cDNA driven by the CMV promoter is amplified and purified by PlasmidFactory (Bielefeld, Germany). The purity (LPS) of this plasmid is ≤ 0.1 EU/μg DNA and the amount of super-coiled DNA $\geq 90\%$ cm^3.

2.6. Measurement of Luciferase Activity

1. Lysis buffer (10×) consists of 15.1 g Tris–HCl in 50 mL distilled water, pH 7.8, and 0.5 g Triton X-100 and one tablet of complete protease inhibitor mix (Roche Molecular Biochemicals, Basel, Switzerland) and is used after 1:10 dilution with water for injection.

2. Luciferin substrate buffer: 60 mM DTT, 10 mM Mg$_2$SO$_4$, 10 mM ATP, 30 μM luciferin in 25 mM glycylglycine buffer, pH 7.8.

3. Methods

In the following section, two independent methods which can be used to increase and localize aerosol deposition in the lungs of mice are presented. Both of the methods exploit nebulization of superparamagnetic iron oxide nanoparticles (SPION) together with application of a magnetic gradient field on the lungs during inhalation. The first method described allows to site-specifically navigate aerosols to focal regions of the lungs. This can be achieved when a solution containing SPIONs is nebulized directly into anesthetized, intubated mice during ventilation and the tip of an electromagnet is positioned as closely as possible above the target lung area. Whereas this method allows to efficiently enrich aerosol deposition in the target lung region, it is limited by the fact that only short-term experiments can be performed because of the lack of animal survival after the ventilation procedure. This may be overcome by using a whole-body aerosol device in which mice can freely move without anesthesia. However, this method does not allow to specifically target a desired lung region because of constraints regarding controlled magnet positioning on the lungs of non-anesthetized, freely moving mice during nebulization but leads to an overall increase of drug deposition.

3.1. Construction of the Electromagnet

To overcome the aerodynamic forces and gravity, a magnet with sufficient flux density is needed. To achieve a high flux density gradient within the whole body of the mouse, a magnet geometry with a closed frame was chosen. At least for successful targeting of magnetosols, a gradient of magnetic flux density of about 100 T/m is necessary for a flow velocity of 0.52 m/s and an aerodynamic particle diameter of 3.5 μm. **Figure 18.2** shows a detailed view of the magnetic system.

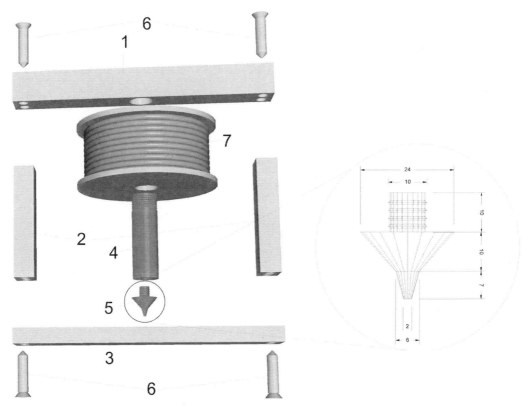

Fig. 18.2. Schematic representation of the construction of the electromagnet. Each part is described in detail under **Section 3.1**.

1. Part #1 – upper bar
   The upper bar is made of Armco Telar 57 N and has a length of 260 mm and a cross-sectional area of 300 mm × 410 mm (width × height). In the middle of the bar, a screw thread (M24) is inserted. To connect this part with the side bars, four M8 screws are used (*see* **Note 3**).

2. Part #2 – side bar
   The two side bars are made of Armco Telar 57 N and have a length of 221 mm and a cross-sectional area of 200 mm × 300 mm (width × depth). Four screw threads are inserted in each bar, two on the top and two on the bottom.

3. Part #3 – lower bar
   The lower bar is made of Armco Telar 57 N and has a length of 260 mm and a cross-sectional area of 400 mm × 260 mm

(width × height). To connect this part with the side bars, four M8 screws are used.

4. Part #4 – bolt
   The bolt is made of Vacuflux50. It has a cylindrical geometry with a diameter of 24 mm. The bolt has a M24 screw thread on the top to connect the bolt with the upper bar and a M10 screw thread on the bottom to connect with the coil tip.

5. Part #5 – coil tip
   The coil tip is made of Vacuflux50. The geometry and the sizes (all dimensions in millimeter) are given in **Fig. 18.2**. The geometry was optimized by means of numerical field calculation for a high flux density gradient of 100 T/m in the lungs of the mice.

6. Part #6 – screws
   All bars are connected using M8 screws made of steel (*see* **Note 4**).

7. Part #7 – coil
   The body of the coil must be made of a non-magnetic material like aluminum or better laminated fabric. One must pay attention to that the distance between wire and bolt must be minimized (in the order of max. 1 mm). The top and the bottom of the coil body are up to 5 mm thick. Eight hundred windings of an isolated lacquer-coated wire is needed (AWG 17 or 18 for up to 5 A) to generate the needed magnetic flux density gradient.

3.2. Preparation of SPION and PEI–pDNA Solution

1. The SPION solution is diluted with water (WFI) to a final concentration of 12.5 mg/mL (referring to Fe content) for injection. At this concentration, each aerosol droplet generated by the nebulizer comprises approximately 2,930 SPIONs, which have been previously shown by computer-aided simulations to result in a sufficiently high magnetic moment to be magnetically attracted within the experimental setup at the tip of the electromagnet (4). This has been further confirmed by preliminary experiments using a system made from plastic tubing in our lab. It is important to dilute SPIONs in WFI and not in saline to avoid colloidal instability of the dispersion (*see* **Note 5**). This is in particular important when pDNA is added to the SPION dispersion. The SPIONs are surface modified with the polyelectrolyte polyethylenimine which tends to aggregate after complex formation with pDNA at concentrations > 200 μg/mL. Before use the SPION dispersion should be sonicated for 1 min in order to disintegrate potential aggregates which are formed during storage. Store the SPION dispersion at 4°C as recommend by the provider.

2. When pDNA is delivered to the lungs of mice, add an equal volume of an aqueous pDNA solution to the SPION dispersion and mix by gently pipetting up and down using the pipettor and incubate for 15 min at ambient temperature before nebulization. We recommend a w/w (SPION/pDNA)=10/1, which results in stable dispersions without precipitation.

3. When SPIONs are co-delivered with PEI–pDNA gene vector nanoparticles, the PEI–pDNA nanoparticles are first generated as follows: Plasmid DNA and PEI are diluted separately in 2.67 mL of double-distilled water, resulting in concentrations of 600 μg/mL pDNA and 870 μg/mL PEI, respectively, corresponding to an N/P ratio of 10 (molar ratio of PEI nitrogen to DNA phosphate). The DNA solution is pipetted into the PEI solution, mixed by vigorously pipetting up and down, to yield a final pDNA concentration of 300 μg/mL. At this concentration, the PEI–pDNA gene vectors are still stable, resulting in spherical particles of 100–200 nm. The resulting PEI–pDNA gene vector solution is then pipetted into 2.67 mL of a SPION solution and mixed vigorously by pipetting up and down, resulting in a final concentration of 12 mg/mL (Fe) with a w/w (SPION/pDNA)=60/1 ratio. Under these conditions, two separate particle populations, i.e., SPIONs and PEI–pDNA gene vectors, coexist in the solution.

4. For aerosol delivery using the whole-body aerosol device, pDNA and PEI are diluted in 4.0 mL of double-distilled water (*see* **Note 6**), resulting in concentrations of 250 μg/mL DNA and 326.3 μg/mL PEI, respectively (corresponding to an N/P ratio of 10) (5). The DNA solution was pipetted into the PEI solution, mixed by vigorously pipetting up and down, to yield a final pDNA concentration of 125 μg/mL. The complexes are incubated for 20 min at ambient temperature before use.

3.3. Intratracheal Aerosol Application

1. Six- to eight-week-old female BALB/c mice (Charles River Laboratories, Sulzfeld, Germany) are maintained under specific pathogen-free conditions. Animals should be acclimatized to the environment of the animal facility for at least 7 days prior to the start of the experiments. The animal procedures have to be approved by the local ethics committee and carried out according to the legal guidelines.

2. Mice are anesthetized intraperitoneally with pentobarbital (80–100 mg/kg of body weight). The trachea is exposed through a skin incision and the blunt end 22-G gauge needle is carefully inserted just below the cricoid cartilage. In order to avoid air flow leakage and removal of the needle, it is

3. Mice are connected to the tubings of the FlexiVent respirator system and ventilated with a tidal volume of 10 μL/g of body weight at a respiration frequency of 120 min^{-1} and a PEEP (positive end expiratory pressure) of 4 cm H_2O.

4. Place the magnet's tip directly above the fur of the target lung area (*see* **Note 7**).

5. The SPION or the SPION/pDNA solution is nebulized to the mice lungs during controlled ventilation (*see* **Note 8**). For this purpose, 200–300 μL of the solution is added to the reservoir of the ultrasonic nebulizer Aeroneb® Lab Micropump Nebulizer which is connected in parallel to the respiration unit by three-way valves which are set in-line during aerosol application (**Fig. 18.3**). Twenty 10-s aerosol boluses of SPION solution can be applied to the lung.

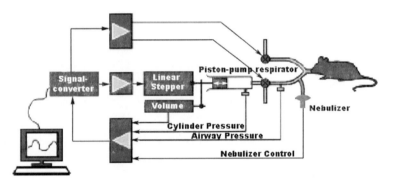

Fig. 18.3. Schematic representation of the FlexiVent respirator system used for ventilation and aerosol application.

6. After aerosol treatment is complete, mice are sacrificed by intraperitoneal pentobarbital overdose injection, the lungs are surgically removed en bloc, and either shock frozen in liquid nitrogen in an Eppendorf tube for subsequent tissue homogenization and analysis of SPION and pDNA tissue content or fixed in 4% paraformaldehyde for histology.

3.4. Whole-Body Aerosol Application

1. A permanent magnet is fixed on the fur covering the thorax of the mice by using either tissue glue or any other instant adhesive (**Fig. 18.4**).

2. Acclimatized mice are placed in the plastic box and the lid is closed by using the screws. To avoid the mice from adhering to their magnets, six small chambers of equal size are inserted into the box made from a fine non-magnetic mesh. The mesh size should allow unrestricted aerosol flow.

tightly fixed using fine cotton. For this purpose, a fine chamfer should be added just beneath the needle's blunt end.

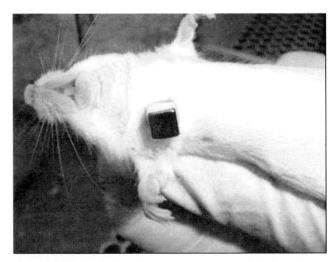

Fig. 18.4. Fixation of a permanent magnet above the thorax of a mouse. The permanent magnet is fixed on the fur covering the thorax of the mice by using either tissue glue or any other instant adhesive.

3. The silica gel is gently, homogenously distributed on the bottom surface of the tube for aerosol drying which is then connected directly to the nebulizer.

4. Four milliliters of gene vector solution is added to the reservoir of the PARI nebulizer and the nebulizer is connected to the drying tube.

5. Before beginning the nebulization process, the compressor of the nebulizer is connected with a gas cylinder containing synthetic air (see **Note 9**) using a tube which is attached to the aspirating port of the compressor and airflow is set to 6 L/min. After the first 4 mL of solution is nebulized, add the second proportion of the solution to the reservoir and repeat the nebulization process.

6. At desired time points, the mice are anesthetized intraperitoneally with pentobarbital and the peritonea are opened by midline incisions. In order to purge blood from the lungs and to avoid interference with the subsequent luciferase assay, a posterior vena cava exit is cut, and 10–15 mL of an heparinized isotonic sodium chloride solution (25,000 IE heparin/1,000 mL) is slowly perfused into the right cardiac ventricles of the mice(see **Note 10**). The lungs are then dissected from animals en bloc and washed in PBS.

3.5. Tissue Homogenization

1. The dissected lungs are placed into an Eppendorf tube and weighed before shock freezing in a Dewar filled with liquid nitrogen. The lungs are stored in a freezer at –80°C until further use.

2. Fill liquid nitrogen into a Styrofoam box and cool down mortar and pestle. After down cooling of mortar and pestle, a homogenous powder of mice lungs can be easily produced.

3.6. Histology

1. For histology the reader is refereed to specialized protocols according to the required research purpose.

3.7. Measurement of Luciferase Activity

1. For luciferase measurement, 400 μL lysis buffer is added to ~25 mg of homogenized lung powder in an Eppendorf tube, briefly vortexed, and then incubated on ice for 15 min.

2. After incubation on ice and another brief vortexing, the samples are centrifuged at 10,000 rcf at 4°C for 10 min.

3. Luminescence expressed as relative light units (RLU) of each sample is determined in duplicates with the Lumat 9,507 tube luminometer (Berthold, Bad Wildbach, Germany). One hundred microliters of the lung tissue supernatant is mixed with 100 μL of luciferin substrate buffer and luciferase activity was measured for 30 s (RLU/s).

4. Notes

1. Unlike humans, mice are compulsive nose breathing animals and aerosol delivery to the deeper compartment of the lungs is strongly reduced due to the physiologic function of the nose to filter hazardous airborne particles from the inhaled air. While particles of an MMAD of 0.27 μm effectively deposit up to 45% in the alveolar region in mice, larger particles of an MMAD of 3.45 μm deposit only up to 0.9% in the alveolar region but the major fraction deposits in the nasopharynx and the gastrointestinal tract (6). Since the MMAD of the aerosol which is generated by the jet nebulizer is about 3–4 μm, only marginal gene vector deposition is expected to occur in the deep areas of the lungs. Interposition of a drying spacer tube induces a ~10-fold reduction in the aerosol diameter and has been demonstrated previously to result in ~10-fold increase in gene expression in the lungs of mice (5).

2. Instead of the custom-made SPIONs previously used, any other type of superparamagnetic SPION that is theoretically equally well suited can be used. Increase in the SPION size will increase their magnetic moment and should therefore allow to even decrease the SPION concentration in the nebulized solution. The Chemicell shelf product

CombiMAG, which is used for plasmid DNA transfection, may be used.

3. When changing the dimensions of the electromagnet, one must be sure that the average magnetic flux density within the bars is smaller than approx. 1.4 T. Other materials than Armco Telar 57 N can be used for the construction of the upper, lower, and side bars when taking the non-linearity of the material into account (e.g., when using simple steel, the average magnetic flux density in the iron frame must be smaller than 0.8 T, which means that the cross-sectional areas of the bars must be increased).

4. The constructor must avoid air gaps, especially at the connecting screws. Holes and the screw threads of the bolt and the coil tip must be constructed in such a way that the screw thread has the same geometry of the blind hole (e.g., conical geometry of the screw thread, not shown in **Fig. 18.2**).

5. In order to prevent colloidal instability of the SPION or PEI–pDNA gene vector solutions, each of the components should be diluted in solvents with low ionic strength. For this purpose, use distilled water (water for injection, WFI) or if isotonicity is necessary, use 5% glucose solution. Avoid saline, which will lead to instant particle aggregation at the high particle concentration used.

6. Distilled water is the preferred solvent for gene vector formulation and aerosol application because of its intrinsic properties to increase gene transfer efficiency in the lungs. It has been previously shown that distilled water inhalation results in transient airway epithelial swelling by a so-called hyposomotic shock (7). Associated swelling and permeabilization of lung tissue have been proposed to be critical for efficient gene transfer to the lungs (8, 9).

7. The extent of aerosol enrichment largely depends on the distance between the tip of the magnet and the target lung tissue due the non-proportional decay of the magnetic gradient field with the distance from the magnetic pole (4). It is therefore recommended to place the tip of the magnet as closely as possible to the target lung region.

8. To test if the PEI–pDNA gene vectors are bound to the SPIONs or exist separately, SPIONs can be separated from PEI–pDNA gene vectors by placing the solution on a permanent magnet (see above). If both of the particles separately coexist, pDNA will be detected in the supernatant only after magnetic separation of the SPIONs. For this purpose, incubate the supernatant with heparin sulfate [w/w (heparin sulfate/pDNA) = 10/1]

and run the sample on an agarose gel electrophoresis. The addition of heparin sulfate is required for the release of the pDNA from the cationic polymer PEI (**Fig. 18.5**).

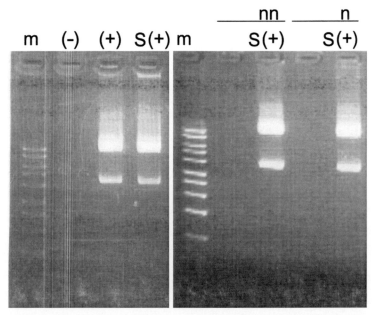

Fig. 18.5. Characterization of the nanomagnetosol solution. The solution comprising SPION and PEI–pDNA particles was prepared as described in **Section 3.2** and analyzed by agarose gel electrophoresis. (Left) Plasmid DNA is tightly bound with the PEI–pDNA gene vectors (–); when heparin sulfate [w/w (heparin sulfate/pDNA) = 10/1] is added to the solution either before (+) or after magnetic separation of the SPIONs from the solution by placing the solution on a permanent magnet (+S), pDNA is detected in equal amounts in the supernatant, indicating the presence of individual PEI–pDNA gene vectors and SPIONs in the solution. (Right) Nebulized (n) and non-nebulized (nn) nanomagnetosol solution is magnetically separated and pDNA released by heparin sulfate addition. The absence of pDNA fragments indicates pDNA integrity after nebulization (M = 1-kb DNA marker).

9. For aerosol application using the whole-body device, it is recommended to operate the nebulizer with air containing 5% carbon dioxide. Carbon dioxide increases tidal volume of inhalation and breathing frequency in mice, which together results in an increase in aerosol deposition (5, 10).

10. Before lungs are excised from the mice, they should be thoroughly purged from blood in order to minimize hemoglobin content of the lung tissue, which has been previously shown to interfere with luciferase activity measurement because of light absorption of light emitted during the luciferase catalytic reaction (11).

Acknowledgments

This work was supported by the German Federal Ministry of Education and Research in the program Nanotechnology, grants 13N8539, 13N8535, 13N8537, 13N9182 and BioFuture [0311898], and LMUexcellent (Investitionsfonds).

References

1. Gkiozos, I., Charpidou, A., and Syrigos, K. (2007) Developments in the treatment of non-small cell lung cancer. *Anticancer Res* 27(4C), 2823–2827.
2. Otterson, G. A., Villalona-Calero, M. A., Sharma, S., Kris, M. G., Imondi, A., Gerber, M., White, D. A., Ratain, M. J., Schiller, J. H., Sandler, A., Kraut, M., Mani, S., and Murren, J. R. (2007) Phase I study of inhaled Doxorubicin for patients with metastatic tumors to the lungs. *Clin Cancer Res* 13(4), 1246–1252.
3. Verschraegen, C. F., Gilbert, B. E., Loyer, E., Huaringa, A., Walsh, G., Newman, R. A., and Knight, V. (2004) Clinical evaluation of the delivery and safety of aerosolized liposomal 9-nitro-20(s)-camptothecin in patients with advanced pulmonary malignancies. *Clin Cancer Res* 10(7), 2319–2326.
4. Dames, P., Gleich, B., Flemmer, A., Hajek, K., Seidl, N., Wiekhorst, F., Eberbeck, D., Bittmann, I., Bergemann, C., Weyh, T., Trahms, L., Rosenecker, J., and Rudolph, C. (2007) Targeted delivery of magnetic aerosol droplets to the lung. *Nat Nanotechnol* 2(8), 495–499.
5. Rudolph, C., Ortiz, A., Schillinger, U., Jauernig, J., Plank, C., and Rosenecker, J. (2005) Methodological optimization of polyethylenimine (PEI)-based gene delivery to the lungs of mice via aerosol application. *J Gene Med* 7(1), 59–66.
6. Raabe, O. G., Al-Bayati, M. A., Teague, S. V., and Rasolt, A. (1988) Regional deposition of inhaled monodisperse coarse and fine aerosol particles in small laboratory animals. *Ann Occup Hyg* 32(Supplement 1), 53–63.
7. Mochizuki, H., Ohki, Y., Arakawa, H., Tokuyama, K., and Morikawa, A. (1999) Effect of ultrasonically nebulized distilled water on airway epithelial cell swelling in guinea pigs. *J Appl Physiol* 86(5), 1505–1512.
8. Lemoine, J. L., Farley, R., and Huang., L. (2005) Mechanism of efficient transfection of the nasal airway epithelium by hypotonic shock. *Gene Ther* 12(16), 1275–1282.
9. Rudolph, C., Schillinger, U., Ortiz, A., Plank, C., Golas, M. M., Sander, B., Stark, H., and Rosenecker, J. (2005) Aerosolized nanogram quantities of plasmid DNA mediate highly efficient gene delivery to mouse airway epithelium. *Mol Ther* 12(3), 493–501.
10. Gautam, A., Densmore, C. L., Xu, B., and Waldrep, J. C. (2000) Enhanced gene expression in mouse lung after PEI-DNA aerosol delivery. *Mol Ther* 2(1), 63–70.
11. Colin, M., Moritz, S., Schneider, H., Capeau, J., Coutelle, C., and Brahimi-Horn., M. C. (2000) Haemoglobin interferes with the ex vivo luciferase luminescence assay: consequence for detection of luciferase reporter gene expression in vivo. *Gene Ther* 7(15), 1333–1336.

Chapter 19

LHRH-Targeted Nanoparticles for Cancer Therapeutics

Tamara Minko, Mahesh L. Patil, Min Zhang, Jayant J. Khandare, Maha Saad, Pooja Chandna, and Oleh Taratula

Abstract

Synthesis and evaluation of a novel cancer cell's receptor-targeted internally quaternized and surface neutral poly(amidoamine) (PAMAM) generation four dendrimer as well as PAMAM–paclitaxel conjugate are described. The advantages of developed nanocarriers include but are not limited to (1) internal cationic charges for the complexation with small interfering RNA or antisense oligonucleotides and their protection from the degradation in systemic circulation; (2) neutral-modified surface for low cytotoxicity of empty unloaded dendrimers; (3) efficient internalization by cancer cells; and (4) preferential accumulation in the tumor and the prevention of adverse side effects of chemotherapy.

Key words: Dendrimer, PAMAM, siRNA, paclitaxel, chemotherapy, tumor targeting, quaternization.

1. Introduction

Modern cancer chemotherapy utilizes two broad approaches: (1) the direct use of simple anticancer drugs and (2) prodrug approach (1–5). The latter is based on the so-called prodrugs – drug precursors that remain inactive during delivery to the site of action and are specifically activated at the target site. The utilization of prodrugs to certain extent allows for the preservation of anticancer activity of active components and targets drug release to tumor cells or their organelles. The most complete realization of the prodrug approach is possible by the use of an advanced type of anticancer prodrug – the tumor-targeted anticancer drug delivery system (DDS) (3, 4, 6, 7). In general, tumor-targeted DDS may include (1) a carrier, which binds its components together and provides solubility for an entire complex; (2) a targeting moiety, which directs DDS specifically to cancer cells, prevents drug accumulation in healthy organs, and facilitates its uptake by cancer cells; and (3) one or more active ingredients, which are responsible for the anticancer effect of DDS. The latter may include one or several anticancer drug(s) and other components for enhancing the cell death-inducing activity of a main drug(s) and suppressing cellular defense. Anticancer drugs, peptides, antisense oligonucleotides (ASO), antibodies or their fragments, short interfering RNA (siRNA), and other moieties are being used as active components of anticancer DDS (8–20). In the present study, we describe several nanocarrier-based delivery systems, which utilize a modified synthetic analog of luteinizing hormone-releasing hormone (LHRH) as a targeting moiety, polyamidoamine (PAMAM)

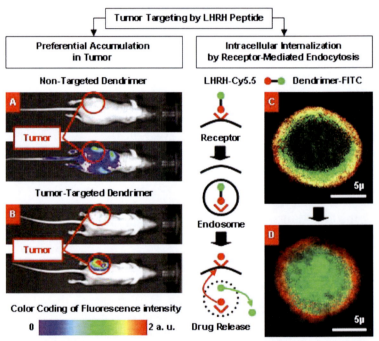

Fig. 19.1. Advantages of tumor targeting by LHRH peptide. (**A**, **B**) Preferential accumulation of targeted dendrimers in the tumor. Animals bearing subcutaneous xenografts of human ovarian carcinoma were treated with dendrimers labeled with a fluorescent dye: nontargeted (**A**) and targeted to LHRH receptors that are overexpressed in the plasma membrane of cancer cells (**B**). The fluorescence was registered using the IVIS imaging system in living animals anesthetized by isoflurane. (**C**, **D**) Intracellular internalization of LHRH–dendrimer complex by receptor-mediated endocytosis. LHRH peptide was labeled with near-infrared dye (Cy5.5, *red fluorescence*). The dendrimer was labeled with FITC (*green fluorescence*). Human cancer cells were incubated for 1 h (**C**) and 24 h (**D**) with LHRH–dendrimer complex, and fluorescence was registered by a confocal microscope. *Green* and *red fluorescence* images were superimposed. *Yellow color* shows colocalization of LHRH and dendrimers in the plasma membrane and cytoplasm on the initial stages of endocytosis (**C**).

generation four dendrimer as a carrier, paclitaxel (TAX) as an anticancer drug, siRNA or ASO targeted to MDR1, and BCL2 mRNA as suppressors of cellular resistance.

The use of LHRH peptide as a tumor-targeting moiety to receptors that are overexpressed in the plasma membrane of many types of cancer cells provides for two main advantages (**Fig. 19.1**). First, in contrast to nontargeted dendrimer-based DDS that accumulates almost equally in a tumor, liver, and kidney (**Fig. 19.1a**), LHRH directs the entire DDS specifically to the tumor and prevents its accumulation in healthy tissues (**Fig. 19.1b**). Second, interacting with receptors in the plasma membrane of cancer cells, LHRH peptide enforces the internalization of DDS by cancer cells via receptor-mediated endocytosis (**Fig. 19.1c, d**). This mechanism of nanocarrier internalization by cancer cells is much more efficient when compared with penetration of free low molecular weight drugs or nontargeted DDS by a "simple" diffusion or endocytosis, respectively. Such a switch of mechanisms substantially enhances intracellular internalization and the anticancer efficacy of the delivered drug and other active components of DDS.

In the proposed DDS, we utilize a novel type of dendrimeric nanocarrier recently developed in our laboratory (21). This carrier possesses two distinct advantages over traditional dendrimeric

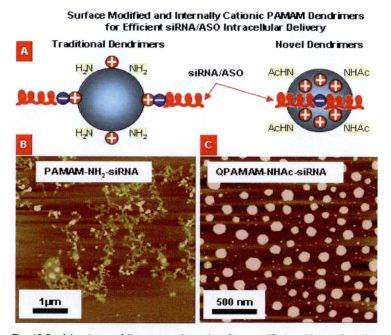

Fig. 19.2. Advantages of the proposed novel surface-modified and internally cationic dendrimers for efficient siRNA/ASO delivery. (**A**) Schematic illustration of siRNA–dendrimer complexes. (**B, C**) Atomic force microscope images of siRNA complexated with traditional (**B**) and modified (**C**) dendrimers.

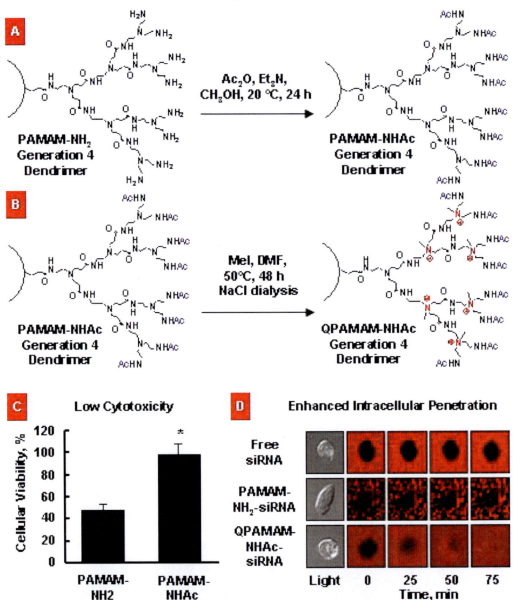

Fig. 19.3. Synthesis and evaluation of surface modified (**A**) and internally quaternized (**B**) dendrimers. (**C**) Cytotoxicity of a traditional (PAMAM-NH$_2$) and novel surface-modified (PAMAM-NHAc) dendrimers. (**D**) Cellular internalization of free siRNA, and dendrimer–siRNA complexes with a traditional (PAMAM-NH$_2$) and internally cationic and surface-modified (QPAMAM-NHAc) dendrimers. siRNA were labeled with a *red fluorescence* dye, conjugated with different dendrimers, and added to the incubation medium containing living cancer cells. Real-time fluorescence was registered using a fluorescent microscope. Free siRNA and traditional non-modified dendrimer–siRNA complexes are poorly internalized by cancer cells, while novel dendrimers provided for an efficient intracellular delivery of siRNA.

carriers suitable for delivering anticancer drugs and/or ASO, DNA, and siRNA (**Fig. 19.2**). First, cationic charges required for complexation with anionic ASO/siRNA are located inside the structure, instead of the outer surface of traditional cationic carriers (**Fig. 19.2a**). Such modification is achieved by internal quaternization of the PAMAM dendrimer. This enforces the formation of well-condensed dendrimer–siRNA nanoparticles (polyplexes) where each molecule of siRNA is covered and protected from the environment and degradation by several dendrimers (**Fig. 19.2c**). In contrast, nonquaternized dendrimers often form microtubule-like structures with noncovered and nonprotected siRNA (**Fig. 19.2b**). Second, it has neutrally modified the (acetylated or hydroxylated) surface leading to the low cytotoxicity of empty dendrimers and enhanced internalization of the entire DDS by cancer cells (**Fig. 19.3c, d**). In the present study, we describe synthesis of several DDS based on such dendrimers and provide some experimental data supporting the advantages of our approach to complex multifunctional tumor-targeted proapoptotic delivery systems.

2. Materials

2.1. Synthesis of Acetylated PAMAM-NHAc Dendrimer

1. Generation four PAMAM-NH$_2$ (Mw ~ 14,214 Da, 64 amine end groups) dendrimer (Sigma-Aldrich Co., St. Louis, MO); anhydrous methanol (Fisher Scientific, Fairlawn, NJ).
2. Triethylamine (Fisher Scientific, Fairlawn, NJ).
3. Acetic anhydride (Sigma-Aldrich Co., St. Louis, MO).
4. Dialysis membrane with molecular mass cutoff at 2,000 Da (Spectrum Laboratories, Inc., Rancho Dominguez, CA).

2.2. Synthesis of Acetylated and Internally Quaternized QPAMAM-NHAc Dendrimer

1. N,N′-Dimethyl formamide (DMF) (Fisher Scientific, Fairlawn, NJ).
2. Methyl iodide (MeI) (Sigma-Aldrich Co., St. Louis, MO).
3. Diethyl ether (Fisher Scientific, Fairlawn, NJ).
4. 2 M solution of sodium chloride (NaCl, Fisher Scientific, Fairlawn, NJ) in deionized water.
5. Dialysis membrane with molecular mass cutoff at 2,000 Da (Spectrum Laboratories, Inc., Rancho Dominguez, CA).

2.3. Synthesis of PAMAM-OH–LHRH Conjugate

1. Synthetic analog of LHRH, Lys6-des-Gly10-Pro9-ethylamide (Gln-His-Trp-Ser-Tyr-D-Lys(D-Cys)-Leu-Arg-Pro-NH-Et), having a reactive amino group only on the side chain of the lysine at position 6 can be synthesized

according to our design by American Peptide Company, Inc. (Sunnyvale, CA); anhydrous pyridine (Fisher Scientific, Fairlawn, NJ).

2. Succinic anhydride (Fisher Scientific, Fairlawn, NJ).
3. N/A.
4. Spectra/Pore dialysis membrane with the molecular weight cutoff at 500 Da (Spectrum Laboratories, Inc., Rancho Dominguez, CA).
5. Anhydrous dichloromethane (5 mL) and anhydrous dimethyl sulfoxide (Fisher Scientific, Fairlawn, NJ).
6. Generation four PAMAM-OH dendrimer (Mw ~ 14,277 Da, 64 hydroxyl end groups, 1,2-diaminoethane dendrimer core) from Sigma-Aldrich Co. (St. Louis, MO).
7. N-(3-Dimethylaminopropyl)-N-ethylcarbodiimide hydrochloride (EDCHCl) and 4-dimethylaminopyridine (DMAP) from Fluka (Allentown, PA).
8. Spectra/Pore dialysis membranes with the molecular weight cutoff at 2,000 Da (Spectrum Laboratories, Inc., Rancho Dominguez, CA); Sephadex™ G-10 column (Sigma-Aldrich Co., St. Louis, MO).

2.4. Synthesis of Internally Quaternized QPAMAM-OH–LHRH Conjugate

1. PAMAM-OH–LHRH synthesized according to Section 3.3; N,N'-dimethyl formamide (DMF) (Fisher Scientific, Fairlawn, NJ).
2. Methyl iodide (MeI) (Sigma-Aldrich Co., St. Louis, MO).
3. N/A.
4. Diethyl ether (Fisher Scientific, Fairlawn, NJ).
5. 2 M solution of sodium chloride (NaCl, Fisher Scientific, Fairlawn, NJ) in deionized water.
6. Dialysis membrane with molecular mass cutoff at 2,000 Da (Spectrum Laboratories, Inc., Rancho Dominguez, CA).

2.5. Synthesis of Tumor-Targeted LHRH–PAMAM Dendrimer–Paclitaxel Conjugate

1. Paclitaxel and succinic acid from Sigma Chemical Co. (Atlanta, GA); anhydrous dimethyl sulfoxide (DMSO) and anhydrous dichloromethane (DCM) from Fischer Scientific (Pittsburgh, PA).
2. N-(3-Dimethylaminopropyl)-N-ethylcarbodiimide HCl (EDCHCl) from Fluka (Allentown, PA); 4-(methylamino)pyridine (DMAP) from Sigma Chemical Co. (Atlanta, GA).
3. Dialysis membrane with molecular mass cutoff at 2,000 Da (Spectrum Laboratories, Inc., Rancho Dominguez, CA).

3. Methods

3.1. Synthesis of Acetylated PAMAM-NHAc Dendrimer

1. Prepare and stir the solution of PAMAM-NH$_2$ generation four dendrimer (172 mg, 0.012 mmol) dissolved in anhydrous methanol (10 mL) (**Fig. 19.3a**).
2. Add 0.17 mL (1.2 mmol) of triethylamine to the stirred solution.
3. Add 0.1 mL (0.96 mmol) of acetic anhydride to the stirred solution.
4. Seal and stir the resulting mixture at room temperature for 24 h.
5. Evaporate methanol under reduced pressure and dissolve the resulting residue in water (2 mL).
6. Purify the dendrimer solution by dialysis against deionizer water using dialysis membrane (molecular mass cutoff at 2,000 Da).
7. Freeze-dry the dialyzed solution to afford acetylated PAMAM dendrimer (PAMAM-NHAc).

3.2. Synthesis of Acetylated and Internally Quaternized QPAMAM-NHAc Dendrimer

1. Dissolve 100 mg (0.0059 mmol) of PAMAM-NHAc (synthesized in **Section 3.1**) in 1 mL of DMF (**Fig. 19.3b**).
2. Add 0.5 mL methyl iodide.
3. Seal the solution off and stir it at 50°C for 48 h.
4. Precipitate the reaction mixture into diethyl ether to obtain a solid, which then should be dried under vacuum and redissolved in water (1 mL).
5. Dialyze the resulting solution against 2 M NaCl and deionized water successively using dialysis membrane (molecular mass cutoff at 2,000 Da) and then lyophilize to afford white solid.

3.3. Synthesis of PAMAM-OH–LHRH Conjugate

1. Dissolve 50 mg (0.036 mmol) of LHRH peptide in 1 mL of anhydrous pyridine and stir the solution (**Fig. 19.4a**).
2. Add 5 mg (0.05 mmol) of succinic anhydride.
3. Seal and stir the reaction mixture at room temperature for 24 h.
4. After the evaporation of solvents under reduced pressure, purify the residue by extensive dialysis against deionized water using dialysis membrane (molecular mass cutoff at 500 Da). Freeze-dry to afford LHRH-hemisuccinate as a white solid.

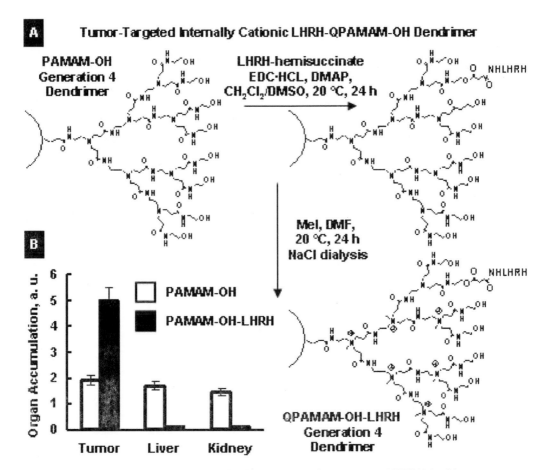

Fig. 19.4. Synthesis (**A**) and organ distribution (**B**) of nontargeted and tumor-targeted PAMAM dendrimers.

5. Prepare the solution of anhydrous dichloromethane (5 mL) and anhydrous dimethyl sulfoxide (5 mL).

6. Dissolve 86 mg (0.006 mmol) of PAMAM-OH generation four dendrimer and 17.2 mg (0.012 mmol) of LHRH-hemisuccinate in this solution.

7. Add 2.5 mg (0.013 mmol) of EDCHCl to the above solution as a condensing agent and 1 mg of DMAP as a catalyst. Stir the reaction mixture for 24 h.

8. After evaporation of the solvent and redissolving in water (1 mL), purify the resulting conjugate by extensive dialysis against deionizer water using dialysis membrane (molecular mass cutoff at 2,000 Da) and passing through a Sephadex column.

9. Lyophilize the solution to afford PAMAM-OH–LHRH conjugate as a pale yellow solid.

3.4. Synthesis of Internally Quaternized QPAMAM-OH–LHRH Conjugate

1. Dissolve 50 mg of PAMAM-OH–LHRH conjugate in 1 mL of N,N'-dimethylformamide and stir the solution (**Fig. 19.4a**).
2. Add 0.5 mL of methyl iodide to a stirred solution.
3. Seal and stir the solution at room temperature for 24 h.
4. Precipitate the reaction mixture into diethyl ether to obtain a solid, which should be dried under vacuum and redissolved in water (1 mL).
5. Dialyze the resulting solution against 2 M NaCl and deionized water successively using dialysis membrane (molecular mass cutoff at 2,000 Da) and then lyophilize it to afford the QPAMAM-OH–LHRH conjugate.

3.5. Synthesis of Tumor-Targeted LHRH–PAMAM Dendrimer–Paclitaxel Conjugate

SA (2) is a bis carboxylic acid moiety and is reacted on equimolar basis with hydroxyl group in paclitaxel (1) to form a paclitaxel–SA conjugate (3) leaving one free carboxyl group for further conjugation with a hydroxyl terminal dendrimer (**Fig. 19.5**).

3.5.1. Synthesis of Paclitaxel–Succinic Acid (SA) Conjugate

1. Dissolve paclitaxel (10.0 mg, 0.0118 mM) and succinic acid (1.4 mg, 0.0118 mM) in 3.0 mL of anhydrous DMSO and 10.0 mL of anhydrous DCM.
2. Add N-(3-dimethylaminopropyl)-N-ethylcarbodiimide HCl (EDCHCl, 2.30 mg, 0.0118 mM) and DMAP (1.0 mg) to the resulting mixture.
3. The reaction is carried out with continuous stirring for 24 h at room temperature. Filter the resulting solution to remove dicyclohexylurea (DCU) obtained as a by-product during the reaction.
4. Precipitate paclitaxel–SA conjugate using diethyl ether and dry it under vacuum.

3.5.2. Synthesis of Tumor-Targeted PAMAM-G4–Succinic Acid–Paclitaxel Conjugate

Conjugation of succinic acid to paclitaxel results in the formation of mono carboxylic acid conjugate (3), which is further conjugated with hydroxyl groups in PAMAM-G4-OH dendrimer (4) (**Fig. 19.5a**).

1. Dissolve tumor-targeted dendrimer (0.0061 mM, actual dendrimer amount in milligram depends on the composition of a dendrimer) and paclitaxel–succinic acid conjugate (6.0 mg, 0.0061 mM) in 4.0 mL of anhydrous DMSO and 10.0 mL of anhydrous DCM. The mole ratio of dendrimer to paclitaxel–SA conjugate is maintained to be 1:1.
2. Add EDCHCl (1.2 mg, 0.0062 mM) and DMAP (1.0 mg) as a coupling agent and a catalyst, respectively. Stir the reaction continuously for 24 h at room temperature.
3. Filter the resulting solution to remove DCU and dialyze the filtrate extensively with anhydrous DMSO using dialysis

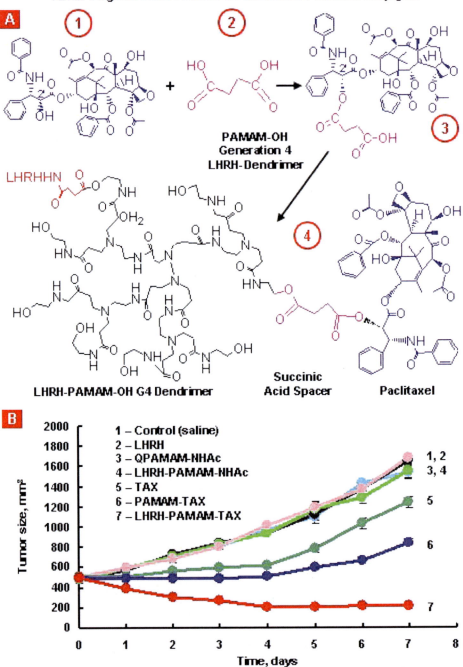

Fig. 19.5. Synthesis and in vivo evaluation of nontargeted and tumor-targeted LHRH–PAMAM–paclitaxel conjugate. (**A**) A synthetic scheme (*1*): paclitaxel (TAX) (*2*); succinic acid (SA) (*3*); TAX–succinic acid conjugate (*4*); resulting LHRH–PAMAM–SA–TAX conjugate. (**B**) Antitumor activity of different substances indicated.

membrane of molecular weight cutoff at 2,000 Da for 24 h to remove unreacted paclitaxel–SA conjugate and EDCHCl.

4. Purify the conjugate by size-exclusion chromatography using a Sephadex column to remove unreacted paclitaxel–SA conjugate and excess EDCHCl.

5. Dry the conjugate under vacuum at room temperature.

4. Notes

1. The synthesized internally quaternized and surface-modified QPAMAM-NHAc dendrimer should have a low cytotoxicity (**Fig. 19.3c**) and provides for an excellent intracellular delivery of complexated siRNA (**Fig. 19.3d**). To measure cytotoxicity one can use a modified MTT assay as previously described (20, 22, 23). In order to evaluate the efficiency of the synthesized dendrimers in delivering siRNA into cellular cytoplasm, siRNA should be labeled with a fluorescent dye, complexated with a dendrimer, and incubated with cancer cells. Fluorescence should be registered periodically (every 1–10 min) within 1–1.5 h by a confocal microscope as previously described (14, 19, 21, 24). Fluorescent RNA duplex – siRNA labeled with Pierce NuLight™ DY-547 fluorophore (si*GLO* Red Transfection Indicator, red fluorescence) can be obtained from Applied Biosystems (Ambion, Inc., Foster City, CA). Mix si*GLO* Red with the dendrimer in water at calculated N/P (amine to phosphate) charge ratio around 3. The charge ratio can be calculated by relating the number of positive charges on dendrimer (primary amine groups of PAMAM-NH$_2$ and quaternary amine groups of QPAMAM-OH and QPAMAM-NHAc) with the number of negatively charged phosphate groups of siRNA. The solution should be incubated for 30 min at room temperature to allow complex formation.

2. The size and shape of synthesized delivery systems should be analyzed by atomic force microscopy (AFM) as previously described (21). The samples of siRNA/dendrimer condensates are imaged with a tapping mode atomic force microscope (Nanoscope III A, Veeco Digital Instruments, Santa Barbara, CA). During imaging, 125 μm long rectangular silicon cantilever/tip assembly is used with a spring constant of 40 N/m, resonance frequency of 315–352 kHz, and a tip radius of 5–10 nm. The images are generated by the change in amplitude of the free oscillation of the cantilever as it interacts with the sample. The height differences on the

surface are indicated in the images by the color code: lighter regions indicate higher heights (**Fig. 19.2b, c**). In order to image siRNA condensates, 5 µL of dendrimer/siRNA solution is deposited on freshly cleaved mica. After 3–5 min of incubation, the mica surface is rinsed with three drops of deionized water four times and dried under a flow of nitrogen.

3. The efficiency of tumor-targeted delivery and cancer treatment can be tested in experiments on nude mice bearing xenografts of human ovarian or lung cancer as previously described (25, 26). Briefly, human cancer cells (2×10^6) are subcutaneously transplanted into the flank of athymic nu/nu mice. The tumor is measured by a caliper every day and its volume is calculated as $d^2 \times D/2$, where d and D are the shortest and longest diameter of the tumor in millimeters, respectively. When the tumor reaches a mean size of 500 mm^3, mice should be treated intravenously (via the tail vein) with different DDS and appropriate control substances.

4. The concentration of cytotoxic DDS for in vivo experiments should be selected close to the maximum tolerated dose. The maximum tolerated dose (MTD) is estimated in separate experiments based on animal weight changes after the injection of increasing doses of the drugs as previously described (7, 25, 27). The minimal dose which leads to the decrease in animal weight 24 h after the treatment should be considered as MTD. The dose selected for animal experiments should be equal or less than MTD.

5. The efficiency of tumor targeting is determined by measuring the distribution of labeled Cy5.5 DDS in the organism of the experimental animals using the IVIS imaging system (Xenogen Corporation, Alameda, CA) as previously described (19, 26, 28). Animals are anesthetized with isoflurane using the XGI-8 Gas Anesthesia System (Xenogen Corporation, Alameda, CA). Visible light and fluorescence images are taken and overlaid using the manufacturer's software to obtain a composite image. The targeted DDS should be found predominately in tumors, while nontargeted dendrimers are almost equally distributed between the tumor, liver, and kidney (**Fig. 19.1a, b**). In addition, total fluorescence level in the tumor should be several times higher for targeted dendrimers when compared with nontargeted delivery systems (**Fig. 19.4b**).

6. The decrease in tumor size is used as an index of the antitumor efficacy of synthesized dendrimers containing anticancer drugs (**Fig. 19.5b**). Saline, LHRH peptide, and

nontargeted and tumor-targeted dendrimers without an anticancer drug should be used as "controls" (**Fig. 19.5b**, curves 1–4). These substances should not influence tumor growth. The antitumor effectiveness of paclitaxel delivered by a dendrimer (**Fig. 19.5b**, curve 6) should be better than that of free paclitaxel (**Fig. 19.5b**, curve 5) and the antitumor efficacy of targeted polymer–paclitaxel conjugate (**Fig. 19.5b**, curve 7) should be the highest when compared with both paclitaxel alone (**Fig. 19.5b**, curve 5) and nontargeted paclitaxel conjugate (**Fig. 19.5b**, curve 6).

Acknowledgments

This research was supported in part by NIH grants CA100098 and CA111766 from the National Cancer Institute.

References

1. Khandare, J. J., Chandna, P., Wang, Y., Pozharov, V. P., and Minko, T. (2006) Novel polymeric prodrug with multivalent components for cancer therapy. *J Pharmacol Exp Ther* **317**, 929–937.
2. Kratz, F., Muller, I. A., Ryppa, C., and Warnecke, A. (2008) Prodrug strategies in anticancer chemotherapy. *ChemMedChem* **3**, 20–53.
3. Minko, T. (2004) Drug targeting to the colon with lectins and neoglycoconjugates. *Adv Drug Deliv Rev* **56**, 491–509.
4. Minko, T., Dharap, S. S., Pakunlu, R. I., and Wang, Y. (2004) Molecular targeting of drug delivery systems to cancer. *Curr Drug Targets* **5**, 389–406.
5. Singh, Y., Palombo, M., and Sinko, P. J. (2008) Recent trends in targeted anticancer prodrug and conjugate design. *Curr Med Chem* **15**, 1802–1826.
6. Allen, T. M. and Cullis, P. R. (2004) Drug delivery systems: entering the mainstream. *Science* **303**, 1818–1822.
7. Chandna, P., Saad, M., Wang, Y., Ber, E., Khandare, J., Vetcher, A. A., Soldatenkov, V. A., and Minko, T. (2007) Targeted proapoptotic anticancer drug delivery system. *Mol Pharm* **4**, 668–678.
8. Betigeri, S., Pakunlu, R. I., Wang, Y., Khandare, J. J., and Minko, T. (2006) JNK1 as a molecular target to limit cellular mortality under hypoxia. *Mol Pharm* **3**, 424–430.
9. Caplen, N. J. and Mousses, S. (2003) Short interfering RNA (siRNA)-mediated RNA interference (RNAi) in human cells. *Ann NY Acad Sci* **1002**, 56–62.
10. Gutierrez-Puente, Y., Tari, A. M., Ford, R. J., Tamez-Guerra, R., Mercado-Hernandez, R., Santoyo-Stephano, M., and Lopez-Berestein, G. (2003) Cellular pharmacology of P-ethoxy antisense oligonucleotides targeted to Bcl-2 in a follicular lymphoma cell line. *Leuk Lymphoma* **44**, 1979–1985.
11. Kang, H., DeLong, R., Fisher, M. H., and Juliano, R. L. (2005) Tat-conjugated PAMAM dendrimers as delivery agents for antisense and siRNA oligonucleotides. *Pharm Res* **22**, 2099–2106.
12. Lukyanov, A. N., Elbayoumi, T. A., Chakilam, A. R., and Torchilin, V. P. (2004) Tumor-targeted liposomes: doxorubicin-loaded long-circulating liposomes modified with anti-cancer antibody. *J Control Release* **100**, 135–144.
13. Pakunlu, R. I., Cook, T. J., and Minko, T. (2003) Simultaneous modulation of multidrug resistance and antiapoptotic cellular defense by MDR1 and BCL-2 targeted antisense oligonucleotides enhances the anticancer efficacy of doxorubicin. *Pharm Res* **20**, 351–359.
14. Pakunlu, R. I., Wang, Y., Saad, M., Khandare, J. J., Starovoytov, V., and Minko, T. (2006) In vitro and in vivo intracellular liposomal delivery of antisense oligonucleotides and anticancer drug. *J Control Release* **114**, 153–162.
15. Pakunlu, R. I., Wang, Y., Tsao, W., Pozharov, V., Cook, T. J., and Minko, T. (2004) Enhancement of the efficacy of chemotherapy for lung cancer by simultaneous suppression of multidrug resistance and

antiapoptotic cellular defense: novel multicomponent delivery system. *Cancer Res* **64**, 6214–6224.
16. Torchilin, V. P. (2006) Multifunctional nanocarriers. *Adv Drug Deliv Rev* **58**, 1532–1555.
17. Torchilin, V. P. (2006) Recent approaches to intracellular delivery of drugs and DNA and organelle targeting. *Annu Rev Biomed Eng* **8**, 343–375.
18. Wang, Y. and Minko, T. (2004) A novel cancer therapy: combined liposomal hypoxia inducible factor 1 alpha antisense oligonucleotides and an anticancer drug. *Biochem Pharmacol* **68**, 2031–2042.
19. Wang, Y., Saad, M., Pakunlu, R. I., Khandare, J. J., Garbuzenko, O. B., Vetcher, A. A., Soldatenkov, V. A., Pozharov, V. P., and Minko, T. (2008) Nonviral nanoscale-based delivery of antisense oligonucleotides targeted to hypoxia-inducible factor 1{alpha} enhances the efficacy of chemotherapy in drug-resistant tumor. *Clin Cancer Res* **14**, 3607–3616.
20. Wang, Y., Pakunlu, R. I., Tsao, W., Pozharov, V., and Minko, T. (2004) Bimodal effect of hypoxia in cancer: the role of hypoxia inducible factor in apoptosis. *Mol Pharm* **1**, 156–165.
21. Patil, M. L., Zhang, M., Betigeri, S., Taratula, O., He, H., and Minko, T. (2008) Surface-modified and internally cationic polyamidoamine dendrimers for efficient siRNA delivery. *Bioconjug Chem* **19**, 1396–1403.
22. Dharap, S. S. and Minko, T. (2003) Targeted proapoptotic LHRH-BH3 peptide. *Pharm Res* **20**, 889–896.
23. Jayant, S., Khandare, J. J., Wang, Y., Singh, A. P., Vorsa, N., and Minko, T. (2007) Targeted sialic acid-doxorubicin prodrugs for intracellular delivery and cancer treatment. *Pharm Res* **24**, 2120–2130.
24. Saad, M., Garbuzenko, O. B., and Minko, T. (2008) Co-delivery of siRNA and an anticancer drug for treatment of multidrug-resistant cancer. *Nanomed* **3**, 761–776.
25. Dharap, S. S., Wang, Y., Chandna, P., Khandare, J. J., Qiu, B., Gunaseelan, S., Sinko, P. J., Stein, S., Farmanfarmaian, A., and Minko, T. (2005) Tumor-specific targeting of an anticancer drug delivery system by LHRH peptide. *Proc Natl Acad Sci USA* **102**, 12962–12967.
26. Saad, M., Garbuzenko, O. B., Ber, E., Chandna, P., Khandare, J. J., Pozharov, V. P., and Minko, T. (2008) Receptor targeted polymers, dendrimers, liposomes: Which nanocarrier is the most efficient for tumor-specific treatment and imaging? *J Control Release* **130**, 107–114.
27. Minko, T., Kopeckova, P., Pozharov, V., Jensen, K. D., and Kopecek, J. (2000) The influence of cytotoxicity of macromolecules and of VEGF gene modulated vascular permeability on the enhanced permeability and retention effect in resistant solid tumors. *Pharm Res* **17**, 505–514.
28. Garbuzenko, O. B., Saad, M., Betigeri, S., Zhang, M., Vetcher, A. A., Soldatenkov, V. A., Reimer, D. C., Pozharov, V. P., and Minko, T. (2008) Intratracheal versus intravenous liposomal delivery of siRNA, antisense oligonucleotides and anticancer drug. *Pharm Res* [Oct 22 Epub ahead of print].

Chapter 20

Antibody Targeting of Nanoparticles to Tumor-Specific Receptors: Immunoliposomes

Miriam Rothdiener, Julia Beuttler, Sylvia K.E. Messerschmidt, and Roland E. Kontermann

Abstract

Immunoliposomes generated by coupling of antibodies to the liposomal surface allow for an active tissue targeting, e.g., through binding to tumor cell-specific receptors. Instead of whole antibodies, single-chain Fv fragments (scFv), which represent the smallest part of an antibody containing the entire antigen-binding site, find increasing usage as targeting moiety. Here we provide protocols for the preparation of type II scFv immunoliposomes by the conventional coupling method as well as the post-insertion method. Furthermore protocols to analyze binding of these immunoliposomes to antigen-expressing cells as well as internalization through receptor-mediated endocytosis are included.

Key words: Antibody, immunoliposomes, nanoparticle.

1. Introduction

The concept of targeting liposomes to cells by attaching antibodies to the liposomal surface is a promising approach for targeted delivery of drugs incorporated or encapsulated into the liposome (1). Several covalent coupling methods are available for the generation of immunoliposomes including the generation of thioether, disulfide, carboxamide, amide, and hydrazone linkages between antibodies and the liposome surface (2). Depending on whether antibodies are coupled to the lipid bilayer or to inserted polyethylene glycol (PEG) chains, immunoliposomes can be grouped into type Ia immunoliposomes (antibody coupled to the lipid bilayer of non-PEGylated liposomes), type Ib immunoliposomes (antibody coupled to the lipid bilayer of PEGylated liposomes), and type II immunoliposomes (antibody coupled to the distal end of the PEG chain incorporated into the lipid bilayer) (**Fig. 20.1**).

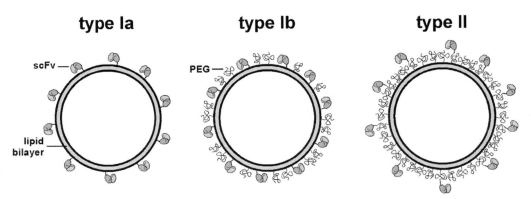

Fig. 20.1. The three types of immunoliposomes: type Ia, antibody (here scFv) coupled to the lipid bilayer; type Ib, antibody coupled to the lipid bilayer of PEGylated liposomes; type II, antibody coupled to the distal end of PEG chains incorporated into the lipid bilayer.

Different antibody formats such as whole antibodies (3), Fab' fragments (4), and scFv (5–8) have been employed for the generation of immunoliposomes. However, immunoliposomes prepared from whole antibodies have been shown to be immunogenic and are rapidly cleared from circulation through Fc-mediated uptake by macrophages, e.g., Kupffer cells of the liver (2). These drawbacks can be circumvented using Fab' or scFv molecules as ligands. ScFv's are small in size and can be easily modified through genetic engineering. For instance, they can be genetically modified to expose an additional cysteine residue (scFv'), e.g., inserted at the C terminus or the linker region connecting the two variable domains (8). Compared to coupling through, e.g., amino or carboxyl groups, this allows a very defined and site-directed coupling, which does not interfere with antigen-binding activity of the antibody fragment. Two approaches to generate immunoliposomes have been described in the literature: (i) the conventional method, coupling the antibody molecules directly to the liposome surface (3), and (ii) the post-insertion method, where the ligands are first coupled to micelles prepared from functionalized lipids which are then inserted into preformed liposomes (9). The post-insertion method offers the advantage of independent liposome preparation (including drug loading) and scFv' coupling, each step performed under optimal conditions or even using commercially available drug-loaded liposomes such as Doxil (liposomal doxorubicin).

2. Materials

2.1. Preparation of Single-Chain Fv' Fragments

1. 2xTY: Add 1 L water, 16 g bacto-tryptone, 10 g yeast extract, 5 g NaCl (Roth, Karlsruhe, Germany).

2. Ampicillin (Roth, Karlsruhe, Germany) stock solution: 100 mg/mL in water.

3. α-D(+)-glucose monohydrate (20%, w/w; Roth, Karlsruhe, Germany) in water.

4. Isopropyl-β,D-thiogalactopyranoside (IPTG) (1 M; GERBU Biotechnik GmbH, Geilberg, Germany) in water.

5. Periplasmatic preparation buffer (PPB): 30 mM Tris–HCl, pH 8.0, 1 mM EDTA, 20% D(+)-sucrose.

6. Lysozyme: 10 mg/mL in water, freshly prepared (Roche Diagnostics Corporation, Indianapolis, USA).

7. $MgSO_4$ (1 M) in water.

8. Dialysis membrane Zellu Trans, MWCO 8–10 kDa (Roth, Karlsruhe, Germany).

9. PBS: 8.06 mM Na_2HPO_4, 1.47 mM KH_2PO_4, 137.93 mM NaCl, 2.67 mM KCl, pH 7.5.

10. Ni-NTA agarose (Qiagen, Hilden, Germany).

11. PolyPrep chromatography columns (Bio-Rad, Hercules, USA).

12. IMAC loading buffer: 50 mM Na phosphate, pH 7.5, 250 mM NaCl, 20 mM imidazole.

13. IMAC wash buffer: 50 mM Na phosphate, pH 7.5, 250 mM NaCl, 35 mM imidazole.

14. IMAC elution buffer: 50 mM Na phosphate, pH 7.5, 250 mM NaCl, 250 mM imidazole.

15. Bradford reagent (Bio-Rad, Hercules, USA), diluted 1:5 in water.

16. SDS-PAGE sample buffer: 30% (v/v) glycerol, 3% (w/v) SDS ultrapure, 0.05% bromophenol blue Na salt (Serva, Heidelberg, Germany), 5% β-mercaptoethanol (Sigma, St. Louis, USA) in 62.5 mM Tris–HCl, pH 6.8.

17. Bio-Rad Mini-PROTEAN 3 Electrophoresis System (Bio-Rad, Hercules, USA).

18. Separation buffer: 1.5 M Tris–HCl, pH 8.8.

19. Acrylamide/bisacrylamide solution (30%), Rotiphorese® (Roth, Karlsruhe, Germany).

20. Ammoniumperoxodisulfate (10%; Merck, Darmstadt, Germany).

21. N,N,N',N'-Tetramethylethylenediamine (TEMED) (Roth, Karlsruhe, Germany).

22. Stacking buffer: 1 M Tris–HCl, pH 6.8.

23. Running buffer: 192 mM glycine, 25 mM Tris, 0.1% SDS, pH 8.3.

24. Prestained molecular weight marker: PageRuler™ Prestained Protein Ladder, #SM0671 (Fermentas, St. Leon-Rot, Germany).

25. Coomassie staining solution: 0.25% (w/v) Coomassie Brilliant Blue R250 (Roth, Karlsruhe, Germany) in destaining solution.
26. Destaining solution: 45% methanol, 10% acidic acid, in ddH$_2$O (Roth, Karlsruhe, Germany).
27. Dialysis tubing, high retention seamless cellulose tubing, size 23, 15 mm, MWCO 7–14 kDa (Sigma, St. Louis, USA).
28. Tris(2-carboxyethyl)phosphine (TCEP) Bond-Breaker, 500 mM stock solution (Pierce, Rockford, IL, USA).
29. Sephadex™ G25 (Amersham, Uppsala, Sweden).
30. HEPES Pufferan® (Roth, Karlsruhe, Germany).
31. Coupling buffer: 10 mM Na$_2$HPO$_4$/NaH$_2$PO$_4$ buffer, 0.2 mM EDTA, 30 mM NaCl, pH 6.7.
32. D-Tube™ Dialyzer Mini, MWCO 6–8 kDa (Calbiochem, Gibbstown, USA).

2.2. Preparation of Immunoliposomes by Conventional Coupling

1. Chloroform (Roth, Karlsruhe, Germany).
2. Egg phosphatidylcholine (EPC) (Lipoid, Ludwigshafen, Germany) dissolved in chloroform at a concentration of 300 mg/mL and stored in a glass vial at −20°C.
3. Cholesterol, (Calbiochem, Gibbstown, USA) dissolved in chloroform at a concentration of 100 mg/mL and stored in a glass vial at −20°C.
4. 1,2-Distearoyl-sn-glycero-3-phosphoethanolamine-N-[maleimide(polyethylene glycol)-2000] (ammonium salt) (Mal-PEG$_{2000}$-DSPE) (Avanti Polar Lipids, Alabaster, USA) dissolved in chloroform at a concentration of 30 mg/mL and stored in a glass vial at −20°C.
5. 1,1′-Dioctadecyl-3,3,3′,3′-tetramethylindocarbocyanine perchlorate (DiI) (Sigma-Aldrich, St. Louis, USA) dissolved in chloroform at a concentration of 3.44 mg/mL and stored in a glass vial at −20°C.
6. 3,3′-Dioctadecyloxacarbocyanine perchlorate (DiO) (Sigma-Aldrich, St. Louis, USA) dissolved in chloroform at a concentration of 4 mg/mL and stored in a glass vial at −20°C.
7. Polycarbonate filter membrane (Avestin, Ottawa, Canada) with a diameter of 19 mm and a pore size of 50 nm.
8. Extruder, LiposoFast Basic (Avestin, Ottawa, Canada).
9. L-Cysteine (Sigma-Aldrich, St. Louis, USA) stock solution: 100 mM in H$_2$O with 2 mM EDTA stored in 10 μL aliquots at −20°C.

2.3. Preparation of Immunoliposomes by the Post-insertion Method

1. 1,2-Distearoyl-sn-glycero-3-phosphoethanolamine-N-[methoxy(polyethylene glycol)-2000] (ammonium salt) (mPEG$_{2000}$–DSPE) (Avanti Polar Lipids, Alabaster, USA) dissolved in chloroform at a concentration of 51 mg/mL and stored in a glass vial at –20°C.
2. Lipids and dyes described under **Section 2.2**.

2.4. Immunoliposome Purification and Characterization

1. Sepharose™ CL4B (Amersham, Uppsala, Sweden).
2. Zetasizer Nano ZS (Malvern Instruments, Herrenberg, Germany).
3. TransBlot SD semi-dry transfer cell (Bio-Rad, Hercules, USA).
4. Blotting buffer: 20% methanol, 192 mM glycine, 25 mM Tris, pH 8.3.
5. Nitrocellulose Transfer Membrane BioTrace NT (Pall Life Sciences, East Hills, USA).
6. Blocking solution: 5% (w/v) milk powder, 0.1% (v/v) Tween 20 in PBS.
7. Anti-His6 HRP-labeled antibody: His-probe (H-3) HRP-conjugated murine monoclonal IgG1, 200 μg/mL, sc-8036 (Santa Cruz Biotechnology, Santa Cruz, USA).
8. PBST: PBS, 0.05% Tween 20.
9. ECL: Solution A: 1.25 mM luminol, 0.1 M Tris–HCL, pH 8.6; Solution B: 0.11% p-hydroxycoumaric acid in dimethyl sulfoxide (DMSO). Mix 4 mL solution A and 400 μL solution B and 1.2 μL 30% H_2O_2.
10. PBA: PBS, 0.2% FCS (PAA Laboratories GmbH, Pasching, Austria), 0.02% Na azide.
11. Ninety-six-well V-bottom tissue culture plate (Greiner Bio-One, Kremsmünster, Austria).
12. Collagen R (Serva Electrophoresis GmbH, Heidelberg, Germany).
13. Microscope slides and coverslips, ø 15 mm (Roth, Karlsruhe, Germany).
14. Twelve-well tissue culture plate (Greiner Bio-One, Kremsmünster, Austria).
15. Paraformaldehyde (Merck, Darmstadt, Germany).
16. DAPI dihydrochloride (Calbiochem, Gibbstown, USA).
17. Mowiol 4.88 (Polysciences, Inc., Warrington, USA).
18. Cell Observer (Zeiss, Jena, Germany).

3. Methods

The scFv molecules used for the generation of immunoliposomes need an additional cysteine residue which will form a stable thioether bond with a maleimide group of functionalized lipids incorporated into the lipid layer. Such genetically engineered scFv' molecules are generated from existing *scFv* genes, e.g., obtained from hybridoma or isolated from phage display libraries as described elsewhere (10), cloned, for instance, as NcoI/NotI fragment into vector pABC4 (**Fig. 20.2**) applying standard protocols. Various maleimide-functionalized lipids are commercially available. To determine the coupling efficiency, SDS-PAGE and western blot are performed. Coupling of Mal–PEG$_{2000}$–DSPE to scFv' is indicated by a shift in the protein band of about 3 kDa (**Fig. 20.3a**).

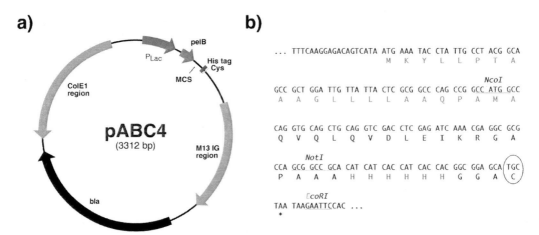

Fig. 20.2. (a) Map of expression plasmid pABC4 and (b) its cloning site showing also the C-terminal His-tag used for purification and the cysteine used for coupling.

Specific binding of immunoliposomes to their target cells can be detected by FACS analysis due to excitation of fluorescent dyes (e.g., DiI, DiO) incorporated into the liposomal bilayer. For binding assays, the immunoliposomes are incubated with the cells at 4°C (**Fig. 20.3b**). In contrast, internalization studies are performed at 37°C to allow receptor-mediated endocytosis. Uptake of fluorescently labeled immunoliposomes can then be visualized by fluorescence microscopy (**Fig. 20.3c**).

3.1. Preparation of Single-Chain Fv' Fragments

1. Make an overnight culture of *Escherichia coli* TG1 transformed with pABC4 scFv' in 10 mL 2xTY, 100 µg/mL ampicillin, 1% glucose, and shake at 180 rpm at 37°C.

2. Inoculate 1 L of 2xTY, 100 µg/mL ampicillin, 0.1% glucose with 10 mL of the overnight culture and incubate

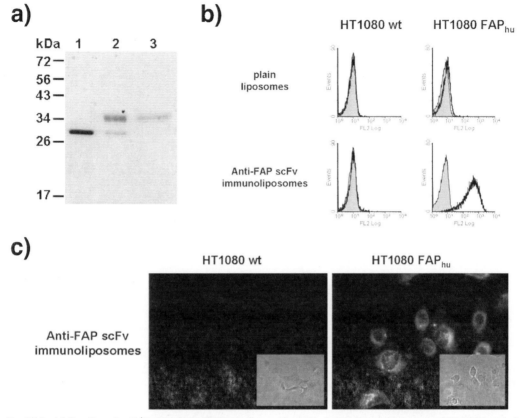

Fig. 20.3. (a) Coupling of scFv' to Mal–PEG–DSPE micelles and insertion into preformed liposomes. SDS-PAGE analysis of scFv' fragment before (1) and after (2) coupling to Mal–PEG–DSPE micelles and after post-insertion (3). Gel was stained with Coomassie. Coupling of the antibody molecule to the lipid is indicated by increased molecular weight. (b) Selective binding of immunoliposomes to FAP-expressing cells. Flow cytometry of plain liposomes and anti-FAP scFv immunoliposomes on FAP-negative (HT1080 wt) and FAP-positive (HT1080 FAP$_{hu}$) cell lines. (Immuno-) Liposomes are shown in *black lines*, cells alone in *grey*. (c) Selective uptake of immunoliposomes in FAP-expressing cells. Fluorescence microscopy images of anti-FAP scFv immunoliposomes on FAP-negative (HT1080 wt) and FAP-positive (HT1080 FAP$_{hu}$) cell lines. Immunoliposomes are labeled with DiO and cells are shown in bright-field images (small image).

at 37°C until culture reaches an OD$_{600}$ of 0.8–1.0 (takes about 2.5–3 h).

3. Add 1 mL of 1 M IPTG (final concentration 1 mM) and incubate for additional 3 h at 180 rpm at room temperature.

4. Centrifuge bacterial suspension at 4,500×g for 10 min at 4°C.

5. Resupend the pellet in 50 mL of PPB.

6. Prepare a 10 mg/mL lysozyme solution in water, add 0.25 mL to the resuspended pellet to a final concentration of 50 μg/mL, and incubate on ice for 15–30 min.

7. To stabilize the spheroplasts, add 0.5 mL of 1 M MgSO$_4$ to 50 mL of solution.

8. Centrifuge at 10,000×g for 15 min at 4°C.
9. Dialyze the supernatant against 5 L PBS overnight at 4°C in a membrane with a cutoff of 8–10 kDa.
10. Centrifuge at 10,000×g for 15 min at 4°C.
11. Add 1 mL Ni-NTA agarose to a PolyPrep column and equilibrate with 5–10 mL IMAC loading buffer.
12. Load the dialyzed supernatant onto the equilibrated column (*see* **Note 1**).
13. Wash the column with 10–20 mL IMAC wash buffer and control the flow-through by Bradford test until unbound proteins are completely washed off (*see* **Note 2**).
14. Elute bound proteins with IMAC elution buffer in fractions of 500 μL.
15. Identify peak fractions either by SDS-PAGE or Bradford test.
16. For SDS-PAGE, mix 30 μL of each fraction including supernatant, flow-through and wash fraction with 7.5 μL five times reducing SDS-PAGE sample buffer and incubate for 10 min at 95°C.
17. For SDS-PAGE, use the Bio-Rad Mini-PROTEAN 3 Electrophoresis System.
18. Prepare a 1.5-mm-thick, 15% gel by mixing 1.9 mL separation buffer, 3.75 mL 30% acrylamide/bisacrylamide solution, 1.7 mL ddH$_2$O, 75 μL ammonium persulfate solution, 75 μL of 10% SDS solution, and 3 μL TEMED.
19. Assemble the glass plates, pour the gel, and overlay it with isopropanol. After polymerization, remove the isopropanol.
20. Prepare the stacking gel (3%) by mixing 315 μL stacking buffer, 415 μL acrylamide/bisacrylamide solution, 1.7 mL ddH$_2$O, 25 μL ammonium persulfate solution, 25 μL of 10% SDS solution, and 2.5 μL TEMED.
21. Pour the stacking gel on top of the separating gel and insert a comb.
22. After assembling the equipment, add the running buffer to the gel unit and remove the comb of the stacking gel.
23. Load the prepared samples and the prestained molecular weight marker into the wells.
24. Run samples at 50 V through the stacking gel and 150 V through the separating gel.
25. To stain the SDS-PAA gel, incubate in Coomassie staining solution on a shaker for 45 min at room temperature.

26. After staining, destain the SDS-PAA gel in destaining solution until definite protein bands are visible.

27. Combine peak fractions and dialyze against 5 L PBS overnight at 4°C in a membrane with a cutoff of 7–14 kDa to remove imidazole.

28. Determine the protein concentration by measuring the OD_{280} in a NanoDrop system.

29. Store protein in aliquots at –20°C.

30. Reduce 100 μg scFv' by adding 5 μL TCEP (625 nmol TCEP per 1 nmol scFv') and incubate under nitrogen atmosphere for 2 h at room temperature.

31. Remove TCEP by dialysis against deoxygenated coupling buffer, pH 6.7, overnight at 4°C. Refresh dialysis buffer after at least 4 h (*see* **Note 3**).

3.2. Preparation of Immunoliposomes by Conventional Coupling to Mal–PEG Liposomes

1. Use the following lipid composition for preparation of liposomes: EPC:cholesterol:Mal–PEG_{2000}–DSPE at a molar ratio of 65:30:5 (for 1 mL of liposomes, combine 16.3 μL EPC, 11.6 μL cholesterol, 46.8 μL Mal–PEG_{2000}–DSPE).

2. For detection purpose the lipid formulation may contain DiI or DiO as fluorescent lipid marker at a molar concentration of 0.3 mol% (for 1 mL total liposome, add 8.1 μL DiI or 6.6 μL DiO stock solution).

3. Rinse a round-bottom flask with chloroform.

4. Put 200 μL chloroform into the round-bottom flask and add the lipid stock solutions.

5. Form a thin lipid film by removing the solvents in a rotary evaporator for 10 min at 42°C (*see* **Note 4**).

6. Dry the lipid film completely in a vacuum drying oven for at least 1 h at room temperature.

7. Hydrate the lipid film in 1 mL of 10 mM HEPES buffer, pH 6.7, and vortex until all components are dissolved. The final lipid concentration is 10 mM (*see* **Note 5**).

8. Extrude the lipid solution 21 times trough 50-nm-pore-size polycarbonate filter membrane using a LiposoFast extruder to obtain small unilamellar vesicles.

9. Incubate the freshly prepared liposomes with reduced scFv' at any adequate molar ratio (e.g., 10 nmol scFv' per 1 μmol lipid). As a negative control, incubate the liposomes with the corresponding volume of PBS (*see* **Note 6**).

10. Overlay the mixed solution with nitrogen and incubate on an orbital shaker for at least 1 h at room temperature.

11. To saturate the unconjugated maleimide groups, add 1 mM L-cysteine to the scFv′-coupled liposomes as well as to the control liposomes and incubate for at least 10 min at room temperature.
12. Continue with **Section 3.4**.

3.3. Preparation of Immunoliposomes by the Post-insertion Method

1. Use the following lipid composition: EPC:cholesterol:mPEG$_{2000}$–DSPE in a molar ratio of 65:30:5 (for 1 mL liposomes, combine 16.3 µL EPC, 11.6 µL cholesterol, 27.5 µL Mal–PEG$_{2000}$–DSPE).
2. For detection purpose the lipid formulation may contain DiI or DiO as fluorescent lipid markers in a molar ratio of 0.3 mol% (for 1 mL liposomes add 8.1 µL DiI or 6.6 µL DiO).
3. Prepare liposomes as described above (Steps 2–8 in **Section 3.2**).
4. For preparation of maleimide-functionalized micelles, transfer 2 µL Mal–PEG$_{2000}$–DSPE solution (30 µg/µL in chloroform) into a 1.5-mL test tube and evaporate the solvent in the open tube at room temperature until a lipid film becomes visible.
5. For the formation of micelles, dissolve the lipid in 6 µL ddH$_2$O (final concentration 4.2 mM) and incubate for 5 min at 65°C in a water bath by shaking from time to time.
6. Mix micellar lipid and reduced scFv′ at a molar ratio of 4.67:1 [add 100 µg (4 nmol) scFv to 5 µL micellar lipid], overlay with nitrogen, and incubate for 30 min at room temperature. As a negative control, mix the liposomes with the corresponding volume of PBS.
7. To saturate the unconjugated coupling groups, add L-cysteine to a final concentration of 1 mM to the scFv′-coupled micelles as well as to the control micelles and incubate for at least 10 min at room temperature.
8. Insert the scFv′-coupled micelles into preformed PEGylated liposomes at any adequate molar ratio (between 0.1 and 2 mol% Mal–PEG–DSPE of total lipid) by incubation for 30 min at 55°C.

3.4. Immunoliposome Purification and Characterization

1. Remove uncoupled scFv′ molecules from immunoliposome preparation by gel filtration using a Sepharose CL4B column (10 mL resin) equilibrated with 10 mM HEPES buffer, pH 7.4. Pool liposome containing fractions visible through incorporated fluorescent dye.
2. Estimate lipid concentration by dividing the initial amount of lipid by the final volume (*see* **Note 7**).

3. Alternatively, remove uncoupled scFv' by ultracentrifugation at 300,000×g for 1 h at 4°C and carefully remove the supernatant.

4. Resuspend the liposomal pellet in a defined volume of 10 mM HEPES, pH 7.4, to achieve an adequate lipid concentration (e.g., 10 mM).

5. To determine the liposome size, dilute liposomal formulations 1:100 in 10 mM HEPES, pH 7.4, in a low-volume disposable cuvette and measure size by dynamic light scattering using a Zetasizer Nano ZS.

6. To determine the coupling efficiency, use 2 μg of scFv' for SDS-PAGE and add PBS ad 30 μL to the sample. Add 7.5 μL of 5× reducing SDS-PAGE sample buffer and incubate for 10 min at 95°C.

7. Accordingly, prepare samples of scFv'-coupled micelles and immunoliposomes containing 2 μg of scFv' (*see* **Note 8**).

8. Perform SDS-PAGE as described above, using one gel for Coomassie staining and another one for Western blotting.

9. For Western blotting, rinse the gel in blotting buffer and transfer to a semi-dry blotter (TransBlot SD, Bio-Rad) onto a nitrocellulose membrane also rinsed in blotting buffer. Arrange the gel on the cathode and the membrane to the anode side of the blotter, between two sheets of Whatman paper rinsed in blotting buffer.

10. The protein is then transferred from the gel to the nitrocellulose membrane at a constant voltage of 10 V for 30 min.

11. Block the blotted membrane in 5% MPBST on a shaker for 1 h at room temperature.

12. After removal of the blocking solution, dilute an anti-His6 HRP-labeled antibody 1:1000 in 5% MPBST and incubate on the membrane on a shaker for 1 h at room temperature.

13. Wash the membrane three times in PBST for 5 min and once in PBS for 5 min.

14. Incubate the membrane in ECL reagent on the shaker at room temperature for 2 min in the dark.

15. Dry the membrane between Whatman papers to completely remove the ECL solution.

16. Detect the protein bands by the luminescence of the HRP-coupled antibody bound to the His-Tag of the scFv' via an X-ray film (**Fig. 20.3a**).

3.5. Analysis of Cell Binding by Flow Cytometry

1. Harvest antigen-expressing and control cell lines and adjust them to a concentration of 2.5×10^6 cells/mL in PBA. For each sample, add 100 μL into a 96-well V-bottom tissue culture plate.

2. As a reference to all the samples, include untreated cells along the whole procedure.
3. Incubate cells with DiI- or DiO-labeled immunoliposomes and control liposomes (e.g., 10–50 nmol lipid) for 1 h at 4°C in the dark.
4. Wash the cells three times by centrifugation at $380 \times g$ for 5 min at 4°C, remove the supernatant, and resuspend the cell pellets in 150 µL PBA.
5. Transfer the cells into FACS tubes in a total volume of 500 µL PBA.
6. The DiI fluorescence intensity of the immunoliposomes bound to cells can be excited at a wavelength of 488 nm and detected at 570 nm. The DiO fluorescence intensity of the immunoliposomes bound to cells can be excited at a wavelength of 484 nm and detected at 501 nm. Compare the fluorescence intensity to the control liposomes and untreated cells. Evaluate the data with WinMDI 2.9, a free analysis software tool (**Fig. 20.3b**).

3.6. Analysis of Internalization by Fluorescence Microscopy

1. Coat autoclaved 15-mm round coverslips in 12-well plate with 800 µL Collagen R for 2 h at 37°C.
2. Rinse the coverslips twice with 1 mL PBS/well.
3. Harvest antigen-expressing and control cell lines and adjust them to a concentration of 5×10^4 cells/mL in medium. For each sample, add 1 mL onto the coverslips and incubate overnight at 37°C in 5% CO_2.
4. Remove the medium and replace it with 1 mL fresh medium.
5. Add adequate amounts of labeled immunoliposomes (e.g., 20 nmol) to the wells and incubate for different time periods (e.g., 1–6 h) at 37°C.
6. After removing the immunoliposomes, rinse the cells rapidly twice with ice-cold PBS.
7. Fix cells by adding 4% paraformaldehyde solution and incubate for 20 min at room temperature.
8. Remove the supernatant and rinse the cells twice with ice-cold PBS.
9. Stain the nuclei in 800 µL DAPI solution for 20 min at room temperature in the dark.
10. Remove the staining solution, rinse the samples twice with PBS, and finally cover them with water.
11. Carefully remove the coverslip from the 12-well plate and invert it into a drop of Mowiol mounting medium on a microscope slide.

12. View the slides under a fluorescent microscope. Excitation at 488 nm induces the DiO fluorescence (green emission) for the immunoliposomes, while excitation at 364 nm induces DAPI fluorescence (blue emission). The cell outlines are visualized in bright-field settings (**Fig. 20.3c**).

4. Notes

1. Collect flow-through of loading and washing and test for remaining scFv' in a SDS-PAGE. If necessary, purify once again after dialysis.
2. For Bradford test, add 10 µL flow-through to 90 µL of 1× Bradford reagent. Protein content is indicated by blue staining.
3. Deoxygenate the coupling buffer by nitrogen aeration for at least 30 min.
4. Be careful to slowly generate vacuum to avoid boiling of the dissolved lipids. In case of boiling, reduce vacuum.
5. To facilitate extrusion, treat the emulsion by sonification for at least 5 min in an ultrasonic cleaning unit.
6. Best coupling efficiency is reached between 10 and 40 nmol scFv' per 1 µmol lipid.
7. For estimation of lipid concentration, it is not taken into account that part of the liposomes might have been lost during the gel filtration step.
8. It is presumed that the total amount of initial scFv' is coupled to micelles and inserted into liposomes.

References

1. Nobs, L., Buchegger, F., Gurny, R., and Allémann, E. (2004) Current methods for attaching targeting ligands to liposomes and nanoparticles. *J Pharm Sci* **93**, 1980–1992.
2. Koning, G. A., Morselt, H. W. M., Gorter, A., Allen, T. M., Zalipsky, S., Scherphof, G. L., and Kamps, J. A. A. M. (2003) Interaction of differently designed immunoliposomes with colon cancer cells and Kupffer cells. An in vitro comparison. *Pharm Res* **20**, 1249–1257.
3. Kontermann, R. E. (2006) Immunoliposomes for cancer therapy. *Curr Opin Mol Ther* **8**, 39–45.
4. Sapra, P., Moase, E. H., Ma, J., and Allen, T. M. (2004) Improved therapeutic responses in a xenograft model of human B lymphoma (Namalwa) for liposomal vincristine versus liposomal doxorubicin targeted via anti-CD19 IgG2a or Fab' fragments. *Clin Cancer Res* **10**, 1100–1111.
5. Marty, C., Scheidegger, P., Ballmer-Hofer, K., Klemenz, R., and Schwendener, R. A. (2001) Production of functionalized single-chain Fv antibody fragments to the ED-B domain of the B-isoform of fibronectin in *Pichia pastoris*. *Protein Exp Purif* **21**, 156–164.
6. Völkel, T., Hölig, P., Merdan, T., Müller, R., and Kontermann, R. E. (2004) Targeting of immunoliposomes to endothelial cells using

a single-chain Fv fragment directed against human endoglin (CD105). *Biochim Biophys Acta* **1663**, 158–166.
7. Park, J. W., Kirpotin, D. B., Hong, K., Shalaby, R., Shao, Y., Nielsen, U. B., Marks, J. D., Papahadjopoulos, D., and Benz, C. C. (2001) Tumor targeting using anti-HER2 immunoliposomes. *J Control Release* **74**, 95–113.
8. Messerschmidt, S. K., Kolbe, A., Müller, D., Knoll, M., Pleiss, J., and Kontermann, R. E. (2008) Novel single-chain Fv′ formats for the generation of immunoliposomes by site-directed coupling. *Bioconjug Chem* **19**(1), 362–369.
9. Iden, D. L. and Allen, T. M. (2001) In vitro and in vivo comparison of immunoliposomes made by conventional coupling technique with those made by a new post-insertion approach. *Biochim Biophys Acta* **1531**, 207–216.
10. Kontermann, R. E. and Dübel, S. (2001) *Antibody Engineering, a Lab Manual.* Springer Verlag, Heidelberg.

Chapter 21

Photoacoustic Tomography for Imaging Nanoparticles

Zhen Yuan and Huabei Jiang

Abstract

Nanotechnology is the key to a new, noninvasive photoacoustic imaging technique that could detect early stages of disease tissues. The combination of photoacoustic imaging with nanotechnology holds promise for determining the structural and functional properties of tissues with enhanced sensitivity and specificity and for monitoring the treatment of diseases. In this chapter, we described in detail photoacoustic reconstruction methods and imaging systems. We also review the recent advances in nanoparticles and their in vivo applications in the field of photoacoustic imaging.

Key words: Nanotechnology, nanoparticles, optical tomography, photoacoustic tomography, imaging methods, reconstruction algorithms.

1. Introduction

Biomedical photoacoustic tomography (PAT), also called optoacoustic tomography or thermoacoustic tomography, is based on the photoacoustic (PA) effect, which was first described in 1880 by Alexander Graham Bell. In PAT, a short-pulsed laser source is typically used to irradiate the tissue of interest. The absorption of the laser pulses gives rise to a rapid temperature rise and subsequent thermo-elastic expansion of the irradiated tissue volume. The pressure distribution induced by tissue expansion prompts acoustic wave propagation toward tissue surfaces where they are detected by one or an array of ultrasound transducers (*see* **Fig. 21.1**). The acquired acoustic data by ultrasound transducers are then used to recover the PA images qualitatively or quantitatively. PAT can capture tissue mechanical properties such as

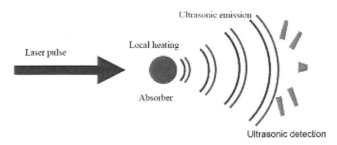

Fig. 21.1. Schematic illustration of PAT imaging.

ultrasound velocity, optical properties such as absorption and scattering coefficients, and physiological or functional parameters such as deoxyhemoglobin (HbR), oxyhemoglobin (HbO_2), and water (H_2O).

Research interest in laser-induced PAT is rapidly growing, largely because of its unique capability of combining high optical contrast and high ultrasound resolution in a single modality. Recent in vivo studies have shown that the optical absorption contrast between tumor and normal tissues in the breast can be as high as 3:1 in the near-infrared region due to the significantly increased vascularity in the tumors (1–3). However, optical imaging has low spatial resolution due to strong light scattering. Ultrasound imaging can provide better resolution than does optical imaging due to less scattering of acoustic wave. However, the contrast for ultrasound imaging is low, making it often incapable of revealing diseases at early stages. In addition, ultrasound imaging cannot provide functional parameters including HbR, HbO_2, and H_2O concentrations. PAT combines the advantages of both optical and ultrasound imaging in a single modality, yet overcomes the limitations associated with optical and ultrasound.

Hence, PAT can be regarded as a hybrid imaging modality that provides the high contrast and specificity of optical imaging along with the high spatial resolution of ultrasound imaging. The latter is depth dependent being limited by the frequency-dependent nature of acoustic attenuation in tissue. For centimeter penetration depths, sub-millimeter spatial resolution is possible. For example, PAT imaging can reach a depth of about 1 cm at the wavelength of 580 nm with an axial resolution of less than 100 μm. PAT has shown the potential to detect breast cancer, to probe brain functioning in small animals, and to assess vascular and skin diseases.

In PAT, the interaction of visible and near-infrared (NIR) light with tissue is dominated by absorbing chromophores including HbR, HbO_2, and H_2O and scattering particles including the cell membranes. The sensitivity and the specificity of PAT to visualize a pathological disorder are governed by its contrast: the ability of the disease to differentially scatter or absorb light compared with healthy tissue and background noise. This native or endogenous contrast may not be sufficient and in any case, the interactions of light with tissue are not disease specific (4). Therefore, there is a role for exogenously administered contrast-enhancing agents that have affinity for the disease site through biochemical interactions, providing not only sensitive but also disease-specific signals. The application of PA contrast agents is able to increase the sensitivity of this modality and render it possible to use photoacoustics for molecular imaging (5). Both organic dyes such as indocyanine green (6) and inorganic nanoparticles (7) are good candidates as PA contrast agents.

Gold nanoparticles (8–10) have become a prime candidate for PAT due to their unusual optical properties and inherent biocompatibility. The intense scattering and absorption of light that occurs under the plasmon resonant condition coupled with the ability to tune the resonance into the NIR by manipulating the aspect ratio, making gold nanoparticles extremely attractive as contrast agents for optical imaging techniques. Further, gold–protein chemistry is well developed and several bioconjugation protocols are available in the literatures, which allows the combination of the targeting functionality of antibodies with such gold nanoparticles. The inertness and the biocompatibility of gold in general hold promise for the use of gold nanoparticles for in vivo imaging applications.

To date, several types of gold nanoparticles including nanoshells, nanotubes, and nanorods have been shown to provide enhanced image contrast for optical imaging methods in biomedical applications. The effect of contrast enhancement is based on the high optical absorption coefficient of these agents (11). For example, optical absorption in metals is governed by plasmon excitation. In a metal nanoparticle, plasmon resonance leads to very highly efficient light absorption. Typically, the absorption cross section of a metal nanoparticle can be an order of magnitude larger than its geometrical cross-sectional area. Its shape plays a crucial role in determining the peak absorption wavelength. For medical imaging applications, the resonance wavelength can be tuned within the "tissue transparent" window of 700–1,000 nm to increase the penetration depth.

In this chapter, we describe two typical reconstruction methods used in PAT, followed by the description of PAT imaging system. Experiments using tissue-like phantom and nanoparticles are presented for validation of PAT imaging methods. In vivo applications using various gold nanoparticles are detailed in the end of the chapter.

2. Methods

2.1. Reconstruction Algorithms

2.1.1. Delay-and-Sum Beam-Forming Algorithm

To form the PA image of an object, an image reconstruction algorithm is required. A simple, yet very effective method is the delay-and-sum beam-forming algorithm that is commonly used in radar signal processing (12). Using this method, the image expression in the case of near field for PA imaging can be stated as

$$S^f(t) = \frac{\sum_i w_i^f S_i(t + \delta_i^f)}{\sum_i w_i^f} \quad [1]$$

where $S^f(t)$ is the image output at a particular focus point f, $S_i(t)$ is the time signal from the ith receiver, δ_i^f is the delay applied to this signal, and w_i^f is an amplitude weighting factor, which is used to enhance the beam shape, to reduce sidelobe effects, or to minimize the noise level. The summed signal is typically normalized to make the output independent of the actual set of transducers. This delay-and-sum algorithm has been tested and evaluated using considerable phantom and in vivo experiments (13).

2.1.2. Finite Element-Based Algorithm

While the delay-and-sum algorithm described above is simple to implement, it does not account for the diffraction effect that is essential to the PA waves. In particular, a major assumption has to be made in this and other linear algorithms seen in the literature [e.g., backprojection (14) or filtered backprojection (15)] that biological tissues are acoustically homogeneous, which is not true in reality. This assumption will certainly affect the accuracy in image reconstruction. In addition, acoustic properties cannot be reconstructed because of this assumption. Importantly, functional parameters such as HbR, HbO_2, and H_2O cannot be obtained with these linear methods.

To overcome the above-mentioned limitations, we have developed a nonlinear reconstruction algorithm which is based on the finite element (FE) solution to the full PA wave equation without the homogeneous acoustic property assumption made thus far in the literature (16, 17). Finite element method (FEM) has been a powerful numerical method for solving the Helmholtz-type equation because of its computational efficiency and unrivaled ability to accommodate tissue heterogeneity and geometrical irregularity as well as allow complex boundary conditions and source representations. The FE-based reconstruction algorithm is implemented based on a dual meshing method, which allows us to use a large mesh for accurate forward solution of the PA wave equation subject to the well-known radiation or absorbing boundary conditions, while a much smaller mesh is used for the inverse solution. This reconstruction approach in PAT is an iterative Newton method with combined Marquardt and Tikhonov regularizations that can provide stable inverse solutions. The approach uses the hybrid regularization-based Newton method to update an initial optical and acoustic property distribution iteratively in order to minimize an object function composed of a weighted sum of the squared difference between computed and measured data. In addition, the adjoint sensitivity method has also been incorporated into the algorithm, which is able to reduce the computational cost dramatically for calculating the Jacobian matrix involved in the nonlinear inverse procedures. Together with an iterative Newton method, this nonlinear algorithm is able to precisely solve the Helmholtz wave equation and fulfill reliable inverse computation for an arbitrary measurement configuration.

Here we detail the FE-based algorithm. The PA wave equation in frequency domain is written if a heterogeneous acoustic field is considered:

$$\nabla^2 P(r,\omega) + k_0^2(1+O)P(r,\omega) = ik_0 v_0 \beta \Psi(r)/C_p \qquad [2]$$

where P is the pressure wave in frequency domain; $k_0 = \omega/v_0$ is the wave number described by the angular frequency, ω and v_0 is the speed of the acoustic wave in a reference or a coupling medium; $\Psi(r)$ is the absorbed optical energy density, which is the product of optical absorption coefficient μ_a and optical fluence or photon density; O is a coefficient that depends on both acoustic speed and attenuation as follows:

$$O = v_0^2/v^2 - 1 + iAv_0/k_0 v^2 \qquad [3]$$

where v is the speed of the acoustic wave in the scattering medium/tissue; A is the acoustic attenuation coefficient. Expanding acoustic pressure, P as the sum of coefficients multiplied by a set of basis functions ψ_j: $P = \sum P_j \psi_j$, the finite element discretization of the Helmholtz wave equation [2] can be written as

$$\sum_{j=1}^{N} P_j \left[\langle \nabla \psi_j \cdot \nabla \psi_i \rangle - \langle k_0^2(1+O)\psi_j \psi_i \rangle - \oint (\eta \psi_j + \gamma \frac{\partial^2 \psi_j}{\partial \varphi^2}) \psi_i \, ds \right]$$
$$= -\langle ik_0 c_0 \beta \Psi / C_P \psi_i \rangle$$
$$\qquad [4]$$

where the following second-order absorbing boundary conditions have been applied for two-dimensional problem (16):

$$\nabla P \cdot \hat{n} = \eta P + \gamma \frac{\partial^2 P}{\partial \varphi^2}$$

where $\eta = (-ik_0 - 3/2\rho + i3/8k_0\rho^2)/(1 - i/k_0\rho)$ and $\gamma = (-i/2k_0\rho^2)/(1 - i/k_0\rho)$; N is the total number of nodes of the finite element mesh, $<(\cdot)>$ indicates the integration over the problem domain, and $\oint$ expresses the integration over the boundary. In both the forward and the inverse calculations, the unknown coefficients O and ψ need to be separated into real (O_R and ψ_R) and imaginary (O_I and ψ_I) parts, both of which are expanded in a similar fashion to P as a sum of unknown parameters multiplied by a known spatially varying basis function. The matrix form of Eq. [4] is expressed as follows:

$$[A]\{P\} = \{B\} \qquad [6]$$

where

$$A_{ij} = \langle \nabla \psi_j \cdot \nabla \psi_i \rangle - k_0^2 \langle \psi_j \psi_i \rangle - k_0^2 \left\langle \sum_k O_{R,k} \psi_k \psi_j \psi_i \right\rangle$$

$$- ik_0^2 \left\langle \sum_l O_{I,l} \psi_l \psi_j \psi_i \right\rangle - \oint (\eta \psi_j + \gamma \frac{\partial^2 \psi_j}{\partial \varphi^2}) \psi_i \, ds$$

$$B_i = -Ik_0 c_0 \beta \left\langle \sum_k \Psi_{R,k} \psi_k \psi_i \right\rangle / C_p + k_0 c_0 \beta \left\langle \sum_l \Psi_{I,l} \psi_l \psi_i \right\rangle / C_p$$

$$\{P\} = \{P_1, P_2, \cdots, P_N\}^T$$

To form an image from a presumably uniform initial guess of the optical and acoustic property distribution, we use iterative Newton's method to update O_R, O_I, ψ_R, and ψ_I from their starting values. In this method, we Taylor expand P about an assumed (O_R, O_I, ψ_R, ψ_I) distribution, which is a perturbation away from some other distribution ($\tilde{O}_R$, $\tilde{O}_I$, $\tilde{\Psi}_R$, $\tilde{\Psi}_I$), such that a discrete set of P values can be expressed as

$$P(\tilde{O}_R, \tilde{O}_I, \tilde{\Psi}_R, \tilde{\Psi}_I) = P(O_R, O_I, \Psi_R, \Psi_I)$$
$$+ \frac{\partial P}{\partial O_R} \Delta O_R + \frac{\partial P}{\partial O_I} \Delta O_I + \frac{\partial P}{\partial \Psi_R} \Delta \Psi_R + \frac{\partial P}{\partial \Psi_I} \Delta \Psi_I + \cdots \qquad [7]$$

where $\Delta O_R = \tilde{O}_R - O_R$, $\Delta O_I = \tilde{O}_I - O_I$, $\Delta \Psi_R = \tilde{\Psi}_R - \Psi_R$, and $\Delta \Psi_I = \tilde{\Psi}_I - \Psi_I$. If the assumed optical and acoustic property distribution is close to the true profile, the left-hand side of Eq. [7]

can be considered as true data (observed or measured), and the relationship can be truncated to yield

$$J\Delta\chi = P^o - P^c \qquad [8]$$

where

$$J = \begin{bmatrix} \partial P_1/\partial O_{R,1} & \cdots & \partial P_1/\partial O_{R,K} & \partial P_1/\partial O_{I,1} & \cdots & \partial P_1/\partial O_{I,L} & \partial P_1/\partial \Psi_{R,1} & \cdots & \partial P_1/\partial \Psi_{R,K} & \partial P_1/\partial \Psi_{I,1} & \cdots & \partial P_1/\partial \Psi_{I,L} \\ \partial P_2/\partial O_{R,1} & \cdots & \partial P_2/\partial O_{R,K} & \partial P_2/\partial O_{I,1} & \cdots & \partial P_2/\partial O_{I,L} & \partial P_2/\partial \Psi_{R,1} & \cdots & \partial P_2/\partial \Psi_{R,K} & \partial P_2/\partial \Psi_{I,1} & \cdots & \partial P_2/\partial \Psi_{I,L} \\ \vdots & \ddots & \vdots & \vdots & \ddots & \vdots & \vdots & \ddots & \vdots & \vdots & \ddots & \vdots \\ \partial P_M/\partial O_{R,1} & \cdots & \partial P_M/\partial O_{R,K} & \partial P_M/\partial O_{I,1} & \cdots & \partial P_M/\partial O_{I,L} & \partial P_M/\partial \Psi_{R,1} & \cdots & \partial P_M/\partial \Psi_{R,K} & \partial P_M/\partial \Psi_{I,1} & \cdots & \partial P_M/\partial \Psi_{I,L} \end{bmatrix}$$

$$\Delta\chi = (\Delta O_{R,1}, \Delta O_{R,2}, \cdots, \Delta O_{R,K}, \Delta O_{I,1}, \Delta O_{I,2}, \cdots,$$
$$\Delta O_{I,L}, \Delta\Psi_{R,1}, \Delta\Psi_{R,2}, \cdots, \Delta\Psi_{R,K}, \Delta\Psi_{I,1}, \Delta\Psi_{I,2}, \cdots, \Delta\Psi_{I,L})^T$$

$$P^o = (P_1^o, P_2^o, \cdots, P_M^o)^T$$

$$P^c = (P_1^c, P_2^c, \cdots, P_M^c)^T$$

and P_i^o and P_i^c are measured and calculated based on the assumed (O_R, O_I, ψ_R, ψ_I) distribution data for $i = 1, 2, \ldots, M$ locations. $O_{R,k}$ ($k = 1, 2, \ldots, K$) and $O_{i,l}$ ($l = 1, 2, \ldots, L$) are the reconstruction parameters for the acoustic property profile, while $\Psi_{R,k}$ ($k = 1, 2, \ldots, K$) and $\Psi_{I,l}$ ($l = 1, 2, \ldots, L$) are the reconstruction parameters for the optical property profile. In order to realize an invertible system of equations for $\Delta\chi$, Eq. [8] is left multiplied by the transpose of J to produce

$$(J^T J + \lambda I)\Delta\chi = J^T(P^o - P^c) \qquad [9]$$

where regularization schemes are invoked in order to stabilize the decomposition of $J^T J$, where I is the identity matrix and λ is the regularization parameter determined by combined Marquardt and Tikhonov regularization schemes. We have found that when $\lambda = \alpha(P^o - P^c)^2 \times \text{trace}[J^T J]$, the reconstruction algorithm generates best results for PAT image reconstruction. The process now involves determining the calculated scattering field data and Jacobian matrix using dual meshing scheme coupled with adjoint sensitivity method. The reconstruction algorithm here uses the hybrid regularization-based Newton method to update an initial (guess) optical and acoustic property distribution iteratively via the solution of Eqs. [6] and [9] so that an object function composed of a weighted sum of the squared difference between computed and measured acoustic pressures for all acoustic frequencies and optical wavelengths can be minimized.

2.2. Imaging System

A typical PAT system consists of a pulsed laser source, a single transducer scanning subsystem or a transducer array, and an acoustic signal detection subsystem (*see* **Fig. 21.2**). In this system, pulsed light from a Nd:YAG, a Ti:Sapphire, or a diode laser is coupled into the phantom via an optical subsystem and generates acoustic pressure wave. A transducer (1 MHz or higher central frequency) is used to receive the acoustic signals. The transducer and the phantom/tissues are immersed in a water tank. A rotary stage rotates the receiver relative to the center of the tank. One set of data is taken at 120/360 positions when the receiver is scanned circularly over 360°. The complex wavefield signal is first amplified by a preamplifier and then amplified further by a pulser/receiver. A data acquisition board converts it into digital one which is fed to a computer. The entire data acquisition is realized through C programming. In this system, data collection for a total of 120 measurements requires about 5 min.

In the typical PAT setup shown above, the mechanical scanning significantly reduces the speed of data acquisition. The use of a transducer array has clear acquisition time advantages over a mechanically scanned system, making real-time data acquisition possible. In addition, a transducer array-based system eliminates the use of water tank and allows the direct contact of the array with the skin (of course ultrasound gel needs to be applied as coupling medium). The major drawback of an array-based system, however, is its significantly added cost.

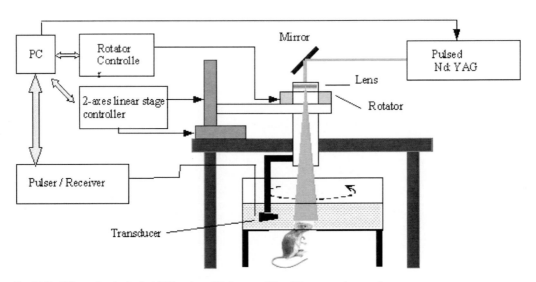

Fig. 21.2. Schematic of a typical PAT system. BS, beam splitter; PC, personal computer.

3. Nanoparticles/Tissue-Like Phantom Experiments

Controlled nanoparticles/tissue-like phantom experiments are necessary before the use of nanoparticles as contrast agents in an in vivo setting. Two representative experiments are presented here. In the experiments, we first embedded one or two nanoparticle-containing objects in a 10- or 25-mm-diameter solid cylindrical Intralipid/Ink phantom. For the two-target case, each target contained 0.5 nM nanoparticles, while for the one-target case, the target had only 0.25 nM nanoparticles. We then immersed the object-bearing solid phantom in a 110-mm-diameter water background. The gold nanoparticles had an average diameter of 20 nm. The molar extinction coefficient of

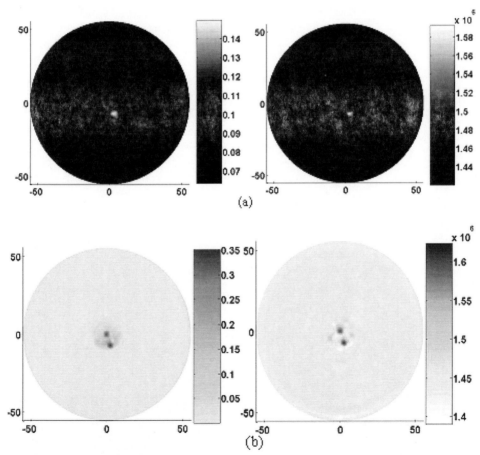

Fig. 21.3. Reconstructed absorbed optical energy density (the first column) and acoustic speed (the second column) images. The axes (*left and bottom*) illustrate the spatial scale, in millimeters, whereas the *gray scale* (*right*) records the acoustic speed, in millimeter per second, or absorbed optical energy density, in a relative unit. (**a**) is for one-target test case and (**b**) is for two-target test case (adapted from Ref. 16).

the nanoparticles was determined to be 1×10^9 M^{-1} cm^{-1}, about three orders of magnitude larger than that of a typical organic molecule. The nanoparticles concentration used in our experiments ranged from 0.25 to 0.5 nM, which gave an absorption coefficient of the object from 0.025 to 0.05 mm^{-1}. **Figure 21.3a, b** presents the reconstructed absorbed optical energy density and acoustic speed images for the one- and two-target cases, respectively. By estimating the full width at half maximum (FWHM) of the acoustic speed, we found that the recovered diameter size of these objects ranges from 2.8 to 3.3 mm, in good agreement with the actual object size of 3 mm. The images were recovered using measured acoustic data at one optical wavelength.

4. In Vivo Applications

Various types of nanoparticles including nanoshells, nanotubes, nanorods, and iron oxide nanoparticles have been successfully used for in vivo PA imaging. In one example, gold nanoparticles served as contrast agent for in vivo tumor imaging. PEGylated gold nanoparticles (50 nm) (200 μL, 10 mg/mL) were administered via tail vein and serial PA images were made of tumors following systemic administration (18). The accumulation of untargeted PEGylated nanoparticles inside tumors following systemic administration is expected and has been demonstrated to occur via a process called "enhanced permeability and retention." In the present case, the accumulation of gold nanoparticles inside tumors can be visualized by PAT and is shown clearly 5 h following systemic administration of gold nanoparticles (*see* **Fig. 21.4**).

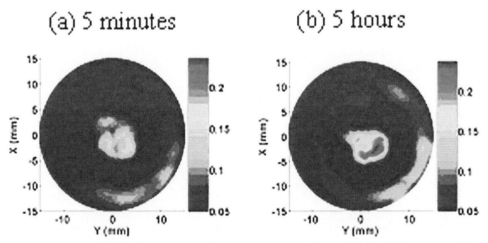

Fig. 21.4. PAT images of tumor following tail vein injection of gold nanoparticles at 5 min following injection (**a**) and 5 h following injection (**b**). The color scale (*right*) represents optical absorption of tissue (arbitrary units).

Metal nanoshells with highly tunable optical properties are synthesized with a dielectric core nanoparticle such as silica surrounded by an ultrathin metal shell, often composed of gold for biomedical applications (19). Depending on the size and composition of each layer of the nanoshell, particles can be designed to either absorb or scatter light over much of the visible and infrared regions of the electromagnetic spectrum, including the NIR region, where penetration of light through tissue is maximal. These shells are also easily conjugated to antibodies and other

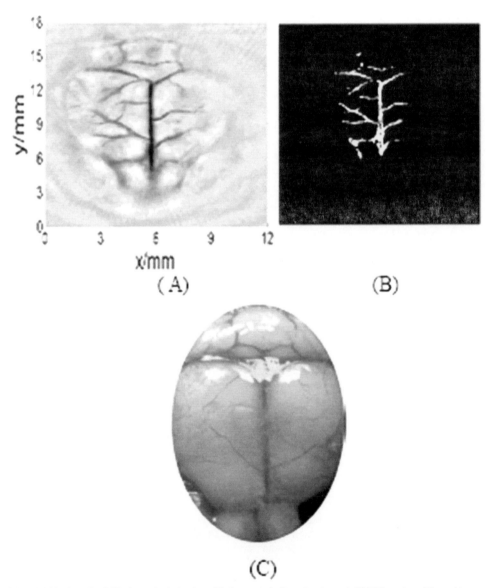

Fig. 21.5. (**a**) Noninvasive PAT of a rat brain in vivo with the nanoshell contrast agent. (**b**) PA imaging of the gold nanoshell distribution in rat brain. (**c**) Open-skull photography of the rat brain cortex obtained after PA imaging. (See also related image in Ref. 19.)

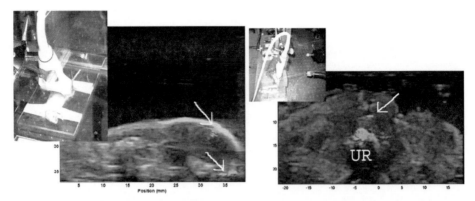

Fig. 21.6. (*Left*) A combined US/PA image of a mouse hind limb with two gold nanorod gelled inclusions implanted in its right hip. *Arrows* show the locations of implanted gelled nanorod solution. (*Left inset*) The mouse was fixed in a water tank with the ultrasonic transducer positioned above its lower body. (*Right*) combined US/PA image of human prostate gland with a gold nanoparticles sample implanted in an incision made on its top part (*marked by arrow*). (*Right insert*) Imaging setup including the ultrasound probe and fiber illumination inserted through the urethra (UR). (See also the related images in reference 20).

biomolecules. Several potential biomedical applications are under investigation, including immunoassays, modulated drug delivery, photothermal cancer therapy, and imaging contrast agents. In an in vivo brain imaging in a small animal study (19), NIR-absorbing gold nanoshells were injected intravenously, and then PAT was used to image the cerebral vasculature. The in vivo rat brain structures with gold nanoshell contrast agents are imaged photoacoustically, as shown in **Fig. 21.5**.

Gold nanorods conjugated with an antibody were also used for targeting cancer cells and for PA imaging of a single layer of cells (20). The specific nanoparticle complex described in this study was designed for peak absorption in the range of 700–840 nm, optimal for in vivo applications. The study validated that gold nanorods produce high contrast between targeted tissue and nontargeted tissue for PAT imaging in an in vitro experiment. The study also showed that nanorod-based PA imaging appear to be attractive for early detection of prostate cancer (**Fig. 21.6**). Using a probe equipped with fiber optic illumination, the physician can image tissue structure and diagnose lesions by their cell type, avoiding unnecessary biopsy procedures. In

Fig. 21.7. (continued) Single-walled carbon nanotube targets tumor in living mice. **a**, Ultrasound (the second row) and photoacoustic (the third to the fifth row) images of one vertical slice (white dotted line) through the tumor. The ultrasound images show the skin and tumor boundaries. Subtraction images were calculated as the 4 h postinjection image minus the pre-injection image. The high PA signal in the mouse injected with plain single-walled carbon nanotubes (indicated with a white arrow) is not seen in the subtraction image, suggesting that it is due to a large blood vessel and not single-walled carbon nanotubes. **b**, Mice injected with SWNT–RGD showed a significantly higher PA signal than mice injected with plain single-walled carbon nanotubes. The error bars represent standard error. (See also related images in reference 21).

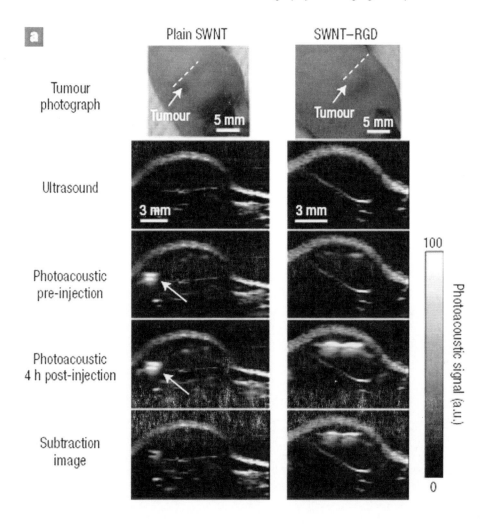
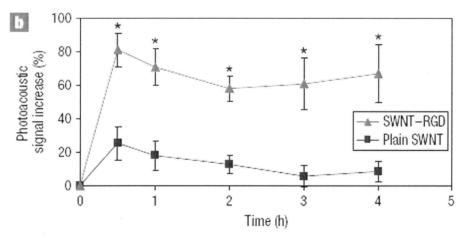

Fig. 21.7. (continued)

cases where biopsy is administered, tissue sampling accuracy can be improved with image guidance.

Recently single-walled carbon nanotubes conjugated with cyclic Arg-Gly-Asp (RGD) peptides were studied as a contrast agent for PAT imaging of tumors (21) (**Fig. 21.7**). Intravenous administration of these targeted nanotubes to mice bearing tumors showed eight times greater PA signal in the tumor than did the administration of nontargeted nanotubes to mice. These results were verified ex vivo using Raman microscopy. This study showed that PAT imaging of targeted single-walled carbon nanotubes may contribute to noninvasive cancer imaging and monitoring of nanotherapeutics in living subjects.

Superparamagnetic iron oxide nanoparticles were also investigated as a contrast agent for PA imaging (5). In this study, the contrast agent consisted of superparamagnetic iron oxide nanoparticle cores coated with carboxydextran (called ferucarbotran; Schering AG, Berlin, Germany, trade name: Resovist) (5, 22). The study demonstrated that in vivo applications with 6 dB signal enhancement may be feasible when local aggregation was four times higher than the average concentration of

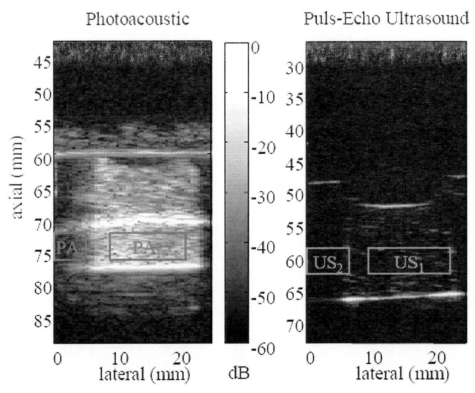

Fig. 21.8. Comparison of PA and pulse-echo ultrasound B-mode images for a concentration of 0.133 mmol Fe/ml. The red boxes depict the regions for the computation of contrast enhancement due to Ferucarbotran. (See also related images in reference 5.)

ferucarbotran in the human liver during conventional clinical applications (**Fig. 21.8**). In addition, ferucarbotran may serve as an inherently multimodal contrast agent for PA and magnetic resonance imaging.

References

1. Jiang, H., Iftimia, N., Xu, Y., Eggert, J., Fajardo, L., and Klove, K. (2002) Near-infrared optical imaging of the breast with model-based reconstruction. *Acad Radiol* **9**, 186–194.
2. Ntziachristos, V., Yodh, A. G., Schnall, M., and Chance, B. (2000) Concurrent MRI and diffuse optical tomography of breast after indocyanine green enhancement. *Proc Natl Acad Sci USA* **97**, 2767–2772.
3. Cerussi, A. E., Berger, A., Bevilacqua, F., Shah, N., Jakubowski, D., Butler, J., Holcombe, R., and Tromberg, B. (2001) Sources of absorption and scattering contrast for near-infrared optical mammography. *Acad Radiol* **8**, 211–218.
4. Rayavarapu, R. G., Petersen, W., Ungureanu, C., Post, J. N., Leeuwen, T. G., and Manohar, S. (2007) Synthesis and bioconjugation of gold nanoparticles as potential molecular probes for light-based imaging techniques. *Int J Biomed Imaging* **2007**, 29817.
5. Mienkina, M. P., Hensel, K., Le, T. N., Gerhardt, N. C., Hansen, C., Hofmann, M., and Schmitz, G. (2006) Experimental characterization of Ferucarbotran as a photoacoustic nanoparticles contrast agent. *IEEE Ultrasonics Symposium* **2006**, 393–396.
6. Wang, X., Ku, G., Wegiel, M. A., Bornhop, D. J., Stoica, G., and Wang, L. (2004) Noninvasive photoacoustic angiography of animal brains in vivo with near-infrared light and an optical contrast agent. *Opt Lett* **29**, 730–732.
7. Copland, J. A., Eghtedari, M., Popov, V. L., Kotov, N., Mamedova, N., Motamedi, M., and Oraevsky, A. A. (2004) Bioconjugated gold nanoparticles as a molecular based contrast agent: implications for imaging of deep tumors using optoacoustic tomography. *Mol Imaging Biol* **6**, 341–349.
8. Lin, A. W. H., Lewinski, N. A., West, J. L., Halas, N. J., and Drezek, R. A. (2005) Optically tunable nanoparticle contrast agents for early cancer detection: model-based analysis of gold nanoshells. *J Biomed Opt* **10**, 064035.
9. Perez-Juste, J., Pastoriza-Santos, I., Liz-Marzan, L., and Mulvaney, P. (2005) Gold nanorods: synthesis, characterization and applications. *Coord Chem Rev* **249**, 1870–1901.
10. Sokolov, K., Follen, M., Aaron, J., et al. (2003) Real-time vital optical imaging of pre-cancer using anti-epidermal growth factor receptor antibodies conjugated to nanoparticles. *Cancer Res* **63**, 1999–2004.
11. Agarwal, A., Huang, S. W., O'Donnell, M., Day, K. C., and Day, M. (2007) Targeted gold nanorod contrast agent for prostate cancer detection by photoacoustic imaging. *J Appl Phys* **102**, 064035.
12. Hoelen, C. G. A. and de Mul, F. F. M. (2000) Image reconstruction for photoacoustic scanning of tissue structures. *Appl Opt* **39**, 5872–5883.
13. Manohar, S., et al. (2007) Initial results of in vivo noninvasive cancer imaging in the human breast using near-infrared photoacoustics. *Opt Express* **15**, 12277–12285.
14. Kruger, R. A., Liu, P., Fang, Y., and Appledorn, C. (1995) Photoacoustic ultrasound (PAUS)-reconstruction tomography. *Med Phys* **22**, 1605–1609.
15. Wang, X., Xu, Y., Xu, M., Yokoo, S., Fry, E., and Wang, L. (2002) Photoacoustic tomography of biological tissues with high cross-section resolution: Reconstruction and experiment. *Med Phys* **29**, 2799–2805.
16. Yuan, Z., Zhang, Q., and Jiang, H. (2006) Simultaneously reconstruction of acoustic and optical properties of heterogeneous medium by quantitative photoacoustic tomography. *Opt Express* **14**, 6749–6753.
17. Yuan, Z. and Jiang, H. (2006) Quantitative photoacoustic tomography: recovery of optical absorption coefficient map of heterogeneous medium. *Appl Phys Lett* **88**, 231101.
18. Zhang, Q., et al. Gold Nanoparticles for Enhanced in Vivo Tumor Imaging with Photoacoustic Tomography (2008) (in review).
19. Xiang, L. Z., Xing, D., Gu, H., Yang, D., Zeng, L., and Yang, S. (2006) Gold nanoshell-based photoacoustic imaging application in biomedicine. *International Symposium on Biophotonics, Nanophotonics and Metamaterials* **2006**, 76–79.
20. Agarwal, A., Huang, S. W., O'Donnell, M., Day, K. C., and Day, M. (2007) Targeted gold nanorod contrast agent for prostate

cancer detection by photoacoustic imaging. *J Appl Phys* **102**, 064035.
21. Zerda, A., Zavalete, C., et al. (2008) Carbon nanotubes as photoacoustic molecular imaging agents in living mice. *Nat Nanotechnol* **3**, 557–561.
22. Reimer, P. and Balzer, T. (2003) Ferucarbotran (Resovist): a new clinically approved RES-specific contrast agent for contrast-enhanced MRI of the liver: properties, clinical development, and applications. *Eur Radiol* **13**, 1266–1276.

Chapter 22

Current Applications of Nanotechnology for Magnetic Resonance Imaging of Apoptosis

Gustav J. Strijkers, Geralda A.F. van Tilborg, Tessa Geelen, Chris P.M. Reutelingsperger, and Klaas Nicolay

Abstract

Apoptosis, or programmed cell death, is a morphologically and biochemically distinct form of cell death, which together with proliferation plays an important role in tissue development and homeostasis. Insufficient apoptosis is important in the pathology of various disorders such as cancer and autoimmune diseases, whereas a high apoptotic activity is associated with myocardial infarction, neurodegenerative diseases, and advanced atherosclerotic lesions. Consequently, apoptosis is recognized as an important therapeutic target, which should be either suppressed, e.g., during an ischemic cardiac infarction, or promoted, e.g., in the treatment of cancerous lesions. Imaging tools to address location, amount, and time course of apoptotic activity non-invasively in vivo are therefore of great clinical use in the evaluation of such therapies. This chapter reviews current literature and new developments in the application of nanoparticles for non-invasive apoptosis imaging. Focus is on functionalized nanoparticle contrast agents for MR imaging and bimodal nanoparticle agents that combine magnetic and fluorescent properties.

Key words: Apoptosis, nanoparticles, magnetic resonance imaging, molecular imaging, optical imaging, cardiovascular disease, atherosclerosis, cancer.

1. Apoptosis

Apoptosis is a distinct form of regulated cell death (1–3). It can be characterized by a sequence of cellular morphological changes, including cellular shrinkage, condensation, and margination of the chromatin as well as budding of the cell membrane followed by formation of the so-called apoptotic bodies (4). In contrast to necrosis, a mode of cell death which is characterized by cellular swelling, lysis, and uncontrolled release of metabolites and electrolytes with concomitant inflammatory reactions, the apoptotic death of cells will not trigger inflammation since the apoptotic bodies are efficiently phagocytized by macrophages or neighboring cells.

The typical morphological manifestation of apoptosis is the result of a highly regulated process that typically involves two major pathways (5). **Figure 22.1** is a simplified schematic drawing of these two pathways involved in the initiation of apoptosis. First, there is an extrinsic pathway that is governed by cell-surface death receptors. Specific cytokines, such as Fas ligand or tumor necrosis factor alpha, released by other cells bind to the receptors, resulting in downstream activation of specialized proteases known as caspases, most notably caspase-3. Caspase activity initiates DNA cleavage in internucleosomal 180–200-base pair fragments (DNA laddering), which ultimately leads to cellular apoptosis (6). Second, in the intrinsic pathway, mitochondria respond to stress factors, such as ischemia and reperfusion injury, cytotoxins, or radiation, by releasing pro-apoptotic factors. Ultimately, the extrinsic pathway converges with the intrinsic pathway through the activation of caspase-3. The two pathways interact via pro- and anti-apoptotic proteins.

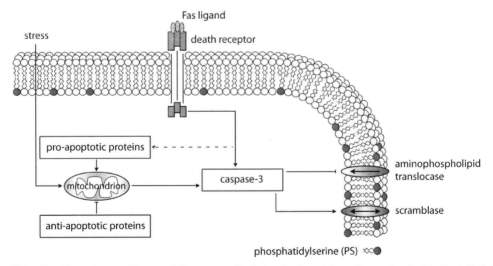

Fig. 22.1. Simplified scheme of the apoptotic process, displaying the two major pathways involved in the initiation of apoptosis, the central role of caspase-3, and the exposure of phosphatidylserine at the outer leaflet of the cell membrane.

A relatively early biochemical hallmark of apoptosis is phospholipid phosphatidylserine (PS) exposure at the outer leaflet of the cell membrane (**Fig. 22.1**). Exposure of PS serves as the main phagocytotic signal for surrounding macrophages and neighboring cells to engulf the apoptotic cell without introducing an inflammatory reaction (7). In most viable cells, PS is predominantly, but not exclusively, located at the inner leaflet of the cellular membrane actively delivered there by an ATP-dependent lipid transporter (aminophospholipid translocase), which rapidly shuttles PS from the outer to the inner leaflet of the cell membrane (8, 9). During the apoptotic process, however, the aminophospholipid translocase activity is inhibited and PS is rapidly exposed on the outer leaflet through activation of the bidirectional Ca^{2+}-dependent lipid tranporter scramblase (10).

Apoptosis plays an important role in tissue development and homeostasis. Insufficient apoptosis is involved in the pathology of various disorders such as cancer and autoimmune diseases, whereas excessive apoptotic activity is associated with neurodegenerative diseases, advanced atherosclerotic lesions (11), and myocardial infarction (12, 13).

Myocyte cell death during the acute stages of myocardial infarction occurs primarily via apoptosis (14, 15). During prolonged ischemia, cell death in the central infarct zone seems to arise mainly from necrosis, while in the ischemic penumbra, apoptosis remains dominant. However, there is controversy about relative contributions (16–18). Formation of reactive oxygen species after reperfusion of ischemic myocardial infarction has been implicated in increased apoptotic rate (19). Apoptosis in areas remote from the infarction plays a negative role in the cardiac remodeling process (16) and has been connected to the pathogenesis of heart failure following ischemic injury (20). Since apoptosis is a highly regulated process, it is recognized as an important therapeutic target. Modulation or inhibition of apoptosis resulting from cardiac ischemia, reperfusion injury, or during the remodeling phase may have a positive clinical impact by preventing a transition to heart failure. To that end, non-invasive imaging tools are desired to assess location and fractions of apoptotic myocytes. In atherosclerosis, a high occurrence of apoptosis and necrosis, as well as high macrophage burden, is believed to contribute significantly to plaque vulnerability and rupture (11, 21–25). Therefore, identification of apoptotic cells by non-invasive diagnostic imaging may contribute in discriminating atherosclerotic lesions with a stable and an unstable phenotype, which would be of great clinical value.

Apoptosis is an efficient defense mechanism to prevent damaged cells from undergoing a transition to malignancy. Insufficient apoptosis may thus be a promoter of tumor development by preventing removal of malignant cells and allowing accumulation of fast dividing cells (26, 27). Many non-surgical anti-cancer treatments, such as hormonal agents, toxins, and radiotherapy, are therefore designed to trigger cancerous cells to undergo apoptosis. Early apoptotic response to treatment is considered a positive prognostic indicator for tumor therapy efficacy (28–30). New non-invasive in vivo imaging methods to assess the amount, the location, and the time course of apoptosis in tumors will therefore be highly useful in the assessment of anti-cancer therapy. Classical evaluation of tumor treatment relies heavily on the observation of tumor regression which may take weeks to become manifest. Apoptosis imaging on the other hand will allow for an early follow-up on the treatment efficacy.

2. Nanoparticle Contrast Agents for MRI

This chapter will concentrate on functionalized nanoparticles that can be used in conjunction with MRI for non-invasive imaging of apoptosis. MRI is an imaging technique that exploits the magnetic properties of hydrogen nuclei (or protons), called spin, present in mainly water and lipids in the human body. When placed in a magnetic field, a tiny imbalance is created between the number of spins that align parallel and anti-parallel with the applied magnetic field, which produces a small net equilibrium magnetization. This magnetization can be excited and manipulated by applying external resonant radiofrequency electromagnetic fields to generate signals that can be recorded and suitably combined to form images. After excitation the magnetization returns back to equilibrium by a process called relaxation.

Contrast in the MR images is mainly obtained by tissue-specific differences in proton density as well as the longitudinal (T_1) and transverse (T_2 and T_2^*) relaxation times. Most contrast agents generate contrast by lowering the T_1 and T_2 relaxation times of water protons surrounding the agent (31). The relaxivity, i.e., the potency to shorten T_1 and T_2, of an MRI contrast agent is defined by the change in longitudinal or transversal relaxation rates per unit concentration of contrast agent. The constant of proportionality is referred to as the relaxivity r_1 or r_2, respectively, expressed in unit of mM^{-1} s^{-1}. Contrast agents with low r_2/r_1 ratio (~1–2) are best visualized using a T_1-weighted MR imaging technique that produces a signal gain at the location of the contrast agent. These contrast agents are therefore often referred to as positive contrast agents. On the other hand, for agents with higher r_2/r_1 ratio, a T_2-weighted imaging technique is more appropriate, resulting in signal loss at the location of the contrast agent. Such agents are referred to as negative contrast agents.

Positive MRI contrast agents are usually Gd^{3+}-based complexes. The Gd^{3+} ion has a strong fluctuating magnetic moment that serves as an efficient pathway for longitudinal relaxation. Most commercially available agents are low molecular weight compounds, such as Gd–DTPA (Magnevist) and Gd–HP–DO3A

(Prohance). They contain a single chelated Gd^{3+} ion requiring rather large concentrations of the order of 0.1 mM to obtain sufficient contrast. To boost the detection sensitivity per particle, multiple Gd chelates can be combined into a single nanoparticle. Such amplification has been employed to produce nanoparticles with multiple Gd chelates linked to polylysine, polyornithine, polysaccharides, and dendrimers (32–36). Nanoparticles of lipidic aggregates were designed to contain thousands of Gd chelates per particle. Aggregate morphology may vary from micelles to liposomes and microemulsions (37–48). By using such strategies the detection sensitivity can be improved down to the low nanomolar concentration regime.

Most commonly used negative MRI contrast agents are based on iron oxide spherical crystals with a diameter of about 5–50 nm (49). The nanoparticles typically have a core-shell structure where the shell sterically or electrostatically stabilizes the particle to prevent aggregation. Based on the hydrodynamic diameter, i.e., the overall core-shell diameter, several types of nanoparticles can be distinguished. These include very small iron oxide particles (VSOPs) of diameter ∼8 nm, ultra small superparamagnetic iron oxide (USPIO) of diameter < 50 nm, superparamagnetic iron oxide (SPIO) typically 50–200 nm in size, and micrometer-sized particles of iron oxide (MPIO). Some specific iron oxide-based agents are referred to as monocrystalline (MION) or cross-linked (CLIO) iron oxide particles (50, 51). Iron oxide nanoparticles contain thousands of magnetically ordered iron atoms, which collectively add up to one large magnetic moment. The particles have no remnant magnetic moment in zero field but are easily magnetized in the large magnetic field of the MRI scanner. The large magnetic moment induces strong field gradients, giving rise to accelerated loss of phase coherence to surrounding water protons, which leads to strong shortening of the $T_2^{(*)}$ relaxation time. Because the collective ordering of the iron atoms within the particle constitutes a single large magnetic moment, the detection sensitivity of such particles is accordingly high.

MRI is one of the most powerful non-invasive imaging techniques in clinical diagnostics and research, capable of producing in vivo high-resolution images in three dimensions and providing a variety of physiological information as well. Nevertheless, for validation of novel (targeted) contrast agents, a complementary technique is highly desirable to, e.g., provide validation for specificity or fate of the agent at the microscopic level once it has interacted with its intended biological target. Therefore, nanoparticle MRI contrast agents, such as the one described above, are often equipped with fluorescent properties as well to allow the use of in vivo intravital microscopy or ex vivo fluorescence histological analysis. Fluorescent properties can be introduced by incorporation of fluorescent dyes, such as rhodamine, fluorescein, near-infrared dye (48), or by the use of fluorescent quantum dots (QD) (47, 52) to create a so-called bi-model nanoparticle with both MRI and fluorescent contrast properties.

3. Imaging of Apoptosis

Figure 22.2 displays schematically a collection of nanoparticles, which are functionalized for binding to apoptotic cells on the basis of phosphatidylserine exposure. In the following sections, a number of studies described in literature are reviewed that have reported on the use of these nanoparticles for in vitro apoptosis detection and for in vivo MR imaging of apoptosis in animal models of ischemic heart disease and cancer.

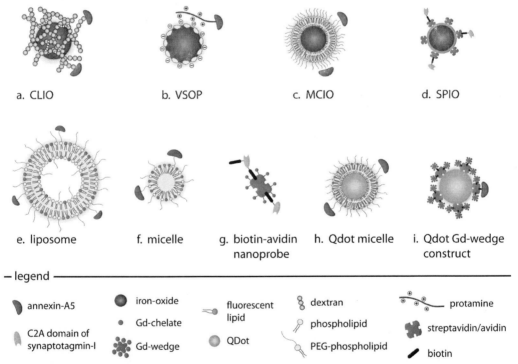

Fig. 22.2. Collection of nanoparticles designed to image apoptosis: (**a**) cross-linked iron oxide (CLIO), (**b**) very small iron oxide particle (VSOP), (**c**) micellular iron oxide (MCIO), (**d**) superparamagnetic iron oxide, (**e**) paramagnetic liposome, (**f**) paramagnetic micelle, (**g**) biotin–avidin nanoprobe, (**h**) quantum-dot micelle, and (**i**) Gd-wedge-coated quantum dot. The nanoparticles are made specific for phosphatidylserine expressed on apoptotic cells by conjugation of either annexin A5 or C2A domain of synaptotagmin I. Nanoparticles **a–d** are negative MR contrast agents, while **e–i** have positive contrast properties. Nanoparticles **c**, **e**, **f**, **h**, and **i** additionally possess fluorescent properties by incorporation of a fluorescent dye or a quantum dot. The *bottom* of the figure shows the legend with the constituents of the nanoparticles. Particles and components are not drawn to scale.

3.1. In Vitro Imaging

Several studies have provided proof of concept for in vitro imaging of apoptosis using targeted nanoparticles. Schellenberger et al. were the first to design a CLIO nanoparticle conjugated with annexin A5 for in vitro detection of apoptosis with MRI (53). Annexin A5 is a 36-kDa protein that binds with high affinity ($K_d < 10^{-9}$ M) to the phosphatidylserine expressed at the outer leaflet of the apoptotic cell membrane in a Ca^{2+}-dependent manner (54, 55). It should be noted that in vivo annexin A5 would also bind to necrotic cells that express phosphatidylserine as well. Previously, annexin A5 assays had been developed for in vitro quantification of apoptosis using predominantly flow cytometry and microscopy (56). **Figure 22.2a** is a schematic drawing of the nanoparticle that was developed by Schellenberger et al. (57). The iron oxide core of the nanoparticle was coated with cross-linked dextran for sterical stabilization. A reaction with ammonia yielded NH_2 functionalization after which a reaction with *N*-succinimidyl 3-(2-pyridyldithio) propionate (SPDP) provided 2-pyridyl disulfide–CLIO. Annexin A5 was reacted with SATA to provide protected sulfhydryl groups, which after deprotection of the thioether groups resulted in thiolated annexin A5. Thiolated annexin A5 was then reacted with the 2-pyridyl disulfide–CLIO to yield the desired annexin A5-functionalized CLIO nanoparticle. The resulting nanoparticles contained on average 2.7 annexin A5 proteins per CLIO and had an average size of approximately 50 nm. The functionality of the nanoparticles was tested by their ability to magnetically separate apoptotic cells from healthy cells and by the ability to detect the apoptotic cells with MRI. To that end, apoptosis was induced in Jurkat T-cell lymphoma cells by treatment with camptothecin. After incubation with the nanoparticles, the apoptotic cell fraction could be removed almost completely from the cell culture by a magnetic separation column, proving specific binding to apoptotic cells. A significant signal decrease was observed in the MR images of camptothecin-treated cells that were incubated with the functionalized nanoparticles, providing first proof of concept for the MR detection of apoptosis.

Schellenberger et al. recently introduced another apoptosis-specific iron oxide nanoparticle (**Fig. 22.2b**), which is based on a VSOP with a hydrodynamic size of about 8 nm (58). Because of its small size, steric stabilization by, e.g., dextran to prevent magnetic aggregation is less effective and therefore VSOPs are citrate monomer coated, which provides a negatively charged particle surface that prevents aggregation by electrostatic repulsion. Specificity for apoptotic cells was introduced by using a protamine–cys-annexin A5 conjugate. Protamine is a naturally occurring positively charged peptide, which binds by electrostatic interaction to the VSOP coating. On average, five annexin A5 proteins could be coupled per VSOP, increasing the total diameter of the nanoparticles to approximately 15 nm. The small size of this particle, compared to the CLIOs, is believed to improve the bioavailability for imaging extravascular apoptotic cells.

Van Tilborg and coworkers have designed a bimodal superparamagnetic micellular iron oxide (MCIO) that allowed detection of apoptosis with both MRI and optical techniques (48). The particle, drawn schematically in **Fig. 22.2c**, consisted of an oleic acid-coated iron oxide core with a diameter of about 5 nm, encapsulated by a PEG2000–DSPE phospholipid micellular shell. The pegylated phospholipid prevents aggregation and is known to increase in vivo circulation times. To enable flow cytometry and imaging of the particles with fluorescence microcopy, 1 mol% PE–carboxyfluorescein was incorporated into the shell. To functionalize the particles for apoptosis imaging, 5 mol% of the phospholipid coating was composed of Mal–PEG2000–DSPE, which allowed conjugation of cys-annexin A5 at the distal end of the PEG. The resulting nanoparticle had an average hydrodynamic diameter of approximately 10 nm. Specificity for anti-Fas-treated apoptotic Jurkat cells was demonstrated by both MRI and confocal fluorescence microscopy. **Figure 22.3a** shows T_2-weighted MR images of a loosely packed pellet of apoptotic Jurkat cells at the bottom of 250-µL PCR tubes (48). The cells were either left untreated (left) or incubated with annexin A5–MCIO (right). Clearly observed is the significant signal drop in the right pellet as a consequence of binding of the MCIOs to the apoptotic cells. The quantitative changes in R_2 ($\equiv 1/T_2$) of the pellets are displayed in **Fig. 22.3b**. Incubation of cells with annexin A5-MCIO in the presence of Ca^{2+} leads to a large R_2 increase as opposed to untreated cells (control) and cells incubated with nonfunctionalized MCIO. When incubations were performed in the presence of excess EDTA to deplete Ca^{2+}, the R_2 increase was lost, which further proves specificity of the annexin A5–MCIO binding.

Commercially available streptavidin-coated SPIO nanoparticles were conjugated with biotinylated C2A–GST fusion proteins (59) (**Fig. 22.2d**). The C2A domain of the protein synaptotagmin I binds to negatively charged phosphatidylserine expressed at the outer leaflet of apoptotic cells with a dissociation constant $K_d \sim 17 \times 10^{-9}$ M in a Ca^{2+}-dependent manner.

The above-described iron oxide-based apoptosis-specific nanoparticles are negative contrast agents, which are best visualized using $T_2^{(*)}$-weighted MRI as areas of signal loss in the images. Accurate detection of areas of signal loss in such images is often compromised by a low signal to noise and other sources of artifact-related signal attenuation. It is therefore in many cases more advantageous to use a T_1-weighted imaging technique in conjunction with a positive Gd-containing contrast agent,

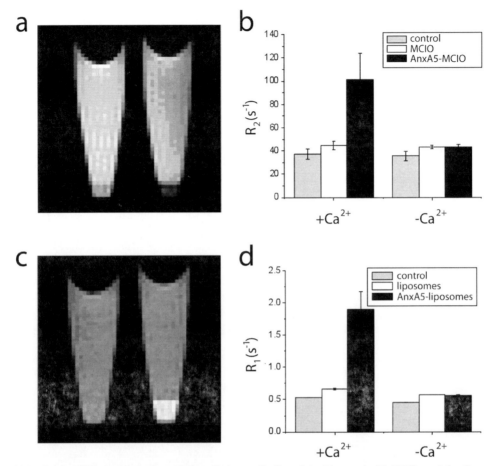

Fig. 22.3. In vitro MRI detection of apoptotic cells by application of (**a, b**) annexin A5–MCIOs and (**c, d**) annexin A5–liposomes. (**a**) Pellet of apoptotic Jurkat cells at the bottom of 250-μL PCR tube either (*left*) untreated or (*right*) incubated with annexin A5–MCIOs. (**b**) Quantification of transverse relaxation rate R_2 for different incubations in either Ca^{2+}-rich environment or buffer depleted of Ca^{2+} by EDTA. (**c**) Pellet of apoptotic Jurkat cells at the bottom of PCR tube either (*left*) untreated or (*right*) incubated with annexin A5–liposomes. (**d**) Quantification of longitudinal relaxation rate R_1 for different incubations with liposomes in either Ca^{2+}-rich environment or buffer without Ca^{2+}. Reproduced with permission from van Tilborg et al. (48). Copyright 2006 American Chemical Society.

leading to signal gain in images that can irrefutably be attributed to the agent.

A liposomal-based positive contrast agent specific for apoptosis (**Fig. 22.2e**) was developed by van Tilborg et al. (48). The liposomes have a diameter of approximately 100 nm, contain about 40,000 Gd–DTPA–bis(stearylamide) entities incorporated in the lipid bilayer, and have a r_2/r_1 ratio of 1.7. The high amount of Gd and the low r_2/r_1 result in an extremely powerful positive contrast agent with nanomolar detection sensitivity. Additional fluorescent lipids were incorporated into the liposomes to allow for parallel detection with fluorescent imaging techniques. Multiple cys-annexin A5 proteins were covalently coupled to Mal–PEG2000–DSPE lipids in the liposomal membrane to introduce specificity for apoptotic cells. **Figure 22.3c** shows a T_1-weighted MR image of two 250-μL PCR tubes with a pellet of apoptotic Jurkat cells at the bottom (48). The pellet that was previously incubated with annexin A5–liposomes (right) clearly shows a large increase in signal in the MR image as opposed to the untreated cells (left). Additionally, increase in R_1 ($\equiv 1/T_1$) was quantified (**Fig. 22.3d**). Significant increase in R_1 was observed only for incubations with annexin A5–liposomes in the presence of Ca^{2+}, proving specificity of the contrast agent.

Extravasation of the above relatively large nanoparticles may be limited due to their size. Therefore, a micellular positive contrast agent based on a 1:1 mixture of Gd–DTPA–bis(stearylamide) and pegylated phospholipids was also developed by the same group (**Fig. 22.2f**). The micelles have a size of approximately 20 nm and therefore more easily extravasate. The drawback of the latter nanoparticles is that they contain significantly less Gd entities (approximately 40 per micelle), which makes them less powerful in terms of detection sensitivity. Nevertheless, this drawback can be compensated for by improved pharmacokinetic behavior.

An even smaller apoptosis-specific positive contrast agent was developed by Neves et al. (60). The nanoparticle of 5 nm in diameter, schematically displayed in **Fig. 22.2g**, is a bivalent probe in which two biotinylated C2A domains are complexed with a single avidin molecule. The nanoparticle bound with high affinity to the phosphatidylserine expressed at the outer leaflet of the apoptotic cell membrane as evidenced by surface plasmon resonance binding experiments and flow cytometry. The probe allowed for detection by MRI as demonstrated by in vitro experiments on apoptotic EL-4 cells.

Finally, in two studies, a fluorescent quantum dot was used as the basis for a positive contrast agent. In the first study by van Tilborg et al. (47), a hydrophobic quantum dot was coated with a mixture of pegylated and Gd-containing lipids to form a micellular quantum dot (**Fig. 22.2h**). Annexin A5 was coupled to the distal end of the PEG chains to introduce specificity for apoptotic cells. The basis of the nanoparticle by Prinzen et al. (**Fig. 22.2i**) was a commercially available quantum dot functionalized with 10 streptavidin proteins (61). The streptavidin allowed for conjugation with multiple wedges, each containing eight Gd complexes and on average 1 annexin A5 protein. Several other groups have synthesized nanoparticles specifically for optical apoptosis imaging (62–67). These nanoparticles lack MRI contrast properties though and therefore will not be elaborated in this review.

3.2. Imaging of Apoptosis in Injured Myocardium

Thus far, only two studies have addressed the potential of using MR contrast agents to image cardiomyocyte apoptosis after myocardial injury. In a seminal study by Sosnovik et al., the ability of annexin A5–CLIO–Cy5.5 bimodal nanoparticles (**Fig. 22.2a**) for imaging apoptosis in a mouse model of transient coronary artery (LAD) occlusion was demonstrated (68). Cy5.5 is a fluorescent dye that allows for fluorescent imaging in the near-infrared wavelength regime. Nonfunctionalized CLIO–Cy5.5 was used as a control. **Figure 22.4a** shows a typical MR image at 9.4 T of the heart of a mouse which was intravenously injected with annexin A5–CLIO–Cy5.5. Injection of the contrast agent took place directly after blood flow to the ischemic myocardium was restored, whereas MR imaging was performed after 24 h. The anatomical MR image is overlaid in color with quantitative T_2^* values in a region of interest in the myocardium defined by the zone of hypokinesis. A significant T_2^* reduction is observed in those regions that correspond with the presence of annexin A5–CLIO–Cy5.5, as evidenced by the presence of near-infrared fluorescence in the same regions (**Fig. 22.4b**). Mice that received nonfunctionalized CLIO–Cy5.5 did not display a significant reduction of T_2^* in the hypokinetic areas of the myocardium (**Fig. 22.4c**), which is corroborated by lack of fluorescent intensity in corresponding regions (**Fig. 22.4d**). This study proved that nanoparticles can be sensitive indicators for the presence of cardiomyocyte apoptosis and suggests that imaging could become

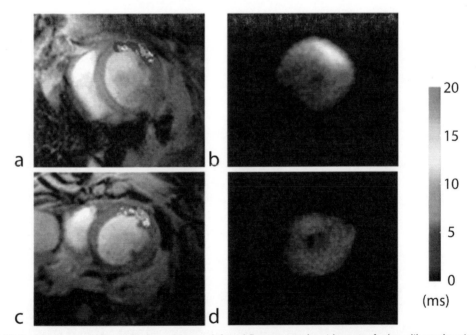

Fig. 22.4. (**a, c**) In vivo MR and (**b, d**) ex vivo near-infrared fluorescence heart images of mice with previous transient ligation of the LAD coronary artery after injection with either (**a, b**) annexin A5–CLIO–Cy5.5 or (**c, d**) CLIO–Cy5.5. MR images are overlaid with a color map according to the scale on the right, indicating significantly lower T_2^* values in the hypokinetic region of the left ventricle for mice injected with annexin A5–CLIO–Cy5.5. Reproduced with permission from Sosnovik et al. (68).

an important tool to assess novel cardioprotective strategies aimed at reducing the extent and amount of cardiomyocyte apoptosis.

Hiller et al. have demonstrated detection of cardiomyocyte apoptosis in isolated rat hearts using positive contrast-generating nanoparticles (69). The nanoparticles consisted of Gd-labeled biotinylated liposomes that were conjugated with biotinylated annexin A5 by an avidin linker. The left coronary artery was transiently ligated and specific binding of the annexin A5–liposome construct was evidenced from T_1 and T_2^*-weighted imaging and quantitative T_1 and T_2^* analysis at 11.7 T.

3.3. Imaging of Apoptosis in Tumors

Magnetic resonance offers a number of different techniques to detect and assess tumors as well as to follow treatment effects (70–73). Tumor location, size, and composition (to some extent) can be measured using T_1- and T_2-weighted imaging, whereas vascular volume, endothelial permeability, and oxygenation can be assessed with dynamic contrast-enhanced MRI and BOLD. ^{1}H magnetic resonance spectroscopy (MRS) allows for quantitative detection of levels and changes in metabolites, e.g., total choline, lactate, lipid, and NAA. Furthermore, pH and energy status can be assessed using ^{31}P MRS. New molecular imaging techniques allow for the detection of sparse receptors expressed in the tumor vasculature (74).

Therapy-induced apoptosis in tumors may induce cell morphological changes, i.e., cell shrinkage and formation of apoptotic bodies, which can be detected and even distinguished from necrosis by regional and specific changes in the tumor T_2-relaxation time and water diffusion constant (75–77), while apoptosis-related metabolic changes may be detected using MRS (73, 78).

Recently, targeted nanoparticles have been employed to detect apoptosis in tumors and to assess treatment efficacy. Potentially, this would provide a more sensitive detection of apoptosis as it relies on an effective amplification via a powerful contrast agent. Brindle and coworkers have pioneered this strategy as described in a number of studies (60, 71, 73, 78–80). **Figure 22.5** shows a collection of MR images of mice with a subcutaneous EL-4 tumor in the flank (80). In **Fig. 22.5a**, a T_1-weighted image is shown, indicating the location of the tumor. **Figure 22.5b** displays a T_1 map in which colors indicate the magnitude of T_1 according to the scale on the right-hand side. To detect cellular apoptosis, a nanoparticle construct that consisted of C2A–GST conjugated with Gd–DTPA and a fluorescein moiety was used. Controls included non-treated tumors as well as a non-binding mutant version of the C2A–GST construct. Tumor cell apoptosis was induced by a single intraperitoneal injection of etoposide and cyclophosphamide. Sixteen hours later, MR images were acquired before and at several time points after contrast agent injection. **Figure 22.5c** shows the T_1 map of a

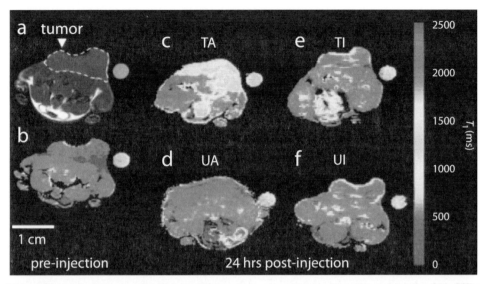

Fig. 22.5. MRI of drug-treated and drug-untreated tumors in mice injected with active and inactive C2A–GST agent. (a) T_1-weighted image indicating location of the tumor. (b) T_1 color map according to the scale on the right-hand side preinjection of contrast agent. (c–f) T_1 color maps 24 h postinjection for (c) treated tumor and active agent, (d) untreated tumor and active agent, (e) treated tumor and inactive agent, and (f) untreated tumor and inactive agent. Reproduced with permission from Krishnan et al. (80).

mouse with a treated tumor 24 h after injection with the active C2A–GST construct (TA). Indeed, massive decrease in the T_1-relaxation time could be observed in the tumor, which correlated with tumor apoptosis as evidenced from ex vivo immunohistology and fluorescence microscopy. For the untreated tumor and the active C2A–GST construct (UA), no significant T_1 decrease was observed (**Fig. 22.5d**), similar as for the treated tumor and the inactive C2A–GST construct (TI) (**Fig. 22.5e**), as well as for the untreated tumor and the inactive C2A–GST construct (UI) (**Fig. 22.5f**). This study convincingly demonstrated that early apoptotic response to tumor treatment, well before any changes in tumor size are expected, can be detected in vivo with MRI using targeted nanoparticles.

4. Summary

In recent years, several kinds of magnetic nanoparticles have been developed to enable MR imaging of the presence of apoptotic cells. Nanoparticles vary in size, from small constructs of several nanometers in size up to relatively large particles with a diameter up to 200 nm. Some of the particles also possess fluorescent properties, which were introduced by including fluorescent dyes or a quantum dot. Specificity for apoptotic cells so far has relied on binding to phosphatidylserine exposed at the outer leaflet of the apoptotic cell membrane. All the apoptosis-specific particles that were developed have been tested extensively and successfully in vitro in cell cultures, which proved the feasibility of apoptosis detection by MRI.

Nevertheless, in vivo MR imaging of apoptosis by these targeted nanoparticles has proven more difficult. Thus far, the presence of apoptotic cells was visualized by the use of functionalized CLIO nanoparticles in a mouse model of transient myocardial infarction as well as with iron oxide nanoparticles and small bimodal positive contrast agents in a mouse tumor model after cytotoxic treatment. Future studies will have to address issues concerning specificity for apoptotic cells detection limits, quantification, and ability to longitudinally follow apoptotic activity. Further down the road, important questions about short- and long-term toxicity have to be addressed, before safe use of nanoparticles can be considered in humans. If successful, the use of magnetic nanoparticles to image in vivo apoptosis will have tremendous diagnostic potential and introduce a powerful tool to assess early drug responses in the management of ischemic heart disease and for anti-tumor treatment clinical studies.

Acknowledgments

This research was supported by the Dutch Technology Foundation STW, applied science division of NWO and the Technology Program of the Ministry of Economic Affairs (grant number 07952). This study was funded in part by the BSIK program entitled Molecular Imaging of Ischemic Heart Disease (project number BSIK03033) and by the EC – FP6-project DiMI, LSHB-CT-2005-512146. This study was performed in the framework of the European Cooperation in the field of Scientific and Technical Research (COST) D38 Action Metal-Based Systems for Molecular Imaging Applications.

References

1. Kerr, J. F., Wyllie, A. H., and Currie, A. R. (1972) Apoptosis: a basic biological phenomenon with wide-ranging implications in tissue kinetics. *Br J Cancer* **26**, 239–257.
2. Samali, A., Gorman, A. M., and Cotter, T. G. (1996) Apoptosis the story so far. *Experientia* **52**, 933–941.
3. Kerr, J. F. (2002) History of the events leading to the formulation of the apoptosis concept. *Toxicology* **181–182**, 471–474.
4. Leist, M. and Jaattela, M. (2001) Four deaths and a funeral: from caspases to alternative mechanisms. *Nat Rev Mol Cell Biol* **2**, 589–598.
5. Van Cruchten, S. and Van Den Broeck, W. (2002) Morphological and biochemical aspects of apoptosis, oncosis and necrosis. *Anat Histol Embryol* **31**, 214–223.
6. van Heerde, W. L., Robert-Offerman, S., Dumont, E., Hofstra, L., Doevendans, P. A.,

Smits, J. F., Daemen, M. J., and Reutelingsperger, C. P. (2000) Markers of apoptosis in cardiovascular tissues: focus on Annexin V. *Cardiovasc Res* **45**, 549–559.

7. Fadok, V. A., de Cathelineau, A., Daleke, D. L., Henson, P. M., and Bratton, D. L. (2001) Loss of phospholipid asymmetry and surface exposure of phosphatidylserine is required for phagocytosis of apoptotic cells by macrophages and fibroblasts. *J Biol Chem* **276**, 1071–1077.

8. Devaux, P. F. (1991) Static and dynamic lipid asymmetry in cell membranes. *Biochemistry* **30**, 1163–1173.

9. Schroit, A. J. and Zwaal, R. F. (1991) Transbilayer movement of phospholipids in red cell and platelet membranes. *Biochim Biophys Acta* **1071**, 313–329.

10. Balasubramanian, K. and Schroit, A. J. (2003) Aminophospholipid asymmetry: a matter of life and death. *Annu Rev Physiol* **65**, 701–734.

11. Kolodgie, F. D., Narula, J., Guillo, P., and Virmani, R. (1999) Apoptosis in human atherosclerotic plaques. *Apoptosis* **4**, 5–10.

12. Haunstetter, A. and Izumo, S. (1998) Apoptosis: basic mechanisms and implications for cardiovascular disease. *Circ Res* **82**, 1111–1129.

13. Korngold, E. C., Jaffer, F. A., Weissleder, R., and Sosnovik, D. E. (2008) Non-invasive imaging of apoptosis in cardiovascular disease. *Heart Fail Rev* **13**, 163–173.

14. Anversa, P., Cheng, W., Liu, Y., Leri, A., Redaelli, G., and Kajstura, J. (1998) Apoptosis and myocardial infarction. *Basic Res Cardiol* **93**(**Suppl 3**), 8–12.

15. Kang, P. M. and Izumo, S. (2003) Apoptosis in heart: basic mechanisms and implications in cardiovascular diseases. *Trends Mol Med* **9**, 177–182.

16. Olivetti, G., Quaini, F., Sala, R., Lagrasta, C., Corradi, D., Bonacina, E., Gambert, S. R., Cigola, E., and Anversa, P. (1996) Acute myocardial infarction in humans is associated with activation of programmed myocyte cell death in the surviving portion of the heart. *J Mol Cell Cardiol* **28**, 2005–2016.

17. Bardales, R. H., Hailey, L. S., Xie, S. S., Schaefer, R. F., and Hsu, S. M. (1996) In situ apoptosis assay for the detection of early acute myocardial infarction. *Am J Pathol* **149**, 821–829.

18. Saraste, A., Pulkki, K., Kallajoki, M., Henriksen, K., Parvinen, M., and Voipio-Pulkki, L. M. (1997) Apoptosis in human acute myocardial infarction. *Circulation* **95**, 320–323.

19. Gottlieb, R. A., Burleson, K. O., Kloner, R. A., Babior, B. M., and Engler, R. L. (1994) Reperfusion injury induces apoptosis in rabbit cardiomyocytes. *J Clin Invest* **94**, 1621–1628.

20. Garg, S., Narula, J., and Chandrashekhar, Y. (2005) Apoptosis and heart failure: clinical relevance and therapeutic target. *J Mol Cell Cardiol* **38**, 73–79.

21. Davies, M. J., Richardson, P. D., Woolf, N., Katz, D. R., and Mann, J. (1993) Risk of thrombosis in human atherosclerotic plaques: role of extracellular lipid, macrophage, and smooth muscle cell content. *Br Heart J* **69**, 377–381.

22. Libby, P., Geng, Y. J., Aikawa, M., Schoenbeck, U., Mach, F., Clinton, S. K., Sukhova, G. K., and Lee, R. T. (1996) Macrophages and atherosclerotic plaque stability. *Curr Opin Lipidol* **7**, 330–335.

23. Kolodgie, F. D., Narula, J., Burke, A. P., Haider, N., Farb, A., Hui-Liang, Y., Smialek, J., and Virmani, R. (2000) Localization of apoptotic macrophages at the site of plaque rupture in sudden coronary death. *Am J Pathol* **157**, 1259–1268.

24. Kolodgie, F. D., Petrov, A., Virmani, R., Narula, N., Verjans, J. W., Weber, D. K., Hartung, D., Steinmetz, N., Vanderheyden, J. L., Vannan, M. A., Gold, H. K., Reutelingsperger, C. P., Hofstra, L., and Narula, J. (2003) Targeting of apoptotic macrophages and experimental atheroma with radiolabeled annexin V: a technique with potential for noninvasive imaging of vulnerable plaque. *Circulation* **108**, 3134–3139.

25. Li, W., Hellsten, A., Jacobsson, L. S., Blomqvist, H. M., Olsson, A. G., and Yuan, X. M. (2004) Alpha-tocopherol and astaxanthin decrease macrophage infiltration, apoptosis and vulnerability in atheroma of hyperlipidaemic rabbits. *J Mol Cell Cardiol* **37**, 969–978.

26. Carson, D. A. and Ribeiro, J. M. (1993) Apoptosis and disease. *Lancet* **341**, 1251–1254.

27. Brown, J. M. and Attardi, L. D. (2005) The role of apoptosis in cancer development and treatment response. *Nat Rev Cancer* **5**, 231–237.

28. Meyn, R. E., Stephens, L. C., Hunter, N. R., and Milas, L. (1995) Apoptosis in murine tumors treated with chemotherapy agents. *Anticancer Drugs* **6**, 443–450.

29. Dubray, B., Breton, C., Delic, J., Klijanienko, J., Maciorowski, Z., Vielh, P., Fourquet, A., Dumont, J., Magdelenat, H., and Cosset, J. M. (1997) In vitro radiation-induced apoptosis and tumour response to radiotherapy:

a prospective study in patients with non-Hodgkin lymphomas treated by low-dose irradiation. *Int J Radiat Biol* **72**, 759–60.
30. Dubray, B., Breton, C., Delic, J., Klijanienko, J., Maciorowski, Z., Vielh, P., Fourquet, A., Dumont, J., Magdelenat, H., and Cosset, J. M. (1998) In vitro radiation-induced apoptosis and early response to low-dose radiotherapy in non-Hodgkin's lymphomas. *Radiother Oncol* **46**, 185–191.
31. Strijkers, G. J., Mulder, W. J., van Tilborg, G. A., and Nicolay, K. (2007) MRI contrast agents: current status and future perspectives. *Anticancer Agents Med Chem* **7**, 291–305.
32. Armitage, F. E., Richardson, D. E., and Li, K. C. (1990) Polymeric contrast agents for magnetic resonance imaging: synthesis and characterization of gadolinium diethylenetriaminepentaacetic acid conjugated to polysaccharides. *Bioconjug Chem* **1**, 365–374.
33. Aime, S., Botta, M., Geninatti Crich, S., Giovenzana, G., Palmisano, G., and Sisti, M. (1999) Novel paramagnetic macromolecular complexes derived from the linkage of a macrocyclic Gd(III) complex to polyamino acids through a squaric acid moiety. *Bioconjug Chem* **10**, 192–199.
34. Wang, S. J., Brechbiel, M., and Wiener, E. C. (2003) Characteristics of a new MRI contrast agent prepared from polypropyleneimine dendrimers, generation 2. *Invest Radiol* **38**, 662–668.
35. Kobayashi, H. and Brechbiel, M. W. (2004) Dendrimer-based nanosized MRI contrast agents. *Curr Pharm Biotechnol* **5**, 539–549.
36. de Lussanet, Q. G., Langereis, S., Beets-Tan, R. G., van Genderen, M. H., Griffioen, A. W., van Engelshoven, J. M., and Backes, W. H. (2005) Dynamic contrast-enhanced MR imaging kinetic parameters and molecular weight of dendritic contrast agents in tumor angiogenesis in mice. *Radiology* **235**, 65–72.
37. Storrs, R. W., Tropper, F. D., Li, H. Y., Song, C. K., Sipkins, D. A., Kuniyoshi, J. K., Bednarski, M. D., Strauss, H. W., and Li, K. C. (1995) Paramagnetic polymerized liposomes as new recirculating MR contrast agents. *J Magn Reson Imaging* **5**, 719–724.
38. Torchilin, V. P. (2002) PEG-based micelles as carriers of contrast agents for different imaging modalities. *Adv Drug Deliv Rev* **54**, 235–252.
39. Glogard, C., Stensrud, G., Hovland, R., Fossheim, S. L., and Klaveness, J. (2002) Liposomes as carriers of amphiphilic gadolinium chelates: the effect of membrane composition on incorporation efficacy and in vitro relaxivity. *Int J Pharm* **233**, 131–140.
40. Glogard, C., Stensrud, G., and Klaveness, J. (2003) Novel high relaxivity colloidal particles based on the specific phase organisation of amphiphilic gadolinium chelates with cholesterol. *Int J Pharm* **253**, 39–48.
41. Hovland, R., Glogard, C., Aasen, A. J., and Klaveness, J. (2003) Preparation and in vitro evaluation of a novel amphiphilic GdPCTA-[12] derivative; a micellar MRI contrast agent. *Org Biomol Chem* **1**, 644–647.
42. Mulder, W. J., Strijkers, G. J., Griffioen, A. W., van Bloois, L., Molema, G., Storm, G., Koning, G. A., and Nicolay, K. (2004) A liposomal system for contrast-enhanced magnetic resonance imaging of molecular targets. *Bioconjug Chem* **15**, 799–806.
43. Nitin, N., LaConte, L. E., Zurkiya, O., Hu, X., and Bao, G. (2004) Functionalization and peptide-based delivery of magnetic nanoparticles as an intracellular MRI contrast agent. *J Biol Inorg Chem* **9**, 706–712.
44. Nitin, N., Santangelo, P. J., Kim, G., Nie, S., and Bao, G. (2004) Peptide-linked molecular beacons for efficient delivery and rapid mRNA detection in living cells. *Nucleic Acids Res* **32**, e58.
45. Morawski, A. M., Winter, P. M., Crowder, K. C., Caruthers, S. D., Fuhrhop, R. W., Scott, M. J., Robertson, J. D., Abendschein, D. R., Lanza, G. M., and Wickline, S. A. (2004) Targeted nanoparticles for quantitative imaging of sparse molecular epitopes with MRI. *Magn Reson Med* **51**, 480–486.
46. Strijkers, G. J., Mulder, W. J., van Heeswijk, R. B., Frederik, P. M., Bomans, P., Magusin, P. C., and Nicolay, K. (2005) Relaxivity of liposomal paramagnetic MRI contrast agents. *MAGMA* **18**, 186–192.
47. van Tilborg, G. A., Mulder, W. J., Chin, P. T., Storm, G., Reutelingsperger, C. P., Nicolay, K., and Strijkers, G. J. (2006) Annexin A5-conjugated quantum dots with a paramagnetic lipidic coating for the multimodal detection of apoptotic cells. *Bioconjug Chem* **17**, 865–868.
48. van Tilborg, G. A., Mulder, W. J., Deckers, N., Storm, G., Reutelingsperger, C. P., Strijkers, G. J., and Nicolay, K. (2006) Annexin A5-functionalized bimodal lipid-based contrast agents for the detection of apoptosis. *Bioconjug Chem* **17**(3), 741–749.
49. Laurent, S., Forge, D., Port, M., Roch, A., Robic, C., Vander Elst, L., and Muller, R. N. (2008) Magnetic iron oxide nanoparticles: synthesis, stabilization, vectorization, physicochemical characterizations, and biological applications. *Chem Rev* **108**, 2064–2110.
50. Shen, T., Weissleder, R., Papisov, M., Bogdanov, A., Jr., and Brady, T. J. (1993)

Monocrystalline iron oxide nanocompounds (MION): physicochemical properties. *Magn Reson Med* **29**, 599–604.

51. Wunderbaldinger, P., Josephson, L., and Weissleder, R. (2002) Crosslinked iron oxides (CLIO): a new platform for the development of targeted MR contrast agents. *Acad Radiol* **9**(**Suppl 2**), S304–S306.

52. Mulder, W. J., Koole, R., Brandwijk, R. J., Storm, G., Chin, P. T., Strijkers, G. J., de Mello Donega, C., Nicolay, K., and Griffioen, A. W. (2006) Quantum dots with a paramagnetic coating as a bimodal molecular imaging probe. *Nano Lett* **6**, 1–6.

53. Schellenberger, E. A., Bogdanov, A., Högemann, D., Tait, J., Weissleder, R., and Josephson, L. (2002) Annexin V-CLIO: a nanoparticle for detecting apoptosis by MRI. *Mol Imaging* **1**, 102–107.

54. Tait, J. F., Gibson, D., and Fujikawa, K. (1989) Phospholipid binding properties of human placental anticoagulant protein-I, a member of the lipocortin family. *J Biol Chem* **264**, 7944–7949.

55. Andree, H. A., Reutelingsperger, C. P., Hauptmann, R., Hemker, H. C., Hermens, W. T., and Willems, G. M. (1990) Binding of vascular anticoagulant alpha (VAC alpha) to planar phospholipid bilayers. *J Biol Chem* **265**, 4923–4928.

56. van Engeland, M., Nieland, L. J., Ramaekers, F. C., Schutte, B., and Reutelingsperger, C. P. (1998) Annexin V-affinity assay: a review on an apoptosis detection system based on phosphatidylserine exposure. *Cytometry* **31**, 1–9.

57. Schellenberger, E. A., Högemann, D., Josephson, L., and Weissleder, R. (2002) Annexin V-CLIO: a nanoparticle for detecting apoptosis by MRI. *Acad Radiol* **9**(**Suppl 2**), S.

58. Schellenberger, E., Schnorr, J., Reutelingsperger, C., Ungethüm, L., Meyer, W., Taupitz, M., and Hamm, B. (2008) Linking proteins with anionic nanoparticles via protamine: ultrasmall protein-coupled probes for magnetic resonance imaging of apoptosis. *Small* **4**, 225–230.

59. Jung, H. I., Kettunen, M. I., Davletov, B., and Brindle, K. M. (2004) Detection of apoptosis using the C2A domain of synaptotagmin I. *Bioconjug Chem* **15**, 983–987.

60. Neves, A. A., Krishnan, A. S., Kettunen, M. I., Hu, D. E., Backer, M. M., Davletov, B., and Brindle, K. M. (2007) A paramagnetic nanoprobe to detect tumor cell death using magnetic resonance imaging. *Nano Lett* **7**, 1419–1423.

61. Prinzen, L., Miserus, R. J., Dirksen, A., Hackeng, T. M., Deckers, N., Bitsch, N. J., Megens, R. T., Douma, K., Heemskerk, J. W., Kooi, M. E., Frederik, P. M., Slaaf, D. W., van Zandvoort, M. A., and Reutelingsperger, C. P. (2007) Optical and magnetic resonance imaging of cell death and platelet activation using annexin a5-functionalized quantum dots. *Nano Lett* **7**, 93–100.

62. Hernandez-Sanchez, B. A., Boyle, T. J., Lambert, T. N., Daniel-Taylor, S. D., Oliver, J. M., Wilson, B. S., Lidke, D. S., and Andrews, N. L. (2006) Synthesizing biofunctionalized nanoparticles to image cell signaling pathways. *IEEE Trans Nanobiosci* **5**, 222–230.

63. Kim, K., Lee, M., Park, H., Kim, J. H., Kim, S., Chung, H., Choi, K., Kim, I. S., Seong, B. L., and Kwon, I. C. (2006) Cell-permeable and biocompatible polymeric nanoparticles for apoptosis imaging. *J Am Chem Soc* **128**, 3490–1.

64. Le Gac, S., Vermes, I., and van den Berg, A. (2006) Quantum dots based probes conjugated to annexin V for photostable apoptosis detection and imaging. *Nano Lett* **6**, 1863–1869.

65. Koeppel, F., Jaiswal, J. K., and Simon, S. M. (2007) Quantum dot-based sensor for improved detection of apoptotic cells. *Nanomedicine (London, England)* **2**, 71–78.

66. Shi, H., He, X., Wang, K., Yuan, Y., Deng, K., Chen, J., and Tan, W. (2007) Rhodamine B isothiocyanate doped silica-coated fluorescent nanoparticles (RBITC-DSFNPs)-based bioprobes conjugated to Annexin V for apoptosis detection and imaging. *Nanomedicine* **3**, 266–272.

67. Yu, K. N., Lee, S. M., Han, J. Y., Park, H., Woo, M. A., Noh, M. S., Hwang, S. K., Kwon, J. T., Jin, H., Kim, Y. K., Hergenrother, P. J., Jeong, D. H., Lee, Y. S., and Cho, M. H. (2007) Multiplex targeting, tracking, and imaging of apoptosis by fluorescent surface enhanced Raman spectroscopic dots. *Bioconjug Chem* **18**, 1155–1162.

68. Sosnovik, D. E., Schellenberger, E. A., Nahrendorf, M., Novikov, M. S., Matsui, T., Dai, G., Reynolds, F., Grazette, L., Rosenzweig, A., Weissleder, R., and Josephson, L. (2005) Magnetic resonance imaging of cardiomyocyte apoptosis with a novel magneto-optical nanoparticle. *Magn Reson Med* **54**, 718–724.

69. Hiller, K. H., Waller, C., Nahrendorf, M., Bauer, W. R., and Jakob, P. M. (2006) Assessment of cardiovascular apoptosis in the isolated rat heart by magnetic resonance molecular imaging. *Mol Imaging* **5**, 115–121.

70. Brindle, K. M. (2003) Molecular imaging using magnetic resonance: new tools for the development of tumour therapy. *Br J Radiol* **76 Spec No 2**, S111–S117.
71. Neves, A. A. and Brindle, K. M. (2006) Assessing responses to cancer therapy using molecular imaging. *Biochim Biophys Acta* **1766**, 242–261.
72. Raman, V., Pathak, A. P., Glunde, K., Artemov, D., and Bhujwalla, Z. M. (2007) Magnetic resonance imaging and spectroscopy of transgenic models of cancer. *NMR Biomed* **20**, 186–199.
73. Brindle, K. (2008) New approaches for imaging tumour responses to treatment. *Nat Rev Cancer* **8**, 94–107.
74. Mulder, W. J., van der Schaft, D. W., Hautvast, P. A., Strijkers, G. J., Koning, G. A., Storm, G., Mayo, K. H., Griffioen, A. W., and Nicolay, K. (2007) Early in vivo assessment of angiostatic therapy efficacy by molecular MRI. *FASEB J* **21**, 378–383.
75. Chenevert, T. L., Meyer, C. R., Moffat, B. A., Rehemtulla, A., Mukherji, S. K., Gebarski, S. S., Quint, D. J., Robertson, P. L., Lawrence, T. S., Junck, L., Taylor, J. M., Johnson, T. D., Dong, Q., Muraszko, K. M., Brunberg, J. A., and Ross, B. D. (2002) Diffusion MRI: a new strategy for assessment of cancer therapeutic efficacy. *Mol Imaging* **1**, 336–343.
76. Ross, B. D., Moffat, B. A., Lawrence, T. S., Mukherji, S. K., Gebarski, S. S., Quint, D. J., Johnson, T. D., Junck, L., Robertson, P. L., Muraszko, K. M., Dong, Q., Meyer, C. R., Bland, P. H., McConville, P., Geng, H., Rehemtulla, A., and Chenevert, T. L. (2003) Evaluation of cancer therapy using diffusion magnetic resonance imaging. *Mol Cancer Ther* **2**, 581–587.
77. Moffat, B. A., Chenevert, T. L., Lawrence, T. S., Meyer, C. R., Johnson, T. D., Dong, Q., Tsien, C., Mukherji, S., Quint, D. J., Gebarski, S. S., Robertson, P. L., Junck, L. R., Rehemtulla, A., and Ross, B. D. (2005) Functional diffusion map: a noninvasive MRI biomarker for early stratification of clinical brain tumor response. *Proc Natl Acad Sci U S A* **102**, 5524–5529.
78. Brindle, K. M. (2002) Detection of apoptosis in tumors using magnetic resonance imaging and spectroscopy. *Adv Enzyme Regul* **42**, 101–112.
79. Zhao, M., Beauregard, D. A., Loizou, L., Davletov, B., and Brindle, K. M. (2001) Non-invasive detection of apoptosis using magnetic resonance imaging and a targeted contrast agent. *Nat Med* **7**, 1241–1244.
80. Krishnan, A. S., Neves, A. A., de Backer, M. M., Hu, D. E., Davletov, B., Kettunen, M. I., and Brindle, K. M. (2008) Detection of cell death in tumors by using MR imaging and a gadolinium-based targeted contrast agent. *Radiology* **246**, 854–862.

Chapter 23

Applications of Gold Nanorods for Cancer Imaging and Photothermal Therapy

Xiaohua Huang, Ivan H. El-Sayed, and Mostafa A. El-Sayed

Abstract

This chapter describes the application of gold nanorods in biomedical imaging and photothermal therapy. The photothermal properties of gold nanorods are summarized and the synthesis as well as antibody conjugation of gold nanorods is outlined. Biomedical applications of gold nanorods include cancer imaging using their enhanced scattering property and photothermal therapy using their enhanced nonradiative photothermal property.

Key words: Gold nanorods, cancer, imaging, photothermal therapy.

1. Optical Properties of Gold Nanorods

1.1. Surface Plasmon Resonance

Gold nanoparticles exhibit enhanced optical properties due to their unique light-particle interactions. In the presence of the oscillating electromagnetic field of the light, the conduction band electrons of the metal nanoparticle undergo a collective coherent resonant oscillation with respect to the ionic metallic lattice, referred to as surface plasmon oscillations (**Fig. 23.1**). The surface plasmon is thus resonant at a specific frequency of the incident light and is called surface plasmon resonance (SPR). The SPR oscillation depends on the particle size, shape, dielectric constant of the metal as well as that of the medium surrounding the nanoparticles. For spherical gold nanoparticles, the SPR can be explained by Mie theory (1) and the SPR frequency is around 520 nm in the visible region, which results in a strong absorption in this region responsible for the intense red color of the particle solution.

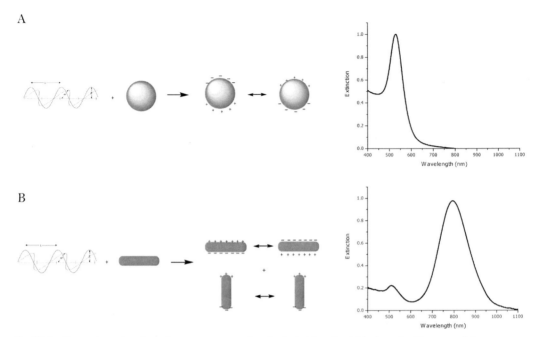

Fig. 23.1. Comparison of surface plasmon resonance in spherical- (**a**) and rod (**b**)-shaped gold nanoparticles.

When the shape of the nanoparticle is changed from spheres to rods, the SPR oscillates along the two directions of the rods: longitudinal and transverse directions. The electron oscillation along the longitudinal direction induces a strong absorption band in the longer wavelength region. The electron oscillation along the transverse direction induces a weak absorption band in the visible region similar to the absorption band of spheres. The SPR of nanorods can be explained by Gans' theory (2), which is an extension of Mie's theory. According to Gans' treatment, the extinction cross section σ_{ext} for elongated ellipsoids is given by the following equation (3):

$$\sigma_{\text{ext}} = \frac{\omega}{3c}\varepsilon_{\text{m}}^{3/2}V\sum_j \frac{(1/P_j^2)\varepsilon_2}{\{\varepsilon_1 + [(1-P_j)/P_j]\varepsilon_{\text{m}}\}^2 + \varepsilon_2^2}, \quad [1]$$

where V is the particle volume, ω is the angular frequency of the exciting light, c is the speed of light, and ε_{m} is the dielectric functions of the surrounding medium, $\varepsilon = \varepsilon_1 + i\varepsilon_2$ is the dielectric constant of the metal, P_j is the depolarization factor along the three axes A, B, and C of the nanorod. With $A > B = C$, P_j is defined as

$$P_A = \frac{1-e^2}{e^2}\left[\frac{1}{2e}\ln\left(\frac{1+e}{1-e}\right)-1\right], \qquad [2]$$

and the aspect ratio R is included in e as follows:

$$e = \left[1-\left(\frac{B}{A}\right)^2\right]^{1/2} = \left(1-\frac{1}{R^2}\right)^{1/2}. \qquad [3]$$

Unlike spheres, the longitudinal SPR band of gold nanorods is very sensitive to the aspect ratio (length/width) of the particle. Slight increase in the aspect ratio greatly red shifts the absorption maximum of the longitudinal band from visible to near-infrared (NIR) region with an increase in the band intensity (**Fig. 23.2**). The absorption maximum of the longitudinal band is linearly dependant on the aspect ratio of the nanorods, while there is no change in the transverse band (4, 5). This optical tunability of the nanorods in the NIR region via the varying of the rod aspect ratio provides great opportunities for in vivo medical applications.

1.2. Radiative and Nonradiative Properties

The surface plasmon oscillation decays by two pathways: radiative decay and nonradiative decay (6) (**Fig. 23.3**). In the radiative decay, photons with the same energy as the incident light are emitted, referred to as Mie scattering, Rayleigh scattering, or surface plasmon resonance light scattering. Due to the surface plasmon excitation, the light scattering intensity of gold nanoparticles is orders of magnitude stronger than that of Rayleigh scattering from polymer bead and dye molecules and therefore they are very useful for biological imaging. The light scattering of gold nanorods is strongly dependent on the aspect ratio of the nanorods (7). With increase in the aspect ratio, the ratio of the light scattering intensity of the longitudinal band to that of the transverse band increases and the scattering maximum wavelength of the longitudinal mode red shifts. This SPR of gold nanorods in the NIR region enables potential noninvasive NIR imaging. In addition to the elastic-type Mie scattering, nanorods are found to give rise to weak inelastic-type scattering (fluorescence) which is also used in two-photon excitation technique of imaging.

The nonradiative decay occurs via electron–hole recombination either within the conduction band (intraband) or between the d band and the conduction band (interband). These excited electrons cool off rapidly within ~1 ps by exchanging energy with the nanoparticle lattice (electron–phonon interaction), resulting in a hot particle lattice (8). This is followed by phonon–phonon interactions, where the nanoparticle lattice cools rapidly by exchanging energy with the surrounding medium on the

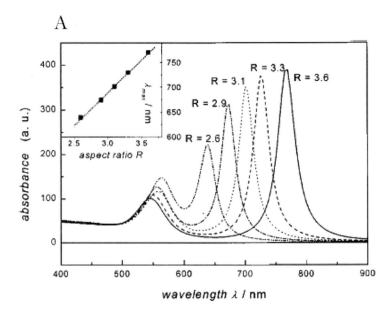

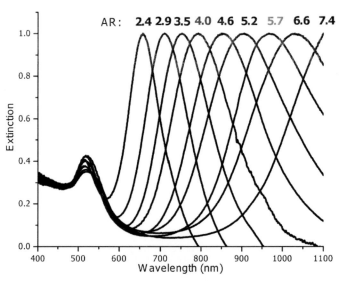

Fig. 23.2. Optical tunability of gold nanorods. (**a**) Calculated absorption spectra of gold nanorods of different aspect ratios according to Gans' theory. Reprinted with permission from Ref. (4). Copyright @ 2006 ACS. (**b**) Experimental absorption spectra of gold nanorods of different aspect ratios by seed-mediated growth method.

timescale of ~100 ps. Such fast energy conversion and dissipation can be readily used for the heating of the local environment by using light radiation with a frequency strongly overlapping with the nanoparticle SPR absorption band. The intense

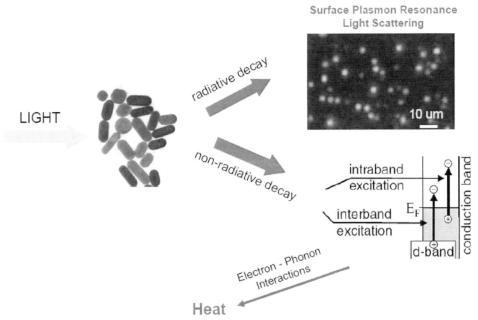

Fig. 23.3. Radiative and nonradiative properties of gold nanorods. Reproduced with permission from Ref. (6). Copyright @ 2007 APS.

SPR-enhanced absorption of gold nanoparticles makes the photothermal conversion process highly efficient. The absorption cross section of gold nanoparticles (9) is typically 4–5 orders of magnitude larger than the strongest absorbing rhodamine 6G dye molecules (10). Hot electron temperatures of several thousand kelvins are easily reached in the nanoparticles even with laser excitation powers as low as 100 nJ and the lattice temperature on the order of a few tens of degrees can be achieved (8). This photothermal property makes the gold nanoparticles greatly promising in the photothermal therapy of cancers and other diseases. The strong absorption of gold nanorods in the NIR region, a region where light penetration is optimal due to minimal absorption from tissue chromophores and water (11), makes NIR-resonant gold nanostructures very useful for clinical therapy applications involving tumors located deep within bodily tissue.

The total extinction efficiency is equal to the sum of the scattering and absorption efficiencies. The absorption and scattering contribution to the total light extinction can be tuned by changing the aspect ratio of the nanorods. **Figure 23.4** shows the calculated size dependence of the absorption and scattering efficiencies on the total extinction using the discrete dipole approximation (DDA) method (12). Increasing aspect ratio increases the contribution of light scattering and decreases that of light absorption. So for imaging applications, larger rods are preferred as they show

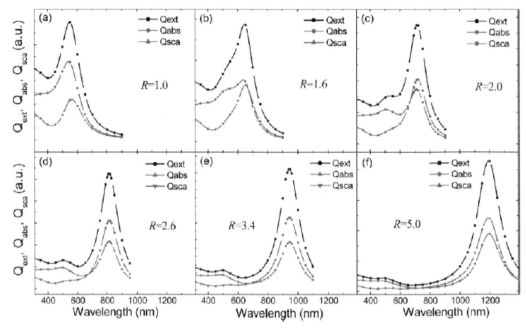

Fig. 23.4. A series of calculated spectra for optical extinction, absorption, and scattering efficiencies for Au nanorods with different aspect ratio R. Reproduced with permission from Ref. (12). Copyright @ 2005 ACS.

large scattering efficiency. For photothermal applications, smaller rods are preferred as they show larger absorption efficiency which correspondingly increases photothermal efficiency.

2. Gold Nanorod Probe

2.1. Nanorod Synthesis

Gold nanorods are synthesized according to the seed-mediated growth method by Nikoobakht and El-Sayed (13). In general, 0.5 mM auric acid (Sigma) in 0.2 M CTAB (cetyltrimethylammonium bromide; Sigma) is reduced at room temperature by ice-cold sodium borohydride (0.01 M) to yield nanospheres with size smaller than 5 nm as seed nanoparticles. A 100 mL growth solution is prepared by the reduction of 1 mM auric acid in a solution containing 0.2 M CTAB and 0.15 M BDAC (benzyldimethylhexadecylammonium chloride; Sigma). Two milliliters of 0.004 M silver salt is added to the gold growth solution and mixed well followed by the addition of 70 μL of 0.0788 M ascorbic acid with stirring to reduce the $HAuCl_4$ to $HAuCl_2$ growth solution. Finally, 8 μL of the seed solution is introduced into the growth solution and the solution is allowed to sit still for nanorod growth. Ascorbic acid could not reduce Au^{3+} to Au^0 directly, but on the surface of gold nanospheres, it can reduce Au^+ to Au^0 due to autocatalysis and thus add gold atom to the nanospheres, leading to nanoparticle growth. The nanorods were obtained after several hours but 24 h are required for the completion of rod formation. The nanorods obtained at 2 mL of silver ions and room temperature around 24°C usually exhibit absorption maximum of 800 nm with aspect ratio of 3.9. Nanorods with various aspect ratios from 2.4 to 7 are obtained by changing the amount of silver ions from 0.8 to 3.6 mL.

The nanorod growth mechanism is still not clear due to complex parameters that control the nanorod formation and growth. It is generally believed that CTAB is preferentially bound to gold (110) or (100) faces to stabilize the faces leaving (111) face for gold atom addition, allowing for nanorod growth along the [100] (14). It is also believed that auric acid binds to CTAB micelles and is then driven to CTAB-capped seed nanoparticles by electric field interactions. The $AuCl_2$–CTAB complex binds to the tip of seed nanoparticles in a faster rate than to side faces and thus lead to nanorod formation and growth (15). The role of silver ions have been explained according to an underpotential model (16). Ag^+ is reduced to Ag atoms on the side (110) face of the nanorods in a faster rate than on the (111) end face. This silver deposition blocks the gold addition to the side faces and thus results in nanorod growth. Completion of silver deposition to the end face will stop the nanorod growth.

2.2. Antibody Conjugation

The antibodies are adsorbed onto rod surface through a polystyrene sulfonate (PSS) polymer layer (17) (**Fig. 23.5**). There are two reasons for the use of this polymer: One is for the charge reversion. The negatively charged PSS molecules are electrostatically adsorbed onto the positively charged CTAB capping layer of the nanorods making the rods negatively charged. This will avoid the aggregation problem if the negatively charged antibodies are directly adsorbed onto positively charged rods as described above. Another reason is that it has been shown that negatively charged polystyrene sulfonate can be nonspecifically adsorbed to negatively charged antibodies through hydrophobic interactions. This hydrophobic interaction has been used to form layer-by-layer structures between negatively charged antibodies and negatively charged PSS polymers.

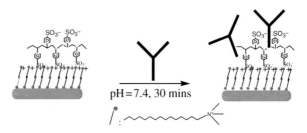

Fig. 23.5. Antibody conjugation of gold nanorods through PSS layer.

3. Gold Nanorods in Cancer Imaging

As described in **Section 1.2**, the nanorods can be used as contrast agents in imaging by using the Mie scattering that is strongly enhanced at the surface plasmon excitation. This light scattering imaging can be realized in dark field with a simple light microscope. The dark field is different from the bright field in the way of light illumination and collection (**Fig. 23.6**). In the bright field, all the light from the white lamp is focused to the sample by a condenser lens. The transmitted light beam after passing through the sample is collected by an objective. The contrast of images originates from the light absorption by the sample, which causes the intensity losses of the illumination beam. In the dark field, a patch stop disc blocks the center transmitted beam, leaving an outer ring of the illumination white light beam. A dark-field condenser focuses the ring illuminating light toward the sample. The objective used in dark field usually has an iris ring on the objective so that the light collection zone can be adjusted by turning the iris. The iris usually closes all the way so that only the scattered light in the center is collected by the objective and the transmitted light on the edge is passed by the objective. In this way, any sample scattering strongly will be lighten up in a dark background.

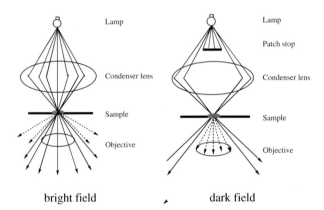

Fig. 23.6. Scheme of bright- (*left*) and dark (*right*)-field imaging.

Figure 23.7 shows the images of control cells and cells treated with antibody-conjugated gold nanorods. The nanorods are synthesized by the seed-mediated growth method by Nikoobakht and El-Sayed (13). The nanorods show absorption maximum of the longitudinal band at around 800 nm with an aspect ratio of 4.0. The nanorods are conjugated with anti-epidermal growth factor receptor (EGFR) antibodies using PSS linker as described in **Section 2.2**. One of the differences between

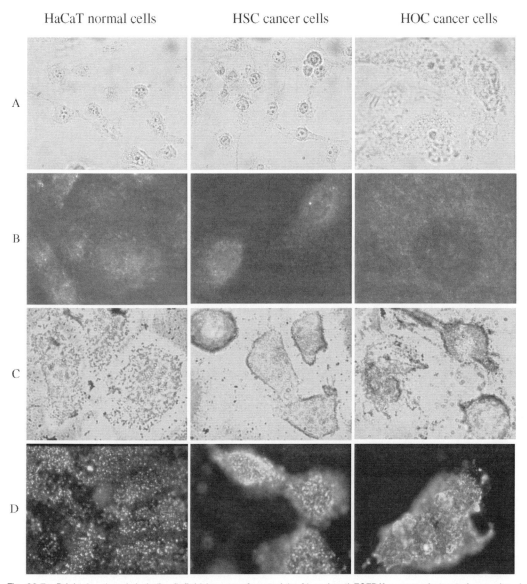

Fig. 23.7. Bright (**a, c**) and dark (**b, d**) field images of control (**a, b**) and anti-EGFR/Au nanorods-treated normal and cancer cells. Bright-field images are taken with a 60× objective and dark-field images are taken with a 100× objective.

cancer and noncancer cells is the overexpression of EGFR on the cytoplasmic membrane of most types of cancer cells. So cancer cells can be targeted and differentiated from normal cells by using the anti-EGFR antibodies conjugated to gold nanoparticles that are used for diagnosis and therapy. The cell lines in **Fig. 23.6** are one normal human skin cell HaCat and two human oral cancer cells HSC 3 and HOC 313. For the nanorod treatment, the cells grown on coverslips are incubated with anti-EGFR-conjugated gold nanorods in PBS buffer solution at pH 7.4 for 30 min. Free nanorods are separated by washing the cells with PBS buffer.

In the bright field, the cells are stained in red color after incubation with anti-EGFR/Au nanorods solution. This is due to the surface plasmon absorption of the nanorods around 800 nm. The dark-field images show much higher resolution than do bright-field images. The cells show some auto-fluorescence in the absence of nanorods. When the antibody-conjugated Au Nps are incubated with the cells, the LS pattern is different between normal and cancer cells. The nanorods are specifically bound to the two types of cancer cells, while they are nonspecifically adsorbed onto the surface of normal cells due to the specific binding of anti-EGFR antibodies to the overexpressed EGFR on the cancer cell surface. The nanoparticles scatter reddish light due to the surface plasmon resonance in the near-infrared region at around 800 nm.

4. Gold Nanorods in Photothermal Therapy

4.1. In Vitro Plasmonic Photothermal Therapy

Gold nanospheres have been shown an efficient and selective photothermal absorbers for destroying cancer cells with a visible argon ion laser without affecting the surrounding nonmalignant cells (18). The laser wavelength at 514 nm overlaps the surface plasmon absorption of the spherical nanoparticles which have an absorption maximum at 520 nm. By conjugation with anti-EGFR monoclonal antibodies that specifically target the molecular marker EGFR, the malignant cells can be destroyed with less than half the laser energy required to kill the normal cells due to the overexpression of the EGFR on the surface of malignant cells. However, at this wavelength, tissue penetration of the light is very low (11) (less than 500 μm). While this may be useful for superficial lesions, to treat cancer in vivo, it is desirable to have deeper tissue penetration. The near-infrared region of the spectrum provides maximal penetration of light due to relatively lower scattering and absorption from the intrinsic tissue chromophores. In this region, the light penetration depth is up to 10 cm depending on the tissue types.

In the in vitro plasmonic photothermal therapy (PPTT), nanorods with an aspect ratio of 3.9 are chosen due to their absorption overlapping with a region of minimum extinction of the human tissues. The absorption band of the nanorods also overlaps the cw Ti:Sapphire red laser wavelength at 800 nm. The laser is focused down to the cells on coverslips which are treated with nanoparticle as described before. The cells are immersed in

PBS buffer and exposed to the laser for 4 min. After irradiation, the cells are stained by trypan blue to test viability. Dead cells will accumulate the dyes making the cells blue, while live cells resist the dye molecules and remain colorless.

Figure 23.8 shows images of irradiated normal and cancer cells at different laser energies. Exposure to the red laser at 800 nm at and above 160 mW (20 W/cm^2) caused photodestruction of all HaCat normal cells (17). The malignant HSC cells suffer photothermal injury at a lower laser power. Cell death occurs within the laser spots after exposure to the laser at and above 80 mW, which corresponds to 10 W/cm^2. The energy threshold for cell death of the HSC cells is about half that needed to cause cell death of the nonmalignant HaCaT cells. The HOC

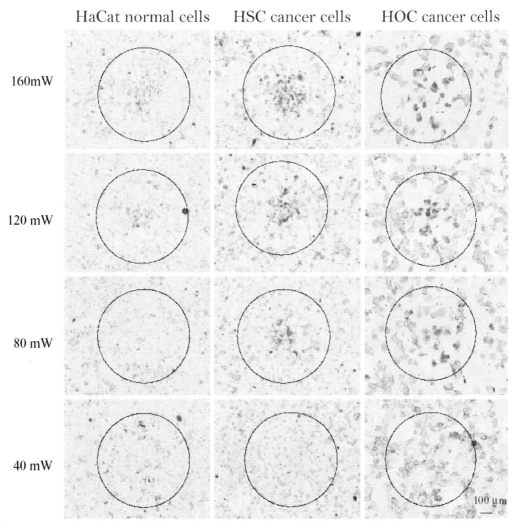

Fig. 23.8. Selective photothermal therapy of cancer cells with anti-EGFR/Au nanorods incubated. The *circles* show the laser spots on the samples. Reproduced with permission from Ref. (17). Copyright @ 2006 ACS.

cancer cells also undergo photothermal destruction at and above 80 mW, while no cell death is observed at lower power. Both types of cancer cells require less than half the energy needed to kill the nonmalignant cells, which is due to the overexpression of EGFR on the cancer cells and the corresponding higher amount of anti-EGFR antibody-conjugated gold nanorods which absorb the light and convert it into heat at the cell surface.

The in vitro results suggest that nanorods conjugated to antibodies can be used as a selective and efficient photothermal agent for cancer cell therapy using low–energy, harmless, near-infrared laser. Thus, for further in vivo applications, it is expected that the tumor tissue will be selectively destroyed at laser energies which will not harm the surrounding normal tissue due to the higher concentration of nanorods selectively bound to the tumor tissue.

4.2. In Vivo Plasmonic Photothermal Therapy

The feasibility of in vivo near-infrared PPTT using gold nanorods is demonstrated in a mice model (19). Subcutaneous squamous cell carcinoma xenografts are grown in nude mice. Gold nanorods are conjugated to mPEG-SH (PEG5000) to increase biocompatibility (20–23), suppress immunogenic responses, and to decrease adsorption to the negatively charged luminal surface of blood vessels. One hundred microliters of pegylated gold nanorods ($OD_{\lambda=800} = 120$) is injected into tail vein and preferential accumulation of pegylated gold nanorods in tumor tissues is achieved due to the enhanced permeability and retention (EPR) effect of tumor tissues (24, 25). Optimized nanorod accumulation in tumor is observed at 24 h after administration by silver staining. In the direct injection, 15 µL of pegylated gold nanorods ($OD_{\lambda=800} = 40$) is directly administered into the tumor interstitium. Control tumor sites are injected with 10 mM PBS. Near-infrared PPTT is performed extracorporeally using a small, portable, inexpensive, continuous-wave diode laser at 808 nm (Power Technologies). For intravenous administration, nanorods are allowed for 24 h circulation to maximize intratumoral particle accumulation and exposed to NIR radiation with intensity of 1.7–1.9 W/cm² for 10 min. For direct administration, mouse tumors are extracorporeally exposed to NIR radiation within 2 min of injection with intensity 0.9–1.1 W/cm² for 10 min.

Nanorod accumulation following direct and intravenous administration is monitored by NIR transmission imaging (**Fig. 23.9**, left image). Intensity line scans of NIR extinction showed marginal diffusion of directly injected particles for over 3 min, with no subsequent change observed for over several hours. Intensity line scans from NIR transmission images of HSC-3 tumor sites injected with 15 µL of 10 mM PBS show nominal extinction due to increased tissue density, while line scans obtained following intravenous delivery at 24 h accumulation showed extinction approximately three times that observed for

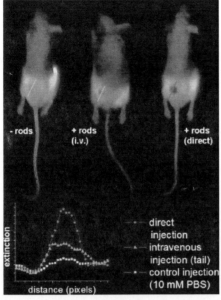
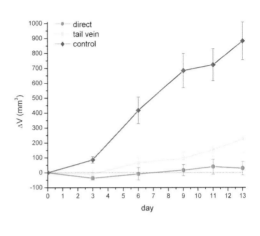

Fig. 23.9. (*Left*) NIR transmission images of mice prior to PPTT treatments and intensity line scans of NIR extinction at tumor sites for control (■), intravenous (▲), and direct (●) administration of pegylated gold nanorods. (*Right*) Average change in tumor volume for HSC-3 xenografts following near-infrared PPTT treatment by control (♦), intravenous (■), and direct (●) injection of pegylated gold nanorods. Error bar is standard error of average value. Reprinted from Ref. (19). Copyright (2008), with permission from Elsevier.

control sites. Directly injected tumor showed NIR extinction more than twice that observed by intravenous delivery and more than seven times that observed at control sites.

Average change in tumor volume, recorded over a 13 day period (**Fig. 23.9**, right graph), shows a >96% decrease in average tumor growth for directly treated tumors and a >74% decrease in average tumor growth for intravenously treated HSC-3 xenografts at day 13 (relative to control tumors). Moreover, resorption of >57% of the directly treated tumors and 25% of the intravenously treated tumors was observed over the monitoring period. In contrast, neither growth suppression nor resorption was observed in any of the control tumors.

Thermal temperature monitoring using a 33-gauge hypodermic thermocouple (Omega) shows that heating efficiencies of PPTT treatments (the ratio of steady-state temperature change in the presence of plasmonic particles to that in its absence) were 3.59 ± 0.5 for direct injection and 1.90 ± 0.4 for intravenous injection of pegylated gold nanorods. The former value is remarkably similar to that observed during in vivo near-infrared PPTT treatments reported by Hirsch et al. (26) by direct injection of gold nanoshells. Observed increases in temperature change for control treatments by direct and intravenous administration correlate well with increases in power density. Disparity of direct and intravenous PPTT heating efficiency is in excellent agreement with intensity line scans obtained from NIR transmission images and is attributed to proportionally decreased particle loading by intravenous delivery. Although particle volume and concentration are significantly higher for intravenous injections, accumulation is likely limited by the extent of tumor angiogenesis and uptake by the reticuloendothelial system (RES). Treatment selectivity and efficacy are most apparent for direct injections; however, both methods showed significantly improved local tumor control.

Acknowledgment

We like to thank the support of the Chemical Science, Geosciences, and Bioscience Division of the Department of Energy (Grant DE-FG02-97ER14799) and the National Cancer Institute Center of Cancer Nanotechnology Excellence Award (U54CA119338).

References

1. Mie, G. (1908) Contribution to the optics of turbid media, especially colloidal metal suspensions. *Ann Phys* **25**, 377–445.
2. Gans, R. (1915) Form of ultramicroscopic particles of silver. *Ann Phys* **47**, 270–284.
3. Papavassiliou, G. C. (1979) Optical properties of small inorganic and organic metal particles. *Prog Solid State Chem* **12**, 185–271.
4. Link, S., Mohamed, M. B., and El-Sayed, M. A. (1999) Simulation of the optical absorption spectra of gold nanorods as a function of their aspect ratio and the effect of the medium dielectric constant. *J Phys Chem B* **103**, 8410–8426.
5. Link, S. and El-Sayed, M. A. (2005) Additions and corrections to simulation of the optical absorption spectra of gold nanorods as a function of their aspect ratio and the effect of the medium dielectric constant. *J Phys Chem B* **109**, 10531–10532.
6. Sönnichsen, C., Franzl, T., Wilk, T., Plessen, G. V., and Feldmann, J. (2002) Drastic reduction of plasmon damping in gold nanorods. *Phys Rev Lett* **88**, 077402–077406.
7. Zhu, J., Huang, L., Zhao, J., Wang, Y., Zhao, Y., Hao, L., and Lu, Y. (2005) Shape dependent resonance light scattering properties of gold nanorods. *Mater Sci Eng B* **121**, 199–203.
8. Link, S. and El-Sayed, M. A. (2000) Shape and size dependence of radiative, non-radiative and photothermal properties of gold nanocrystals. *Int Rev Phys Chem* **19**, 409–453.
9. Jain, P. K., Lee, K. S., El-Sayed, I. H., and El-Sayed, M. A. (2006) Calculated absorption and scattering properties of gold nanoparticles of different size, shape, and composition: applications in biological imaging and biomedicine. *J Phys Chem B* **110**, 7238–7248.
10. Du, H., Fuh, R. A., Li, J., Corkan, A., and Lindsey, J. S. (1998) PhotochemCAD††: a computer-aided design and research tool in photochemistry. *Photochem Photobiol* **68**, 141–142.
11. Weissleder, R. (2001) A clearer vision for in vivo imaging. *Nat Biotechnol* **19**, 316–317.
12. Lee, K. S. and El-Sayed, M. A. (2005) Dependence of the enhanced optical scattering efficiency relative to that of absorption for gold metal nanorods on aspect ratio, size, end-cap shape, and medium refractive index. *J Phys Chem B* **109**, 20331–20338.
13. Nikoobakht, B. and El-Sayed, M. A. (2003) Preparation and growth mechanism of gold nanorods using seed-mediated growth method. *Chem Mater* **15**, 1957–1961.

14. Murphy, C. J., Sau, T. K., Gole, A. M., Orendorff, C. J., Gao, J., Gou, L., Hunyadi, S. E., and Li, T. (2005) Anisotropic metal nanoparticles: synthesis, assembly, and optical applications. *J Phys Chem B* **109**, 13857–13870.
15. P'erez-Juste, J., Pastoriza-Santos, I., Liz-Marz'an, L. M., and Mulvaney, P. (2005) Gold nanorods: synthesis, characterization and applications. *Coord Chem Rev* **249**, 1870–1901.
16. Orendorff, C. J. and Murphy, C. J. (2006) Quantitation of metal content in the silver-assisted growth of gold nanorods. *J Phys Chem B* **110**, 3990–3994.
17. Huang, X., El-Sayed, I. H., and El-Sayed, M. A. (2006) Cancer cell imaging and photothermal therapy in the near-infrared region by using gold nanorods. *J Am Chem Soc* **128**, 2115–2120.
18. El-Sayed, I. H., Huang, X., and El-Sayed, M. A. (2006) Selective laser photo-thermal therapy of epithelial carcinoma using anti-EGFR antibody conjugated gold nanoparticles. *Cancer Lett* **239**, 129–135.
19. Dickerson, E. B., Dreaden, E. C., Huang, X., El-Sayed, I. H., Chu, H., Pushpanketh, S., McDonald, J. F., and El-Sayed, M. A. (2008) Gold nanorods assisted near-infrared plasmonic photothermal therapy (PPTT) of squamous cell carcinoma in mice. *Cancer Lett* **269**, 57–66.
20. Harris, J. M. and Chess, R. B. (2003) Effect of pegylation on pharmaceuticals. *Nat Rev Drug Discov* **2**, 214–221.
21. Huff, T. B., Hansen, M. N., Zhao, Y., Cheng, J. X., and Wei, A. (2007) Controlling the cellular uptake of gold nanorods. *Langmuir* **23**, 1596–1599.
22. Liao, H. W. and Hafner, J. H. (2005) Gold nanorod bioconjugates. *Chem Mater* **17**, 4636–4641.
23. Niidome, T., Yamagata, M., Okamoto, Y., Akiyama, Y., Takahashi, H., Kawano, T., Katayama, Y., and Niidome, Y. (2006) PEG-modified gold nanorods with a stealth character for in vivo applications. *J Control Release* **114**, 343–347.
24. Maeda, H. (2001) The enhanced permeability and retention (EPR) effect in tumor vasculature: the key role of tumor-selective macromolecular drug targeting. *Adv Enzyme Regul* **41**, 189–207.
25. Jain, R. K. (1987) Transport of molecules in the tumor interstitium: a review. *Cancer Res* **47**, 3039–3051.
26. Hirsch, L. R., Stafford, R. J., Bankson, J. A., Sershen, S. R., Rivera, B., Price, R. E., Hazle, J. D., Halas, N. J., and West, J. (2003) Nanoshell-mediated near-infrared thermal therapy of tumors under magnetic resonance guidance. *Proc Natl Acad Sci USA* **100**, 13549–13554.

Chapter 24

Use of Nanoparticles for Targeted, Noninvasive Thermal Destruction of Malignant Cells

Paul Cherukuri and Steven A. Curley

Abstract

Shortwave (MHz range) radiofrequency (RF) energy is nonionizing, penetrates deeply into biological tissues with no adverse side effects, and heats metallic nanoparticles efficiently. Targeted delivery of these nanoparticles to cancer cells should result in hyperthermic cytotoxicity upon exposure to a focused, noninvasive RF field. We have demonstrated that gold nanoparticles conjugated with cetuximab (C225) are quickly internalized by Panc-1 (pancreatic adenocarcinoma) and Difi (colorectal adenocarcinoma) cancer cells overexpressing epidermal growth factor receptor (EGFR). Panc-1 or Difi cells treated with naked gold nanoparticles or nonspecific IgG-conjugated gold nanoparticles demonstrated minimal intracellular uptake of gold nanoparticles by transmission electron microscopy (TEM). In contrast, there were dense concentrations of cytoplasmic vesicles containing gold nanoparticles following treatment with cetuximab-conjugated gold nanoparticles. Exposure of cells to a noninvasive RF field produced nearly 100% cytotoxicity in cells treated with the cetuximab-conjugated gold nanoparticles, but significantly lower levels of cytotoxicity in the two control groups ($p < 0.00012$). Treatment of a breast cancer cell line (CAMA-1) that does not express EGFR with cetuximab-conjugated gold nanoparticles produced no enhanced cytotoxicity following treatment in the RF field. Conjugation of cancer cell-directed targeting agents to gold nanoparticles may represent an effective and cancer-specific therapy to treat numerous types of human malignant disease using noninvasive RF hyperthermia.

Key words: Gold nanoparticles, carbon nanotubes, radiofrequency, hyperthermia.

1. Introduction

Hyperthermic cancer therapy was first described in Egyptian papyri over 4000 years ago by applying hot oil or cautery to tumors (1). Modern hyperthermic treatments are now applied to both premalignant and malignant tumors in various locations such as the gut, liver, kidneys, lungs, and prostate. Hyperthermia also potentiates the effects of cytotoxic chemotherapeutic agents and improves the response of tumors to ionizing radiation. Thus, regional or systemic hyperthermia has been induced as part of a treatment regimen in patients with certain types of malignancies. Hyperthermic isolated limb perfusion with melphalan with or without dactinomycin is performed to treat in-transit melanoma metastases and is being investigated as a treatment for advanced extremity soft-tissue sarcoma (2). Over the last several years there has been a growing number of reports on hyperthermic intraperitoneal chemotherapy combined with cytoreductive surgery for patients with diffuse peritoneal spread of colorectal cancer, gastric cancer, mesothelioma, or pseudomyxoma peritoneii (3–5).

Although effective at treating several cancer types, recent studies have shown that some mammalian cancer cells are sensitive, whereas others are significantly more resistant to hyperthermia compared to healthy cells (6). The reasons for the variable sensitivity to hyperthermia in cancer are multifactorial, but are primarily due to the role of heat-shock proteins (HSPs) in cancer's resistance to the physical stress of increasing temperature (7). Mammalian cancer cells that are heat sensitive frequently have mutated or underexpressed HSPs, whereas deregulation in some malignant cells leads to increased expression of HSPs, which confers increased thermal protection and reduces apoptosis following thermal stress.

Many hyperthermic devices have been designed to produce low-level total-body hyperthermia (42–46°C) and have been used to treat a wide variety of advanced malignancies combined with systemic cytotoxic agents (8–10). Both regional and systemic hyperthermic treatment systems elevate tissue temperatures from 3 to 7°C above normal over a 1–12-h period. Some populations of malignant cells are sensitive to relatively long durations of exposures to low-level hyperthermia, but results to date suggest that these regional and systemic hyperthermic treatments have produced little benefit in overall patient outcomes at the expense of major regional and systemic toxicities and side effects. Interestingly, exposure of mammalian cells to temperatures of 55–60°C for periods of a few seconds to less than a minute has been shown to produce apoptosis and necrosis, so a treatment system that can achieve such brief periods of heating in cancer cells would be highly desirable (11).

Thermal tumor ablation is routinely practiced, particularly for malignant liver tumors, through direct intratumoral insertion of radiofrequency (RF) needle electrodes, microwave-emitting probes, or end- and side-firing laser fibers (12). RF ablation therapy is an invasive treatment that is implemented by inserting needle electrodes directly into the tumor(s) to be treated and applying RF current through the wire into the tumor, resulting in local tumor and adjacent tissue necrosis (**Fig. 24.1**). The basis for the observed heating phenomena is understood by the rotational response of the charged ions and proteins in the tissue under the RF field. This rapid molecular rotation results in local frictional heating of the aqueous environment of the tumor and death of tumor cells through protein denaturation, melting of lipid bilayers, and destruction of nuclear DNA.

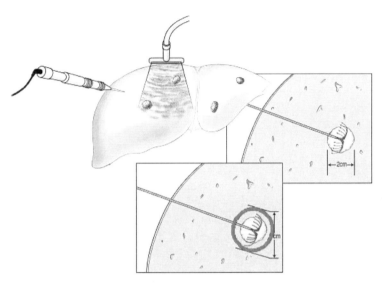

Fig. 24.1. Schematic illustration demonstrating invasive radiofrequency ablation of malignant liver tumors. A multiple array needle electrode is inserted directly into the tumor to be treated using ultrasound guidance to assure proper placement of the needle. An alternating current is then passed across the array resulting in frictional ionic heating in the tumor and tissue surrounding the array.

Although RFA has demonstrated efficacy in cancer therapy, there are several limitations to this approach. First, clinical studies have shown incomplete tumor destruction in 5–40% of the treated lesions, allowing significant probability of local cancer recurrence and metastasis. Another limitation of RFA is that the treatment is not targeted (i.e., nonspecific). Placement and insertion of the needle electrode is usually guided by an imaging system with poor spatial resolution (e.g., ultrasonography $\sim$ mm) and therefore this method is dependent on the experience of the physician that implements RFA. Furthermore, RFA treatments result in significant complications in approximately 10% of patients due to thermally induced necrosis of healthy noncancerous tissues. The final and most problematic limiting factor with respect to wire-based RFA is that it is a clinical treatment that is indicated for just a few select organ sites and specific tumor types (e.g., liver, kidney, breast, lung). On the other hand, tissue penetration by noninvasive RF energy fields is known to be excellent (13). Theoretically, noninvasive RF treatment of malignant tumors at any site in the body should be possible if agents that preferentially respond to RF energy with intracellular release of heat can be delivered to the malignant cells.

Nanotechnology is a term used to describe the engineering of materials that utilize the unique physical properties of nanometer scale matter. Nanomaterials have been used across all the major scientific disciplines including chemistry, physics, and medicine (14). It is in the medical realm that nanotechnology is widely heralded as one of the most promising and important approaches to diagnose and treat cancer (15–18). Some nanoscale materials are already FDA approved and are used clinically. For example, iron oxide nanoparticles (Feridex^{TM}) have been shown to enhance the diagnostic capability of magnetic resonance imaging (MRI) to detect cancer (19, 20). Conjugating iron nanoparticles to antibodies that target proteins expressed on the surface of human cancer cells may further enhance the accuracy of MRI to diagnose early-stage cancer (21).

Other nanoparticles such as carbon or polymeric nanoparticles labeled with fluorine-18 deoxyglucose have been studied in preclinical models to enhance tumor diagnosis and detection rates using positron emission tomography (22, 23). Surface modification of quantum dots, which are semiconducting nanocrystals that fluoresce upon absorption of visible light, is being investigated to better detect lymph nodes and other sites of metastases during surgical procedures (24, 25). Additionally, conjugation of quantum dots with tumor-specific peptides or antibodies may improve targeting of cancer cells and thus improve the diagnostic accuracy of this technique. Optimal imaging techniques using fluorescent nanoparticles targeted to a variety of types of human cancer with immunoconjugation of targeting antibodies is being studied to permit in vivo localization of malignant cells (26, 27). It is hoped that such imaging techniques will improve the diagnostic accuracy in numerous types of imaging modalities used to detect and follow patients with cancer. It is possible that these techniques may also allow earlier detection of cancer in high-risk populations and guide the duration and type of therapy in patients with more advanced stages of malignant disease. Finally, immunocomplexes consisting of gold nanoparticles and labeled antibodies have been demonstrated to improve the detection of several known serum tumor markers, including carcinoembryonic antigen, carcinoma antigen 125, and carbohydrate antigen 19-9, in a more rapid and accurate fashion than currently available techniques (28).

Nanoparticles are being used as intravascular carriers to enhance delivery of anticancer agents to malignant cells. Given that most anticancer drugs have a narrow therapeutic index with significant acute and cumulative toxicities in normal tissues, a variety of types of nanoparticles are being studied in preclinical and in vitro experiments to increase the delivery of cytotoxic chemotherapy drugs to cancer cells while reducing toxicity by limiting exposure of the drug to normal tissues. For example, nanoparticles loaded with hydroxycamptothecin (29), 5-fluorouracil (30), docetaxel (31), and gemcitacine (32) have been used in preclinical studies to improve chemotherapy-induced cytotoxicity in lung, colon, squamous, and pancreas cancers.

Colloidal gold nanoparticles bearing tumor necrosis factor-α (TNF-α) molecules are being used in early-phase human clinical trials to treat several types of cancer. Preclinical studies demonstrated that delivery of TNF-α to malignant tumors was enhanced using the nanoparticle delivery system, while avoiding the systemic toxicities that usually limit the clinical utility of this biological agent (33, 34). Nanoparticles conjugated with targeting agents are also being investigated to deliver gene therapy payloads to malignant cells (35, 36). Carbon nanotubes have been used to deliver genes or proteins through nonspecific endocytosis in cancer cells (37). Similar to some cytotoxic chemotherapy drugs, gold or other metal nanoparticles have been shown to improve the therapeutic efficacy of external beam ionizing radiation in preclinical models (38). In addition to being used to deliver pharmaceutical agents, nanoparticles may be used as intrinsic chemotherapeutic agents. Gold nanoparticles 5–10 nm in diameter have been shown to have antiangiogenic properties in solid tumors and appear to induce apoptosis in B chronic lymphocytic leukemia cells through mechanisms not elucidated entirely (39, 40).

Recent studies have shown that nanoscale materials are capable of enhancing thermal deposition in cancer cells by absorbing optical energy. Gold–silica nanoshells 150 nm in diameter have a particular plasmon resonance in near-infrared (NIR) wavelengths (650–950 nm) of light and release significant heat when exposed to NIR laser sources (**Fig. 24.2**) (41). A clinical trial using gold–silica nanoshell hyperthermia following NIR light exposure has been initiated for patients with oropharyngeal malignancies. Thermal therapy with NIR energy is limited to the treatment of superficial tumors (<1–2 cm deep) due to the significant attenuation of NIR light by biological tissues (42). Iron oxide nanoparticles are also being evaluated to produce alternating magnetic field-based hyperthermia in tumors, but the limited thermal enhancement of these nanoparticles in a magnetic field requires extremely high concentrations of iron oxide (43). These high concentrations and the difficulty targeting the iron oxide nanoparticles to only cancer cells lead to destruction of normal (nonmalignant) cells surrounding the tumor.

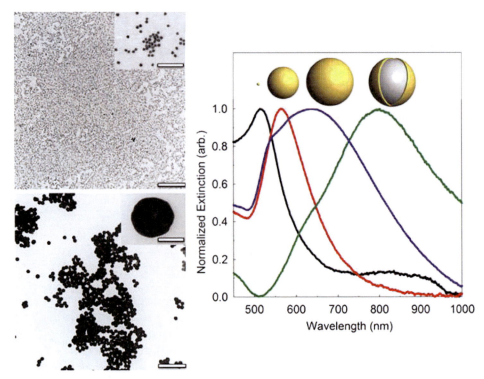

Fig. 24.2. *Left column* – Transmission electron micrographs of 10 nm diameter solid gold nanoparticles (*top*) and 150 nm diameter gold nanoshells (*bottom*). TEM images are 20,000× magnification and 500,000 × (*inset*) magnification and scale bars = 1,000 nm (*main*) and 100 nm (*inset*). *Right column* – Diameter-dependent visible spectra of solid gold nanoparticles (*black* = 10 nm, *red* = 100 nm, *blue* = 150 nm) and the red-shifted gold nanoshell spectrum (*green* = 150 nm). Nanoparticle illustrations above each corresponding spectra are drawn to scale. Note, spectra have been normalized and background subtracted to ease viewing of relative peak positions.

2. Materials

2.1. Human Cancer Cells and Cell Culture

Panc-1, Difi, SN12PM6, and CAMA-1 cells utilized for all experiments were obtained from the American Type Culture Collection (Bethesda, MD). Cells were maintained in DMEM culture media with 10% fetal calf serum and penicillin/streptomycin at 37°C in a 21% O_2 incubator. Each cell line was utilized only from passages 2 to 9 for experiments performed in this study.

2.2. Gold Nanoparticle Production

The ~5 nm gold nanoparticles used in this study were prepared using previously described methods (44). Briefly, 50 mL of an aqueous solution containing 4.3 mg of solid sodium borohydride ($NaBH_4$) was added to 100 mL of 100 μmol/L aqueous solution of tetrachloroauric acid ($HAuCl_4$) under vigorous stirring for 12 h. Nanoscale gold particles were then filtered through a 0.22 μm filter. Sodium borohydride and tetrachloroauric acid were purchased from Sigma-Aldrich Chemicals (St. Louis, MO). Optical extinction spectra were obtained on 500 μL gold nanoparticle suspensions dispensed into a 1 × 1 cm PNMA cuvette using a Nanospectralyzer-1 fluorometer (Applied NanoFluorescence, Inc., Houston, TX). The diameters of gold nanoparticles used in these experiments were measured by transmission electron microscopy.

2.3. Shortwave Radiofrequency Field Heating System

A 13.56 MHz RF power generator (Therm Med LLC, Erie, PA) was coupled to a high Q circuit (Therm Med LLC, Erie, PA), which consists of a transmission head (Tx, focused end-fired antenna circuit) and reciprocal receiving (Rx) head mounted on a swivel bracket allowing the direction of the RF field to be oriented in either a horizontal or a vertical direction. The spacing between both heads was also adjustable. The coaxial Tx head produced a local RF field of 15 cm in diameter. Each time the RF generator was activated, the couplers were checked and fine-tuned to assure that there was no reflective power between the Rx and Tx heads. The electromagnetic field strength between the Tx and Rx head was measured in a Faraday-shielded room to exclude any interference from external RF sources. The field was measured using a Hewlett Packard Spectrum Analyzer (model 8566B, Agilent, Santa Clara, CA) and an isotropic field monitor probe (models FM2004 and FP2000, Amplifier Research Inc., Souderton, PA). In our instrument, output powers of 600 W were used, giving a maximum measured electric field strength (E_p) 2.5 cm from the Tx head of 12.4 kV/m.

3. Methods

3.1. Gold Nanoparticle Antibody Conjugates

The synthesis of IgG or C225 gold nanoparticle antibody conjugates was performed by incubating either the IgG or the C225 antibody with nanoparticle suspensions at a pH of 7.8. The saturation concentration of antibodies conjugated to 5 nm gold nanoparticles has been previously determined to be 4 μg/mL (32). A solution of gold nanoparticles was incubated with IgG or C225 concentration of 4 μg/mL for 1 h, followed by slow addition of a NaCl solution to a final concentration of 140 mmol/L. Fifteen minutes after addition of the NaCl, the UV–vis spectra of the antibody–gold nanoparticle conjugates were recorded using a Shimadzu spectrophotometer (UV 2401PC, Columbia, MD). Saturation of the gold nanoparticles by IgG or C225 was confirmed along with the characteristic red shift in the λ_{max} value with an increase in plasmon resonance characteristic of protein binding to gold nanoparticles (32). Binding of antibody to the gold nanoparticles was finally confirmed and measuring an increase in the dielectric constant of the media surrounding the gold nanoparticle antibody conjugates (45).

3.2. RF Field Treatment of Cancer Cells

Each of the four cell lines were grown to near confluence on 60 mm Pyrex dishes. Cells were incubated for 120 min with media alone or media containing naked gold nanoparticles, IgG-conjugated gold nanoparticles, or C225-conjugated gold nanoparticles at a dose of 12.5, 25, or 50 mg/L, respectively. Following incubation with the gold nanoparticles, the medium was aspirated and the cells were gently washed three times with phosphate-buffered saline (PBS) and then 3 mL of fresh medium without any gold nanoparticles was added to each dish. The cell cultures were then placed on a Teflon stand 2.5 cm below the Tx head with a 10 cm air space between the Tx and Rx heads. Cell cultures were treated at 600 W of power for 2 min, after which the cell cultures were returned to the incubator at 37°C for 24 h. All treatments were performed in triplicate.

3.3. Assessment of Apoptosis and Cytotoxicity

Cells from all four human cancer cell lines were harvested from the culture dishes by trypsinization, washed gently with PBS, and centrifuged at 1,500 rpm for 5 min. The resultant cell pellet was resuspended during gentle vortexing while adding 5 mL of 95% ethanol. Cells were fixed overnight at room temperature and then stored at 4°C until specimens were ready for staining. Cells were stained with propidium iodide (PI) and annexin (Sigma-Aldrich Corp, St. Louis, MO). Following addition of the PI and annexin, the cells were centrifuged in the ethanol fixative at 1,500 rpm for 5 min and then resuspended in a Tris buffer solution (stock solution: 24 g Tris, 12 g sodium chloride, 160 mL 1 N HCl in a total volume of 2 L at pH 7.4). The cell pellets were resuspended in 500 µL of Tris buffer and 1 mL of PI and annexin (500 µg/mL). Thirty minutes before flow cytometric analysis, 100 µL of 1 mg/mL RNase (DNase-free, Sigma-Aldrich Corp, St. Louis, MO) was added and the fixed cells were incubated at 37°C. Cell viability, including the apoptotic and necrotic fractions, was assessed in a fluorescence-activated cell sorter (FACS) Calibur unit (BD Biosciences, San Jose, CA) with analysis and graphing using a Cell Quest Pro software (BD Biosciences, San Jose, CA). All experiments were performed in triplicate.

3.4. Transmission Electron Microscopy

Samples were fixed with a solution containing Trumps fixative for 1 h. Samples were postfixed with 1% buffered osmium tetroxide for 1 h, then stained en-bloc with 1% Millipore-filtered uranyl acetate. The samples were dehydrated in increasing concentrations of ethanol, infiltrated, and embedded in Spurr's low-viscosity medium, which underwent polymerization in a 70°C oven for 2 days. Ultra-thin sections were cut in a Leica Ultracut microtome (Leica, Deerfield, IL) stained with uranyl acetate and lead citrate in a Leica EM stainer and examined using a JEM 1010 transmission electron microscope (JEOL, USA, Inc., Peabody, MA) at an accelerating voltage of 80 kV. Digital images were obtained using AMT Imaging System (Advanced Microscopy Techniques Corp., Danvers, MA).

We have recently demonstrated that gold or carbon nanoparticles and a confined, noninvasive shortwave RF field produces significant local heat release that can be used to produce thermal cytotoxicity in cancer cells in vitro and in vivo with RF field treatments of 2 min or less (46, 47). The heat release from gold nanoparticles exposed to shortwave RF fields is particularly impressive and is dependent on both the concentration and the diameter of gold nanoparticles (**Fig. 24.3**) (48). Solid gold nanoparticles smaller in diameter (5–10 nm) heated at a more rapid rate than gold nanoparticles 50–250 nm in diameter.

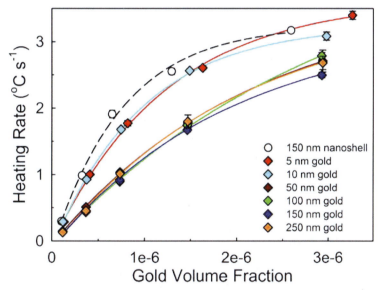

Fig. 24.3. At gold nanoparticle concentrations less than 10 ppm, the heating rate of deionized water in a 13.56 MHz RF field was almost 3°C/s. This remarkable heating rate at very low concentrations of gold nanoparticles represents a heating efficiency of >30,000 W/g of nanoparticles and indicates the generation of elevation temperatures in the nanoscale environment surrounding the gold nanoparticles sufficient to denature proteins, melt lipid bilayers, and produce irreparable damage to intracellular structures and organelles.

In addition, our method does not suffer the limitations of other nanoparticle-based hyperthermia systems given that shortwave radiofrequency (RF) energy has excellent deep tissue penetration, low tissue-specific absorption rates (SAR), and documented safety for brief exposures of humans to this form of electromagnetic radiation (13, 49, 50). Concerns have been expressed about possible mutagenic alterations in cells exposed to nonionizing electromagnetic radiation in the GHz range (51, 52). However, studies of shortwave RF from 10 to 100 MHz has not been associated with any cytogenetic or cytotoxic damage (53–55). Exposure of volunteer test subjects to prolonged periods of shortwave RF irradiation can produce minimal thermoregulatory effects (vasodilation, sweating) but has not been found to cause any acute or long-term damage to normal cells and tissues. Thus, our finding that gold nanoparticles release heat in response to shortwave RF exposure for durations of seconds to a few minutes has important implications. We are investigating the physical nature of this phenomenon and our data suggest that conductive polarizations of metal nanoparticles may explain the high thermal efficiency and tremendous heat release at low concentrations of nanoparticles exposed to the RF field (48, 56). Importantly, since tissue penetration by shortwave RF fields is excellent with low attenuation of the signal, it should be possible to treat tumors at almost any site in the body. The crucial component of this treatment will be successful delivery of adequate numbers of gold nanoparticles to cancer cells to produce intracellular temperatures of at least 55°C following an RF field exposure of no more than a few minutes duration, while ideally limiting uptake of the nanoparticles by normal cells.

We have shown that by directly conjugating 5 nm gold nanoparticles to cetuximab to target epidermal growth factor receptors (EGFR) expressed on cancer cells there is enhanced uptake of the gold nanoparticles (**Fig. 24.4**).

In contrast, cells expressing little or no EGFR should have no enhanced uptake of cetuximab-conjugated gold nanoparticles and, thus, should not be significantly affected by treatment in the RF field. Targeting gold nanoparticles approximately 5–10 nm in diameter to cancer cells to create RF-induced hyperthermic cytotoxicity has several advantages: Gold nanoparticles are simple and inexpensive to synthesize; they are easily characterized due to the presence of a characteristic surface plasmon resonance band, their surface chemistry permits manipulation of charge and shape relatively easily; attaching cancer cell targeting molecules, including antibodies, peptides, or pharmacological agents, is easily achieved; and they are biocompatible and not associated with any acute or chronic toxicities in preclinical studies (40, 57–59). In addition to producing significant heat upon exposure to shortwave RF fields, 5–10 nm gold nanoparticles easily penetrate through pores and fenestrations in the neovasculature of solid tumors (40). This method may be promising for focused local or regional application of a noninvasive RF field to treat primary or established metastatic malignant tumors overexpressing EGFR, but would be problematic for whole-body RF therapy to treat diffuse micrometastatic disease. Constitutive expression of

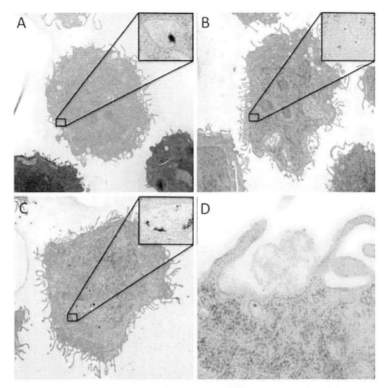

Fig. 24.4. (a) Transmission electron microscope (TEM) image of Panc-1 human pancreatic adenocarcinoma cells (7,500 × magnification) that were incubated for 30 min with unconjugated, nontargeted 5 nm gold nanoparticles (control group). Almost no gold nanoparticles are seen within the cytoplasm of the cell and it is only at a magnification of 100,000 × (*inset upper right*) that an intracytoplasmic vesicle containing a small number of gold nanoparticles is seen. Incubation of Panc-1 cells for 60 or 120 min with the unconjugated gold nanoparticles also produced only a few scattered vesicles in the cytoplasm containing gold nanoparticles. (b) TEM image of Panc-1 cells incubated for 30 min with nonspecific IgG-conjugated gold nanoparticles (control group). Similar to the unconjugated gold nanoparticles, the nonspecific IgG-conjugated gold nanoparticles were not readily taken into the Panc-1 cells. The larger image (7,500 × magnification) demonstrates few or no obvious intracytoplasmic vesicles containing gold nanoparticles. At higher magnification (100,000 ×, *inset upper right*), an occasional intracytoplasmic vesicle with a few gold nanoparticles is evident. (c) TEM image of a Panc-1 pancreatic adenocarcinoma cells incubated for 30 min with C225-conjugated 5 nm gold nanoparticles. At 30 min, a number of intracytoplasmic vesicles (dense black vesicles) containing gold nanoparticles are evident in the larger image (7,500 × magnification). At a higher magnification (100,000 ×), numerous vesicles containing dense collections of gold nanoparticles are found throughout the cytoplasm. At 60 and 120 min of incubation with the C225-targeted gold nanoparticles, the number of intracytoplasmic vesicles containing gold nanoparticles was seen to increase. (d) A higher magnification TEM image (100,000 ×) showing details of the cell surface of Panc-1 cells incubated for 30 min with C225-conjugated gold nanoparticles. Numerous gold nanoparticles are seen at the surface of the cell consistent with binding of the C225 to epidermal growth factor receptor (EGFR). Pretreatment of the cells with C225 alone completely blocked any binding of targeted gold nanoparticles to the cell surface and led to no gold nanoparticles appearing in intracytoplasmic vesicles 30, 60, or 120 min after incubation.

EGFR at normal levels occurs throughout many tissues in the body (60, 61), and our results in SN12PM6 renal cancer cells (low-level expression of EGFR) show that even with low levels of EGFR expression, there is enough uptake of cetuximab-targeted gold nanoparticles to produce low levels of thermal apoptosis following exposure to the RF field. It may be possible to modulate or minimize effects on normal tissues expressing a target molecule like EGFR by use of brief-duration-pulsed RF therapy or repeated short-duration exposures, but these effects must be studied in greater detail to confirm this theoretical consideration. Nonetheless, our results indicate that it is possible to use overexpression of a specific cell-surface moiety, e.g., EGFR, to enhance delivery and uptake of gold nanoparticles to produce thermal cytotoxicity in the malignant cells following brief exposure to a noninvasive RF field.

There are numerous other possibilities for targeted delivery of nanoparticles into malignant cells. Radiolabeled carbon nanotubes have been conjugated with rituximab and lintuzumab to diagnose and potentially treat lymphoma cells (62). Recently, aptamers, nucleic acid ligands much smaller than monoclonal antibodies, have been shown to target specific molecules in the neovasculature of tumors or on the surface of prostate cancer cells (63–65). These aptamers have been conjugated to gold nanoparticles initially for use as an improved diagnostic technique. However, co-conjugation of cytotoxic agents, or use of our noninvasive RF field treatment technique, could be used as an actual anticancer therapy using this targeting technique. The so-called cell-penetrating peptides, generally less than 100 amino acids in length, also have been shown to target certain types of cancer cells. The 86 amino acid HIV-1 Tat protein has been conjugated to gold nanoparticles, with subsequent rapid intracellular uptake of the nanoparticles and localization to the nucleus (66, 67). Our monoclonal antibody-conjugated gold nanoparticles are found in the cytoplasm of cells within 30 min of adding these nanoparticle conjugates to cancer cells in culture. Localization of the nanoparticles to the nucleus with thermal destruction of DNA following RF field exposure must be investigated as a technique to enhance cancer cell destruction. Chlorotoxin is another small peptide (36 amino acids) cancer cell agent that can be easily conjugated with gold nanoparticles and is currently being investigated as a cancer cell targeting agent in several human malignant cell lines (68). Identification of cancer-specific ligands not expressed on normal cells will permit targeting of gold nanoparticles to only malignant cells for treatment in our noninvasive RF field generator and should allow treatment of measurable tumors and micrometastatic disease with minimal therapy-related toxicities. Targeting ligands, such as EGFR, that are overexpressed but not unique to cancer cells is feasible but will require careful evaluation to determine acute and long-term thermal effects in normal cells and organs following RF field therapy.

Nanoscale thermal therapy of targeted cancer cells is a promising new weapon in the battle against cancer. By combining nonionizing radiation and targeted metallic nanoparticles, noninvasive-targeted thermal therapy has the promise of benefiting cancer patients that need a nontoxic alternative to the debilitating effects of conventional chemotherapeutics. Using noninvasive RF fields to heat nanoscale materials that are internalized into cancer cells has the promise of reducing toxicity and maximizing therapeutic benefit for cancer patients.

References

1. Frey, E. F. (1985) The earliest medical texts. *Clio Med* **20**, 79–90.
2. Beasley, G. M., Ross, M. I., and Tyler, D. S. (2008) Future directions in regional treatment strategies for melanoma and sarcoma. *Int J Hyperthermia* **24**, 301–309.
3. Di Carlo, I., Pulvirenti, E., Sparatore, F., Toro, A., and Cordio, S. (2007) Treatment of peritoneal carcinomatosis from colorectal cancer with cytoreductive surgery and perioperative intraperitoneal chemotherapy: state of the art and future prospects. *Surg Oncol* **16 Suppl 1**, S145–S148.
4. Stewart, J. H. T., Shen, P., Russell, G., et al. (2008) A phase I trial of oxaliplatin for intraperitoneal hyperthermic chemoperfusion for the treatment of peritoneal surface dissemination from colorectal and appendiceal cancers. *Ann Surg Oncol* **15**, 2137–2145.
5. Baratti, D., Kusamura, S., Sironi, A., et al. (2008) Multicystic peritoneal mesothelioma treated by surgical cytoreduction and hyperthermic intra-peritoneal chemotherapy (HIPEC). *In Vivo* **22**, 153–157.
6. Kampinga, H. H. (2006) Cell biological effects of hyperthermia alone or combined with radiation or drugs: a short introduction to newcomers in the field. *Int J Hyperthermia* **22**, 191–196.
7. Calderwood, S. K. and Ciocca, D. R. (2008) Heat shock proteins: stress proteins with Janus-like properties in cancer. *Int J Hyperthermia* **24**, 31–39.
8. Fatehi, D., van der Zee, J., van der Wal, E., Van Wieringen, W. N., and Van Rhoon, G. C. (2006) Temperature data analysis for 22 patients with advanced cervical carcinoma treated in Rotterdam using radiotherapy, hyperthermia and chemotherapy: a reference point is needed. *Int J Hyperthermia* **22**, 353–363.
9. Sumiyoshi, K., Strebel, F. R., Rowe, R. W., and Bull, J. M. (2003) The effect of whole-body hyperthermia combined with 'metronomic' chemotherapy on rat mammary adenocarcinoma metastases. *Int J Hyperthermia* **19**, 103–118.
10. Ismail-Zade, R. S. (2005) Whole body hyperthermia supplemented with urotropin in the treatment of malignant tumors. *Exp Oncol* **27**, 61–64.
11. Lounsberry, W., Goldschmidt, V., and Linke, C. (1995) The early histologic changes following electrocoagulation. *Gastrointest Endosc* **41**, 68–70.
12. Arciero, C. A. and Sigurdson, E. R. (2008) Diagnosis and treatment of metastatic disease to the liver. *Semin Oncol* **35**, 147–159.
13. Durney, C. H., Massoudi, H., and Iskander, M. E. (1986) Radiofrequency Radiation Dosimetry Handbook. 4th ed, U.S. Air Force School of Aerospace Medicine Press, Brooks City, Texas.
14. Link, S. and El-Sayed, M. A. (2003) Optical properties and ultrafast dynamics of metallic nanocrystals. *Annu Rev Phys Chem* **54**, 331–366.
15. Hartman, K. B., Wilson, L. J., and Rosenblum, M. G. (2008) Detecting and treating cancer with nanotechnology. *Mol Diagn Ther* **12**, 1–14.
16. Sumer, B. and Gao, J. (2008) Theranostic nanomedicine for cancer. *Nanomedicine* **3**, 137–140.
17. Cho, K., Wang, X., Nie, S., Chen, Z. G., and Shin, D. M. (2008) Therapeutic nanoparticles for drug delivery in cancer. *Clin Cancer Res* **14**, 1310–1316.
18. Hartman, K. B. and Wilson, L. J. (2007) Carbon nanostructures as a new high-performance platform for MR molecular imaging. *Adv Exp Med Biol* **620**, 74–84.

19. Kou, G., Wang, S., Cheng, C., et al. (2008) Development of SM5-1-conjugated ultrasmall superparamagnetic iron oxide nanoparticles for hepatoma detection. *Biophys Res Commun* **374**, 192–197.
20. Barcena, C., Sra, A. K., Chaubey, G. S., Khemtong, C., Liu, J. P., and Gao, J. (2008) Zinc ferrite nanoparticles as MRI contrast agents. *Chem Commun (Camb)*, **19**, 2224–2226.
21. Neumaier, C. E., Baio, G., Ferrini, S., Corte, G., and Daga, A. (2008) MR and iron magnetic nanoparticles. Imaging opportunities in preclinical and translational research. *Tumori* **94**, 226–233.
22. Liu, Z., Cai, W., He, L., et al. (2007) In vivo biodistribution and highly efficient tumour targeting of carbon nanotubes in mice. *Nat Nanotechnol* **2**, 47–52.
23. Matson, J. B. and Grubbs, R. H. (2008) Synthesis of fluorine-18 functionalized nanoparticles for use as in vivo molecular imaging agents. *J Am Chem Soc* **130**, 6731–6733.
24. Zhang, H., Yee, D., and Wang, C. (2008) Quantum dots for cancer diagnosis and therapy: biological and clinical perspectives. *Nanomedicine* **3**, 83–91.
25. Misra, R. D. (2008) Quantum dots for tumor-targeted drug delivery and cell imaging. *Nanomedicine* **3**, 271–274.
26. Curry, A. C., Crow, M., and Wax, A. (2008) Molecular imaging of epidermal growth factor receptor in live cells with refractive index sensitivity using dark-field microspectroscopy and immunotargeted nanoparticles. *J Biomed Opt* **13**, 014022.
27. Kelly, K. A., Setlur, S. R., Ross, R., et al. (2008) Detection of early prostate cancer using a hepsin-targeted imaging agent. *Cancer Res* **68**, 2286–2291.
28. Wu, J., Yan, F., Zhang, X., Yan, Y., Tang, J., and Ju, H. (2008) Disposable reagentless electrochemical immunosensor array based on a biopolymer/sol–gel membrane for simultaneous measurement of several tumor markers. *Clin Chem* **54**, 1481–1488.
29. Wang, A. and Li, S. (2008) Hydroxycamptothecin-loaded nanoparticles enhance target drug delivery and anticancer effect. *BMC Biotechnol* **8**, 46.
30. Li, S., Wang, A., Jiang, W., and Guan, Z. (2008) Pharmacokinetic characteristics and anticancer effects of 5-fluorouracil loaded nanoparticles. *BMC Cancer* **8**, 103.
31. Hwang, H. Y., Kim, I. S., Kwon, I. C., and Kim, Y. H. (2008) Tumor targetability and antitumor effect of docetaxel-loaded hydrophobically modified glycol chitosan nanoparticles. *J Control Release* **128**, 23–31.
32. Patra, C. R., Bhattacharya, R., Wang, E., et al. (2008) Targeted delivery of gemcitabine to pancreatic adenocarcinoma using cetuximab as a targeting agent. *Cancer Res* **68**, 1970–1978.
33. Visaria, R. K., Griffin, R. J., Williams, B. W., et al. (2006) Enhancement of tumor thermal therapy using gold nanoparticle-assisted tumor necrosis factor-alpha delivery. *Mol Cancer Ther* **5**, 1014–1020.
34. Farma, J. M., Puhlmann, M., Soriano, P. A., et al. (2007) Direct evidence for rapid and selective induction of tumor neovascular permeability by tumor necrosis factor and a novel derivative, colloidal gold bound tumor necrosis factor. *Int J Cancer* **120**, 2474–2480.
35. Richard, C., de Chermont Qle, M., and Scherman, D. (2008) Nanoparticles for imaging and tumor gene delivery. *Tumori* **94**, 264–270.
36. Opanasopit, P., Apirakaramwong, A., Ngawhirunpat, T., Rojanarata, T., and Ruktanonchai, U. (2008) Development and characterization of pectinate micro/nanoparticles for gene delivery. *AAPS PharmSciTech* **9**, 67–74.
37. Kam, N. W., Liu, Z., and Dai, H. (2006) Carbon nanotubes as intracellular transporters for proteins and DNA: an investigation of the uptake mechanism and pathway. *Angew Chem Int Ed Engl* **45**, 577–581.
38. Chang, M. Y., Shiau, A. L., Chen, Y. H., Chang, C. J., Chen, H. H., and Wu, C. L. (2008) Increased apoptotic potential and dose-enhancing effect of gold nanoparticles in combination with single-dose clinical electron beams on tumor-bearing mice. *Cancer Sci* **99**, 1479–1484.
39. Mukherjee, P., Bhattacharya, R., Bone, N., et al. (2007) Potential therapeutic application of gold nanoparticles in B-chronic lymphocytic leukemia (BCLL): enhancing apoptosis. *J Nanobiotechnol* **5**, 4.
40. Mukherjee, P., Bhattacharya, R., Wang, P., et al. (2005) Antiangiogenic properties of gold nanoparticles. *Clin Cancer Res* **11**, 3530–3534.
41. Gobin, A. M., Lee, M. H., Halas, N. J., James, W. D., Drezek, R. A., and West, J. L. (2007) Near-infrared resonant nanoshells for combined optical imaging and photothermal cancer therapy. *Nano Lett* **7**, 1929–1934.
42. Arnfield, M. R., Mathew, R. P., Tulip, J., and McPhee, M. S. (1992) Analysis of tissue optical coefficients using an approximate equation valid for comparable absorption and scattering. *Phys Med Biol* **37**, 1219–1230.

43. Kalambur, V. S., Longmire, E. K., and Bischof, J. C. (2007) Cellular level loading and heating of superparamagnetic iron oxide nanoparticles. *Langmuir* **23**, 12329–12336.
44. Bhattacharya, R., Patra, C. R., Verma, R., Kumar, S., Greipp, P. R., and Mukherjee, P. (2007) Gold nanoparticles inhibit the proliferation of multiple myeloma cells. *Adv Mater* **19**, 711–716.
45. Mangeney, C., Ferrage, F., Aujard, I., et al. (2002) Synthesis and properties of water-soluble gold colloids covalently derivatized with neutral polymer monolayers. *J Am Chem Soc* **124**, 5811–5821.
46. Gannon, C. J., Cherukuri, P., Yakobson, B. I., et al. (2007) Carbon nanotube-enhanced thermal destruction of cancer cells in a noninvasive radiofrequency field. *Cancer* **110**, 2654–2665.
47. Gannon, C. J., Patra, C. R., Bhattacharya, R., Mukherjee, P., and Curley, S. A. (2008) Intracellular gold nanoparticles enhance noninvasive radiofrequency thermal destruction of human gastrointestinal cancer cells. *J Nanobiotechnol* **6**, 2.
48. Moran, C. H., Wainerdi, S. M., Cherukuri, T. K., Kittrell, C., Wiley, B. J., Nicholas, N. W., Curley, S. A., Kanzius, J. S., Cherukuri, P. C. (2009) Size dependent joule heating of gold nanoparticles using capacitively coupled radiofrequency fields. *Nano Res* **2**, 400–405.
49. Erdreich, L. S. and Klauenberg, B. J. (2001) Radio frequency radiation exposure standards: considerations for harmonization. *Health Phys* **80**, 430–439.
50. Adair, E. R., Blick, D. W., Allen, S. J., Mylacraine, K. S., Ziriax, J. M., and Scholl, D. M. (2005) Thermophysiological responses of human volunteers to whole body RF exposure at 220 MHz. *Bioelectromagnetics* **26**, 448–461.
51. Diem, E., Schwarz, C., Adlkofer, F., Jahn, O., and Rudiger, H. (2005) Non-thermal DNA breakage by mobile-phone radiation (1800 MHz) in human fibroblasts and in transformed GFSH-R17 rat granulosa cells in vitro. *Mutat Res* **583**, 178–183.
52. Tice, R. R., Hook, G. G., Donner, M., McRee, D. I., and Guy, A. W. (2002) Genotoxicity of radiofrequency signals. I. Investigation of DNA damage and micronuclei induction in cultured human blood cells. *Bioelectromagnetics* **23**, 113–126.
53. Lantow, M., Viergutz, T., Weiss, D. G., and Simko, M. (2006) Comparative study of cell cycle kinetics and induction of apoptosis or necrosis after exposure of human mono mac 6 cells to radiofrequency radiation. *Radiat Res* **166**, 539–543.
54. Adey, W. R. (1981) Tissue interactions with nonionizing electromagnetic fields. *Physiol Rev* **61**, 435–514.
55. Klima, J. and Scehovic, R. (2006) The field strength measurement and SAR experience related to human exposure in 110 MHz to 40 GHz. *Meas Sci Rev* **6**, 40–44.
56. Tripathi, V. and Loh, Y. L. (2006) Thermal conductivity of a granular metal. *Phys Rev Lett* **96**, 046805.
57. Whitesides, G. M., Kriebel, J. K., and Love, J. C. (2005) Molecular engineering of surfaces using self-assembled monolayers. *Sci Prog* **88**, 17–48.
58. Daniel, M. C. and Astruc, D. (2004) Gold nanoparticles: assembly, supramolecular chemistry, quantum-size-related properties, and applications toward biology, catalysis, and nanotechnology. *Chem Rev* **104**, 293–346.
59. Hainfeld, J. F., Slatkin, D. N., Focella, T. M., and Smilowitz, H. M. (2006) Gold nanoparticles: a new X-ray contrast agent. *Br J Radiol* **79**, 248–253.
60. Hidalgo, M. (2008) Clinical development of epidermal growth factor receptor (EGFR) tyrosine kinase inhibitors: what lessons have we learned? *Adv Exp Med Biol* **610**, 128–143.
61. Ferguson, K. M. (2008) Structure-based view of epidermal growth factor receptor regulation. *Annu Rev Biophys* **37**, 353–373.
62. McDevitt, M. R., Chattopadhyay, D., Kappel, B. J., et al. (2007) Tumor targeting with antibody-functionalized, radiolabeled carbon nanotubes. *J Nucl Med* **48**, 1180–1189.
63. Simberg, D., Duza, T., Park, J. H., et al. (2007) Biomimetic amplification of nanoparticle homing to tumors. *Proc Natl Acad Sci USA* **104**, 932–936.
64. Javier, D. J., Nitin, N., Levy, M., Ellington, A., and Richards-Kortum, R. (2008) Aptamer-targeted gold nanoparticles as molecular-specific contrast agents for reflectance imaging. *Bioconjug Chem* **19**, 1309–1312.
65. Farokhzad, O. C., Jon, S., Khademhosseini, A., Tran, T. N., Lavan, D. A., and Langer, R. (2004) Nanoparticle–aptamer bioconjugates: a new approach for targeting prostate cancer cells. *Cancer Res* **64**, 7668–7672.
66. Berry, C. C. (2008) Intracellular delivery of nanoparticles via the HIV-1 tat peptide. *Nanomedicine* **3**, 357–365.
67. Berry, C. C., de la Fuente, J. M., Mullin, M., Chu, S. W., and Curtis, A. S. (2007) Nuclear localization of HIV-1 tat functionalized gold nanoparticles. *IEEE Trans Nanobiosci* **6**, 262–269.
68. Mamelak, A. N. and Jacoby, D. B. (2007) Targeted delivery of antitumoral therapy to glioma and other malignancies with synthetic chlorotoxin (TM-601). *Expert Opin Drug Deliv* **4**, 175–186.

Chapter 25

Colloidal Gold: A Novel Nanoparticle for Targeted Cancer Therapeutics

Anathea C. Powell, Giulio F. Paciotti, and Steven K. Libutti

Abstract

Since their initial description in 1857, gold nanoparticles have been used extensively in the fields of diagnostics and therapeutics. Now, gold nanoparticles are engineered to target the delivery of potent anti-cancer therapeutics to solid tumors to improve either their safety or efficacy or both. Described in this chapter is the development of one such nanotherapeutic, termed CYT-6091, that targets the delivery of tumor necrosis factor alpha (TNF) to solid tumors. Outlined in the presentation is a discussion of nanoparticles and specifically colloidal gold, an historical review on the biology of TNF and its limited use in the clinic when administered systemically, and finally, how gold nanoparticles bound with TNF may improve the safety and efficacy profiles of TNF.

Key words: Tumor necrosis factor, colloidal gold, colloidal gold nanoparticles, pegylated colloidal gold, tumor necrosis factor conjugated to colloidal gold.

1. Overview of Nanoparticle-Based Drug Delivery Systems

Applications of nanotechnology in cancer detection and treatment are rapidly evolving. Nanoparticles are commonly defined as man-made particles (1) ranging in size from 1 to 100 nm (1, 2). The large surface area of these particles provides a broad platform upon which to attach agents for targeted approaches to cancer informatics, detection, diagnostics, therapeutics, and imaging (3). Targeted therapeutic strategies are of great interest as they may provide increased efficacy of anti-cancer agents with decreased toxicity. In order to provide this benefit, the engineering goals of targeted nanoparticles have been described as twofold: first, to increase target, or tumor, specificity and second, to formulate the agent in such a way as to overcome non-specific biologic barriers (1). The three main components of such nanoparticles are a core material, the active agent, and modifiers to assist in biological barrier evasion (1).

Nanoparticles may home to tumors based on either passive or active targeting mechanisms. Passive targeting relies on changes that occur in the tumor microenvironment during tumor growth and angiogenesis. Under the influence of such regulators as vascular endothelial growth factor (VEGF), tumor vasculature becomes disorganized and chaotic. Vessels become more permeable, blood flow patterns through the tumor may be disrupted, and lymphatic drainage may be impaired (4). As a result of these and other changes in the tumor microenvironment, nanoparticles may sequester within the tumor (2, 3). In contrast to passive targeting, active targeting uses a targeting moiety conjugated to the nanoparticle (2). These moieties are directed toward specific interactions with cell surface molecules, receptors, or antigens that direct the nanoparticle to the tumor (1–3).

Cells of the reticuloendothelial system (RES), such as macrophages, are immunologic scavengers that can derail nanoparticle treatment by sequestering nanoparticles and preventing them from reaching tumor cells (1). Plasma proteins may also adsorb nanoparticles, causing aggregation or ligand dissociation (3). Particle size limits and hydrophilic coats have been shown to help minimize this non-specific uptake. The experience with liposomes has demonstrated the utility of polyethylene glycol (PEG) for this purpose. Amphipathic PEG preparations, such as PEG conjugated to a phospholipid (5), cause the PEG-conjugated nanoparticles to form micellar structures in aqueous solution (6). The combination of steric interference and surface hydrophilicity (5) permits particles to avoid the RES (5–7). Additionally, particles of less than 100 nm have been shown to exist longer in circulation due to diminished uptake by hepatic and splenic circulation (5).

These advances in the understanding of the biologic fate of systemic administration of nanoparticles have greatly increased the interest in the use of these platforms for drug delivery. Two main categories of constituent materials have been described: liposomes and degradable polymers (1). Metal nanoparticles are also under investigation (3); we have been studying colloidal gold as the platform for targeted delivery of therapeutic agents to tumor cells (8, 9).

2. Colloidal Gold

From a practical standpoint, colloidal gold nanoparticles represent an ideal technology for developing tumor-targeting nanotherapies as they represent a biocompatible platform with a well-established record of safety. Gold preparations have a varied therapeutic history in the treatment of human diseases. Michael Faraday first described the synthesis of nanoparticles of Au^0 from gold chloride and sodium citrate in 1857 (10). Water-soluble gold compounds, such as gold sodium thiosulfate, containing between 37 and 50% gold by weight, have been administered by intravenous, intramuscular, and oral routes in the treatment of rheumatoid arthritis (RA) (11). Interestingly, colloidal gold preparations have not been shown to be efficacious in RA (11).

Radioactive conjugates of colloidal gold have been used in the treatment of human cancers since the 1940s (12). Systemic administration of colloidal radiogold was first used in the treatment of leukemias and lymphomas because it was shown that the majority of these systemically administered particles were taken up by the RES cells in the liver, the spleen, and the bone marrow (12, 13). After these observations, systemic colloidal radiogold was used experimentally in primary and metastatic liver cancers. Intraperitoneal administration of colloidal gold was also explored for metastatic endometrial and ovarian cancers (14, 15). Little therapeutic benefit was realized in any of these histologies (12, 13). Toxicities of intraperitoneal administration appeared to be related to radiation and not the gold particles (14). Major toxicity of systemic administration consisted of bone marrow depression; this was also attributed to radiation effect and not the gold particles themselves (12, 13).

Given the lack of demonstrated toxicity associated with the colloidal gold particles, colloidal gold appeared to offer a neutral nanoplatform for drug delivery. More recent studies of colloidal gold particles have demonstrated particle uptake by Kupffer cells in the liver by electron microscopy (16, 17); this uptake is consistent with data regarding the clearance of nanoparticles by the RES. Overall, the long-term safety data, combined with the observations that the particles are eventually eliminated from the body, provide a practical advantage to the use of gold nanoparticles in drug delivery.

3. Tumor Necrosis Factor

It is now well established that the toxicity of many existing cancer therapies is in large part due to their indiscriminate actions on both healthy and malignant tissues. In many cases, such lack of specificity has led to the failure of many cancer therapies that show promise in pre-clinical settings. A prime example of this failure was the inability to re-create, in a clinical setting, the remarkable anti-tumor responses obtained with human cytokines, such as tumor necrosis factor alpha (TNF-α), interleukin-2 (IL-2), and interleukin-12 (IL-12) in pre-clinical cancer models. These protein-based therapies were at the heart of the biologic treatment of cancer and targeted such pathways as direct tumor apoptosis, obliteration of the tumor neovasculature, and/or the recruitment of the immune system as means of generating a tumor-specific immune response. Although initial efforts to harness this cytokine in the treatment of cancer failed, several key studies yielded clues on how to address these failures.

TNF was first identified in 1975 during investigations of antitumor properties of normal serum (18). The cytokine is secreted by activated macrophages (19, 20) and mediates the inflammatory response (21); other effects of TNF include induction of apoptosis in cancer cells (21), activation of hematopoietic cells, effects on the immune system, and activation of the coagulation system (21, 22). The gene for human TNF, a protein of 157 amino acid subunits (21), was cloned in 1984, and recombinant human TNF has been available since that time (20). Two cell surface receptors TNF-R1 and TNF-R2 have been described; TNF-R1 has been shown to be the most significant biologic pathway for TNF effects, leading to cellular apoptosis and other downstream protein activation (21).

TNF has been investigated as an anti-tumor agent through a variety of administration routes. Subcutaneous (23) and intramuscular administration (24) of TNF were attempted but abandoned due to local toxicity at the site of injection. Extensive clinical trials of systemic administration of TNF have been conducted in multiple cancer histologies. Phase I (19, 25–27) trials in patients with advanced-stage solid malignancies demonstrated the dose-limiting toxicity of systemic TNF to be due to vascular collapse; other toxicities included constitutional symptoms such as fever and rigors, as well as transient leucopenia and elevations in liver function tests. Objective responses in Phase II trials were rare (28–31); although the biology behind the lack of response is unclear, it is possible that the doses administered based on toxicity data were insufficient to cause response.

Despite these data, work has demonstrated tumor regression with intratumoral injection of TNF (32). Some postulated that the vasculature of tumors may be sensitive to TNF but require higher concentrations than can be achieved with safe systemic doses (22). Isolated limb perfusion allows TNF to be given in combination with other active agents in a setting where the agents were sequestered to the affected limb. Regimens that combined TNF with interferon gamma and melphalan for intransit melanoma metastases have shown complete local responses

(33, 34) but the contribution of each agent to the outcome has been unclear.

Collectively, these data demonstrate that limiting the distribution of TNF to solid tumors not only is critical to improve the safety of TNF administration but also may improve efficacy. Our attempts to mimic the localized delivery of the ILP have focused on using colloidal gold nanoparticles to target the delivery of TNF to solid tumors.

4. Developing CYT-6091 (TNF Conjugated to Colloidal Gold)

The physical properties of colloidal gold nanoparticles make them especially well suited for developing tumor-targeting nanotherapies. As described in the first section, the size of the nanoparticles can be customized to passively target the tumor neovasculature and gain initial entry into the tumor interstitium (35–38). The newly formed blood vessels of tumors are immature and are composed of loosely junctioned endothelial cells. These open junctions, known as fenestrae, have diameters that range from 100 to 400 nm (35–39). Given that the diameter of the fenestrae of normal blood vessels ranges from 2 to 7 nm, the larger 27-nm colloidal gold nanoparticle, bound with anti-cancer therapeutics such as TNF, may redistribute its therapeutic payload away from healthy tissues and passively accumulate within solid tumors. It is also postulated that the well-described interaction between TNF and its receptor TNF-R1 may assist with active targeting of the nanoparticle delivery system to the tumor cells.

In order to avoid the systemic toxicity that hampered prior formulations of TNF, it is imperative that the therapeutic payload is not released from the particle once the nanotherapy is injected into the circulation. For TNF, this is achieved by the formation of a dative covalent bond (8, 40) that is formed between the sulfur atoms present on cysteine residues on TNF and the empty electronic orbitals present on the atoms of gold at the surface of the particle. Dative covalent bonds formed by free sulfhydryl or disulfide groups on the biomolecule and gold atoms are nearly as strong as a carbon–carbon bond and keep the TNF tightly bound to the particle as it circulates in the body. Interestingly, the formation of the dative covalent bond does not destroy the biologic activity of TNF, as once bound to the particle surface, TNF is equipotent, on a mole-to-mole basis, to a soluble TNF reference standard (8).

5. Pre-Clinical Studies

Initial formulations of this novel vector included TNF conjugated to the colloidal gold platform (cAu–TNF) without a hydrophilic shield. Unsurprisingly, as described in the first section, this vector was not successful at evading the RES (8). This initial formulation was re-engineered by interspersing molecules of a thiol-derivatized polyethylene glycol (PEG–THIOL) in between the molecules of TNF. Similar to TNF, the thiolated polymer is covalently linked to the surface of the particles by a dative covalent bond. In vivo testing of this new formulation, termed CYT-6091, revealed that the presence of the PEG–THIOL polymer dramatically reduced RES uptake and clearance of the gold nanoparticles. These data are consistent with the known ability of hydrophilic polymers, such as PEG–THIOL, to hydrate nanoparticles and in doing so sterically and electrostatically (i.e., the zeta potential is near 0) block their interaction with blood-borne opsins. By blocking this interaction, the PEG–THIOL increases the circulatory half-life of TNF, allowing it to passively accumulate with the tumors over time. Furthermore, once inside the tumor interstitium, TNF is thought to anchor the particle in the tumor microenvironment by binding to its receptor and acting as a tumor-targeting ligand (8).

Systemic administration of the new pegylated colloidal gold–TNF construct (CYT-6091) was compared with the non-pegylated construct (cAu–TNF), a pegylated control conjugated to an inactive agent (murine serum albumin; PT–cAu–MSA), and rhTNF in mice burdened with TNF-sensitive colon cancer xenografts. This pre-clinical model allowed characterization and evaluation of the experimental colloidal gold construct (8).

Pharmacokinetic analysis revealed the CYT-6091 construct to remain in systemic circulation significantly longer than rhTNF and the non-pegylated cAu–TNF construct, with 20 times more TNF found in the blood at 3 and 6 h after injection in the PT–cAu–TNF animals vs. rhTNF alone. Intratumoral levels of CYT-6091 were significantly higher than rhTNF. Electron micrographs demonstrating gold particles in the CYT-6091-treated tumors visually confirmed these findings (8).

Efficacy and toxicity studies were also carried out in the colon cancer xenograft model with a dose-escalation strategy for both CYT-6091 and recombinant TNF. Doses of 7.5 and 15 µg of TNF were administered either in native formulation or in conjugation with the colloidal gold nanoparticle platform. The 7.5 and 15 µg doses of recombinant TNF caused tumor regression in 51 and 79% of cases, but also caused death of the animal in 11 and 40% of cases, respectively. In contrast, none of the animals receiving either dose of the colloidal gold–TNF construct became sick or died, and tumor regression occurred in 72 and 82% of animals at the respective dose levels (8).

CYT-6091 causes the accumulation of TNF in both TNF-sensitive and TNF-insensitive murine tumor models. The relative sensitivity of these tumors was determined by whether TNF inhibited cell proliferation in vitro. In TNF-sensitive models, the accumulation of TNF results in a potent anti-tumor response with a single injection. In contrast, in TNF-insensitive models, such as B16/F10 melanoma tumors, the accumulation results in only a transient inhibition of tumor growth (data not yet published). In a series of follow-up studies, we determined that these resistant tumors could be sensitized by repeated administration of CYT-6091. In effect, the repeated administration of CYT-6091 blocked tumor growth. Immunohistological examination revealed that repeated administration of CYT-6091 caused an immediate loss of vascular endothelial cell marker, CD34, and over time resulted in a breakdown of the vascular integrity as evidenced by a lack of association of CD31-positive cells with the tumor blood vessel lumen (9). Furthermore, CYT-6091 has been reported to cause vascular leak at the boundary of the tumor and the normal vasculature (9). Such vascular disruption is consistent with the destruction of the tumor vasculature described with ILP.

6. Phase I Clinical Trial of CYT-6091

As described, pre-clinical studies with the CYT-6091 construct support the idea of improved targeting with decreased toxicity of TNF, or an improved therapeutic index, within the colloidal gold nanoparticle platform. In order to explore the construct within human cancers, we have recently completed a phase I, open-label trial of the CYT-6091 construct (CYT-6091) within the Tumor Angiogenesis Section of the Surgery Branch of the National Cancer Institute, in collaboration with CytImmune Sciences (41).

Patients with advanced-stage solid malignancies were eligible for the trial. The trial was conducted as a dose-escalation trial. Three patients were assigned to each dose cohort; the beginning dose was 50 $\mu g/m^2$ and increased by 50 $\mu g/m^2$ as the trial progressed. Patients were admitted to the NIH Clinical Center and received two systemic injections of CYT-6091 on days 0 and 14; they were monitored for at least 48 h following each injection. As this is a phase I trial, the primary end point was to determine the maximum tolerated dose of CYT-6091. Secondary end points consisted of pharmacokinetic data, disease response (assessed at 45 days after the second injection), and assessment of gold particles in the tumor and adjacent normal tissue (procured through biopsy).

Complete data is available for seven patients thus far. Similar to the pre-clinical data, no patient experienced a dose-limiting toxicity following administration of CYT-6091. The three patients in the first, and lowest, dose cohort (50 $\mu g/m^2$) experienced fever; subsequently, this reaction was prevented with acetaminophen and indomethacin pre-treatment. No other physiologic parameters showed significant or sustained changes from baseline following treatment. Electron micrographs demonstrated up to a 10-fold increase in the number of gold nanoparticles in tumors from 5 to 6 patients as compared to adjacent normal tissue. The data from this trial are continuing to be analyzed.

7. Conclusion

Both pre-clinical and early clinical data support the use of the novel nanotechnology of colloidal gold as a platform for delivery of anti-cancer agents. Although efficacy data is not yet available, TNF-bound colloidal gold does accumulate preferentially within tumors and appears to do so via an active mechanism. The use of the hydrophilic thiol-derivatized pegylated particle allows TNF to persist in circulation by reducing uptake by the RES. Finally, in contrast to systemic administration of recombinant TNF, there appear to be no significant toxicities associated with colloidal gold delivery of TNF. Thus, all goals of nanoparticle therapy are satisfied with the use of the pegylated colloidal gold platform. Further investigation is ongoing to elucidate the mechanism of the TNF accumulation within the tumor but currently is believed to be due to an anchoring of the gold nanoparticle on the tumor surface via the TNF–TNFR1 ligand–receptor interaction.

The lessons of limb perfusion trials are helpful in directing further therapy. Improved responses were seen with combination therapy in those trials. Future applications of the colloidal gold technology may include conjugating other active agents onto the gold nanoparticle. In such a construct, the delivery system of the gold particle, the possible anchoring mechanism of the TNF molecule or other active accumulation strategies, and the anti-tumor efficacy of another chemotherapy agent could all be leveraged in synergy to extend the therapeutic indices of treatment agents.

References

1. Ferrari, M. (2005) Cancer nanotechnology: opportunities and challenges. *Nat Rev Cancer* **5**(3), 161–171.
2. Sinha, R., Kim, G. J., Nie, S., and Shin, D. M. (2006) Nanotechnology in cancer therapeutics: bioconjugated nanoparticles for drug delivery. *Mol Cancer Ther* **5**(8), 1909–1917.
3. Nie, S., Xing, Y., Kim, G. J., and Simons, J. W. (2007) Nanotechnology applications in cancer. *Annu Rev Biomed Eng* **9**, 257–288.
4. Carmeliet, P. and Jain, R. K. (2000) Angiogenesis in cancer and other diseases. *Nature* **407**(6801), 249–257.
5. Nagayasu, A., Uchuyama, K., and Kiwada, H. (1999) The size of liposomes: a factor which affects their targeting efficiency to tumors and therapeutic activity of liposomal antitumor drugs. *Adv Drug Deliv Rev* **40**(1–2), 75–87.
6. Klibanov, A. L., Maruyama, K., Beckerleg, A. M., Torchilin, V. P., and Huang, L. (1991) Activity of amphipathic poly(ethylene glycol) 5000 to prolong the circulation time of liposomes depends on the liposome size and is unfavorable for immunoliposome binding to target. *Biochim Biophys Acta* **1062**(2), 142–148.
7. Park, J. W. (2002) Liposome-based drug delivery in breast cancer treatment. *Breast Cancer Res* **4**(3), 95–99.
8. Paciotti, G. F., Myer, L., Weinrich, D., et al. (2004) Colloidal gold: a novel nanoparticle vector for tumor directed drug delivery. *Drug Deliv* **11**(3), 169–183.
9. Farma, J., Puhlmann, M., Soriano, P. A., et al. (2007) Direct evidence for rapid and selective induction of tumor neovascular permeability by tumor necrosis factor and a novel derivative, colloidal gold bound tumor necrosis factor. *Int J Cancer* **120**(11), 2474–2480.
10. Faraday, M. (1857) Experimental relations of gold (and other metals) to light. *Philos Trans R Soc Lond B Biol Sci* **14**, 145–181.
11. Gottlieb, N. L. and Gray, R. G. (1981) Pharmacokinetics of gold in rheumatoid arthritis. *Agents Actions Suppl* **8**, 529–538.
12. Rubin, P. and Levitt, S. H. (1964) The response of disseminated reticulum cell sarcoma to the intravenous injection of colloidal radioactive gold. *J Nucl Med* **5**, 581–594.
13. Root, S. W., Andrews, G. A., Kniseley, R. M., and Tyor, M. P. (1954) The distribution and radiation effects of intravenously administered colloidal Au198 in man. *Cancer* **7**(5), 856–866.
14. Holbrook, M. A., Welch, J. S., and Childs, D. S. (1964) Adjuvant use of radioactive colloids in the treatment of carcinoma of the ovary. *Radiology* **83**, 888–891.
15. Fountain, K. S. and Malkasian, G. D. (1981) Radioactive colloidal gold in the treatment of endometrial cancer. *Cancer* **47**, 2430–2432.
16. Renaud, G., Hamilton, R. L., and Havel, R. J. (1989) Hepatic metabolism of colloidal gold-low-density-lipoprotein complexes in the rat: evidence for bulk excretion of lysosomal contents into bile. *Hepatology* **9**(3), 380–392.
17. Hardonk, M. J., Harms, G., and Koudstaal, J. (1985) Zonal heterogeneity of rat hepatocytes in the in vivo uptake of 17 nm colloidal gold granules. *Histochem* **83**, 473–477.
18. Carswell, E. A., Old, L. J., Kassel, R. L., et al. (1975) An endotoxin-induced serum factor that causes necrosis of tumors. *Proc Natl Acad Sci USA* **72**(9), 3666–3670.
19. Selby, P., Hobbs, S., Jackson, E., et al. (1987) Tumour necrosis factor in man: Clinical and biological observations. *Br J Cancer* **56**(6), 803–808.
20. Pennica, D., Nedwin, G. E., Hayflick, J. S., et al. (1984) Human tumour necrosis factor: precursor structure, expression and homology to lymphotoxin. *Nature* **312**(5996), 724–729.
21. Chen, G. and Goeddel, D. V. (2002) TNF-R1 signaling: a beautiful pathway. *Science* **296**(5573), 1634–5.
22. Frei, E., 3rd and Spriggs, D. (1989) Tumour necrosis factor: still a promising agent. *J Clin Oncol* **7**(3), 291–294.
23. Chapman, P. B., Lester, T. J., Casper, E. S., et al. (1987) Clinical pharmacology of recombinant human tumor necrosis factor in patients with advanced cancer. *J Clin Oncol* **5**(12), 1942–1951.
24. Jakubowski, A. A., Casper, E. S., Gabrilove, J. L., et al. (1989) Phase I trial of intramuscularly administered tumor necrosis factor in patients with advanced cancer. *J Clin Oncol* **7**(3), 298–303.
25. Gamm, H., Lindemann, A., Mertelsmann, R., and Herrmann, F. (1991) Phase I trial of recombinant human tumour necrosis factor alpha in patients with advanced malignancy. *Eur J Cancer* **27**(7), 856–863.
26. Creaven, P. J., Plager, J. E., Dupere, S., et al. (1987) Phase I Clinical Trial of recombinant human tumor necrosis factor. *Cancer Chemother Pharmacol* **20**(2), 137–144.
27. Taguchi, T. (1988) Phase I study of recombinant human tumor necrosis factor

28. Kemeny, N., Childs, B., Larchian, W., et al. (1990) A phase II trial of recombinant tumor necrosis factor in patients with advanced colorectal carcinoma. *Cancer* **66**(4), 659–663. (rHu-TNF:PT-050). *Cancer Detect Prev* **12**(1–6), 561–572.

29. Lenk, H., Tanneberger, S., Muller, U., et al. (1989) Phase II clinical trial of high-dose recombinant human tumor necrosis factor. *Cancer Chemother Pharmacol* **24**(6), 391–2.

30. Feldman, E. R., Creagan, E. T., Schaid, D. J., and Ahmann, D. L. (1992) Phase II trial of recombinant tumor necrosis factor in disseminated malignant melanoma. *Am J Clin Oncol* **15**(3), 256–259.

31. Budd, G. T., Green, S., Baker, L. H., et al. (1991) A southwest oncology group phase ii trial of recombinant tumor necrosis factor in metastatic breast cancer. *Cancer* **68**(8), 1694–5.

32. Haranaka, K., Satomi, N., and Sakurai, A. (1984) Antitumor activity of murine tumor necrosis factor (TNF) against transplanted murine tumors and heterotransplanted human tumors in nude mice. *Int J Cancer* **34**(2), 263–267.

33. Lienard, D., Ewalenko, P., Delmotte, J. J., et al. (1992) High-dose recombinant tumor necrosis factor alpha in combination with interferon gamma and melphalan in isolation perfusion of the limbs for melanoma and sarcoma. *J Clin Oncol* **10**(1), 52–60.

34. Fraker, D. L., Alexander, H. R., Andrich, M., and Rosenberg, S. A. (1996) Treatment of patients with melanoma of the extremity using hyperthermic isolated limb perfusion with melphalan, tumor necrosis factor, and interferon gamma: results of a tumor necrosis factor dose-escalation study. *J Clin Oncol* **14**(2), 479–489.

35. Dvorak, A. M., Kohn, S., Morgan, E. S., et al. (1996) The vesiculo-vacuolar organelle (VVO): a distinct endothelial cell structure that provides a transcellular pathway for macromolecular extravasation. *J Leukoc Biol* **59**(1), 100–115.

36. Feng, D., Nagy, J., Hipp, J., et al. (1996) Vesiculo-vacuolar organelles and the regulation of venule permeability to macromolecules by vascular permeability factor, histamine, and serotonin. *J Exp Med* **183**(5), 1981–1986.

37. Hashizume, H., Baluk, P., Morikawa, S., McLean, J. W., Thurston, G., Roberge, S., Jain, R. K., and McDonald, D. M. (2000) Openings between defective endothelial cells explain tumor vessel leakiness. *Am J Pathol* **156**(4), 1363–1380.

38. Jain, R. K. (2003) Molecular regulation of vessel maturation. *Nat Med* **9**(6), 685–693.

39. Folkman, J. (1971) Tumor angiogenesis: therapeutic implications. *New Engl J Med* **285**(21), 1182–1186.

40. Hermanson, G. T. (1996) Preparation of colloidal-gold labeled proteins. in *Bioconjugate Techniques.* Academic Press, Inc., San Diego, pp. 594–597.

41. Libutti, S. K., Paciotti, G. F., Myer, L., et al. Preliminary results of a phase I clinical trial of CYT-6091: A pegylated colloidal-gold TNF. J Clin Oncol, 2007 ASCO Annual Meeting Proceedings, Part I. Vol 25, No. 18S (June 20 Supplement), 3603.

Chapter 26

Liposomal Doxorubicin and *nab*-Paclitaxel: Nanoparticle Cancer Chemotherapy in Current Clinical Use

Alexander Gaitanis and Stephen Staal

Abstract

Liposomal doxorubicin and *nab*-paclitaxel are nanoparticle formulations of traditional cancer chemotherapy drugs which have ample clinical experience both pre- and post-nanoparticle modification. The alterations in pharmacokinetics, pharmacodynamics, efficacy, and toxicity compared with their parent compounds are instructive for future development of nanoparticle-based therapies. In this article we review the current status of these agents, emphasizing the alterations in clinical behavior resulting from the nanoparticle formulation of the parent compound.

Key words: Nanoparticle, chemotherapy, doxorubicin, paclitaxel.

1. Introduction

There are currently nanoparticle formulations of two widely used traditional cancer chemotherapy drugs available to medical oncologists. The experience of using these drugs, contrasted with their traditionally formulated precursors, provides insights into what may be expected as additional such agents are developed. Nanoparticle formulations can be expected to alter the following features of drug action and metabolism :(1) drug preparation and delivery, (2) pharmacokinetics blood and tissue levels over time, (3) pharmacodynamics – the mechanisms by which the drug interacts with the cancer cell to arrest its growth or kill it, (4) tissue distribution, which will affect both targeting of the cancer cells and side effects, and (5) toxicity, which classically has limited the dosing of cancer chemotherapy drugs. In this chapter we will contrast liposomal doxorubicin and *nab*-paclitaxel with their respective parent compounds, doxorubicin and paclitaxel.

2. Doxorubicin and Liposomal Doxorubicin

Doxorubicin (Adriamycin, Rubex) (DOX) (1) has been in clinical use since the 1970s. Originally isolated from a strain of *Streptomyces* along with other anthracyclines, it is one of the most widely active and effective anti-cancer agents. It binds to DNA and interacts with topoisomerases, the DNA-unwinding enzyme necessary for transcription and replication of the genetic material, to produce stabilized DNA strand breaks which trigger cell death. It is administered intravenously after aqueous reconstitution, typically by bolus injection. Side effects are hair loss, bone marrow suppression, nausea, and cardiac damage, which occur with increasing frequency above a cumulative dose of 550 mg/m^2. Heart damage (2) may result from oxidative stress, is usually irreversible, and was a significant cause of morbidity and mortality in the early drug trials (earning DOX the rueful sobriquets, "killer red" and the "red death"). The cumulative dose of DOX is limited to 400–550 mg/m^2 in an attempt to avoid this side effect.

Pegylated liposomal doxorubicin (PLD) (Doxil, Caelyx) is a nanoparticle formulation of doxorubicin (3). DOX is encapsulated in a polyethylene glycol-coated lipid membrane with a vesicle size of 80–90 nm and a drug concentration which can reach 15,000 molecules per vesicle. Pharmacokinetics is drastically altered with a circulation half-life of 2–3 days for PLD versus less than 5 min for DOX. Prolonged survival in the circulation gives it an opportunity to take advantage of the increased permeability of tumor blood vessels and accumulate in tumor tissues. This preferential accumulation in tumor versus surrounding normal tissues, which does not occur with DOX, has been documented in AIDS-related Kaposi's sarcoma (ARKS) (4) and breast cancer patients (5). It is thought that DOX is released locally via disruption of the liposome. Concentration of drug within the tumor can be up to six times greater with PLD than with DOX, likely accounting for the ability of PLD to kill DOX-resistant cells.

PLD has been approved for clinical use against ARKS. Clinical trials showed a superior outcome with PLD alone versus DOX at the same dose combined with two other chemotherapy agents. The highly vascular nature of ARKS, and the tendency of PLD to accumulate in the skin where ARKS arises, may account for the particular effectiveness of the drug against this tumor. PLD has also been approved for use as second-line therapy against ovarian cancer, where it was shown to be at least as effective as another standard agent topotecan, but less toxic. A phase III clinical trial involving over 500 metastatic breast cancer patients compared PLD to DOX at standard doses of 50 mg/m^2 every 4 weeks or

60 mg/m² every 3 weeks, respectively (6). The benefits were similar in the two arms but there were less long-term side effects with PLD. Further studies may give insight as to why breast cancer outcome is not improved despite the improved pharmacokinetic parameters associated with PLD.

The most striking clinical advantage of PLD is a reduction in toxicity. The primary dose-limiting side effects of PLD are mucositis and a painful reddening, swelling, and potentially desquamating skin condition – palmar plantar erythrodysesthesia (PPE). This is in marked contrast to DOX which is limited by bone marrow suppression and cumulative cardiac toxicity. PLD is also less likely to cause nausea and hair loss than does DOX, and the risk of significant cardiac toxicity is less. In the breast cancer study above, 10 PLD patients and 48 DOX patients experienced a decline of more than 20% in their cardiac function, as measured by the left ventricular ejection fraction. Ten of the DOX patients developed clinical symptoms of congestive heart failure versus none of the PLD patients. Although DOX doses are typically limited to 450–550 mg/m², PLD doses up to 1,500 mg/m² have been given to individual patients with little or no significant cardiac consequences. Low peak plasma levels of free drug and reduced cardiac muscle penetration due to the liposomal formulation best explain the reduced cardiac risk with PLD.

A recent expert panel has recommended that the dose intensity of PLD should not exceed 10 mg/m² weekly to limit the risk of PPE (7). This recommendation had already entered clinical practice based on the clinical judgment of treating physicians. Given the ability of PLD to concentrate at tumor sites, it seems likely that a similar efficacy with reduced toxicity may be achieved with a lowering of the dose, but this has not been formally tested. The usual approach to dosing cytotoxic chemotherapy is to recommend the maximum tolerated dose. With the potential for improved targeting of the tumor tissue with nanoparticle formulations, along with the concept of a "threshold" dose and little additional benefit to increased dosing beyond this, nanoparticle formulations of traditional chemotherapy drugs may find their best benefit from an improved benefit/toxicity ratio. This benefit will be discovered only by careful testing of efficacy rather than the traditional paradigm of toxicity as the end point of dosing studies, i.e., application of the maximally tolerated dose.

3. Paclitaxel and nab-Paclitaxel

Like DOX, paclitaxel (PXL) is one of the most broadly effective chemotherapy agents. PXL was extracted in the 1960s from the bark of the Pacific yew tree, *Taxus brevifolia,* a product of a combined NCI–USDA effort to discover natural products useful against cancer (8, 9). It inhibits cell growth by interacting with and stabilizing microtubules which are necessary for successful cell division. Due to its poor aqueous solubility, it was necessary to prepare the drug in cremophor, a polyethoxylated derivative of castor oil (c-PXL) (10). The concentration of this vehicle necessary to solubilize PXL for clinical use is the highest of any marketed drug and requires the use of specialized tubing and in-line filters. Cremophor is toxic and was responsible for an early suspension of trials due to an infusion-related anaphylactic death. Prolonged infusions and pre-medication made delivery of PXL feasible and its efficacy manifest, although the risks of infusion persisted albeit to a lesser extent. It was approved for the treatment of refractory ovarian cancer in 1992 followed by approvals in breast and lung cancer and ARKS treatments. Interestingly, there is some data to support cremophor acting to reverse drug resistance to paclitaxel in those cancer cells that have developed the multi-drug-resistant phenotype (11). In initial evaluation of vehicles, polyethylene glycol 400, which would have been preferred from a pharmaceutical point of view, was less efficacious than the cremophor formulation. Inadvertently, the prolonged infusion required because of the cremophor may also have aided acceptance of the drug. PXL is toxic only during certain phases of the cell cycle and longer infusions allow more cells to enter the susceptible phase of the cell cycle (12).

Albumin-bound *nab*-paclitaxel (n-PXL)(Abraxane) is a polymeric nanoparticle developed as a superior drug delivery vehicle compared to cremophor-formulated PXL (13). It was first approved by the FDA in 2005 for the treatment of previously treated metastatic breast cancer. It is prepared by high-pressure homogenization of PXL in the presence of human serum albumin at a concentration of 3–4%, resulting in a nanoparticle colloidal suspension (14). The resultant nanoparticles have a mean particle diameter of 130–150 nm and are readily soluble, avoiding the need for premedication, specialized tubing, or prolonged infusions necessary for c-PXL.

The pharmacokinetics of c-PXL and n-PXL has been directly compared (15, 16). C-PXL displays non-linear pharmacokinetics due to interference with clearance and tissue distribution by the cremophor formulation. Clearance and volume of distribution were about 50% greater for n-PXL than c-PXL. The maximum tolerated dose for n-PXL was likewise increased by 50% compared to c-PXL. In the most recent study involving a crossover design where the same patient received c-PXL and n-PXL successively or vice versa, the peak plasma concentrations of PXL was 3.8-fold higher with n-PXL, but due to more rapid clearance, total drug exposure between the two agents was similar (17).

Studies in mice with equivalent doses of PXL and n-PXL demonstrated a more rapid and higher concentration of paclitaxel in the tumor with n-PXL, resulting in a 33% higher cumulative intratumor accumulation of the drug compared to PXL (15). The albumin-based formulation of n-PXL potentially exploits a mechanism favoring uptake of this drug. Albumin can carry hydrophobic substances and is well known to serve as a carrier for many molecules which can be non-covalently bound and transported to cells where they are released as effectors. The intra- and transcellular transport of albumin-bound drugs can be facilitated by binding to a cell-surface glycoprotein, gp60, and invagination and transport via intracellular vesicles called caveolae. Comparison of c-PXL and n-PXL showed that the latter was more effectively transported across an endothelial membrane, providing a mechanistic explanation for the more rapid and complete accumulation of n-PXL in tumor tissues. PXL is eventually released from cremophor and binds to albumin in vivo; the level of tumor tissue penetration is significantly higher than would be predicted from the demonstrated transport across normal endothelium, suggesting that other mechanisms for entry of drug into tumor cells, such as passive diffusion, are also operative.

The recommended dose of n-PXL is 260 mg/m^2, whereas the usual dose of c-PXL is 175 mg/m^2. Although it could be argued that treatment outcome was affected by this dose difference, when c-PXL dose was escalated in an earlier study, there was no improvement in response rate or overall survival but toxicity increased markedly (18). In the study leading to the FDA approval of n-PXL, previously treated patients with metastatic breast cancer were randomly assigned to an every 3-week IV infusion of n-PXL or c-PXL. The outcome was significantly improved with n-PXL. Response rates went from 19% with c-PXL to 33% with n-PXL, and there was also a longer time to tumor progression, 23 weeks with n-PXL and 16.9 weeks with c-PXL (19).

The major side effects of PXL are bone marrow suppression, hair loss, a transient generalized arthritic syndrome, and nerve damage. The nerve damage is often the most significant clinical problem since it is dose related and cumulative, and can be long lasting or permanent. In the comparison trial in breast cancer above, n-PXL was more neurotoxic than c-PXL, with a 10% incidence of Grade III neurotoxicity (which interfere with the activities of daily living) versus 2% with PXL. This toxicity reversed to a manageable grade in most of the n-PXL patients such that by 28 days after its first occurrence, there were equivalent numbers with Grade III neuropathy in both arms. There was also a significant increase in the incidence of nausea and diarrhea with n-PXL, but less bone marrow suppression. There is data demonstrating neurotoxicity associated with cremophor alone, so c-PXL initiated neurotoxicity is likely triggered both by the chemotherapy drug and the solubilizing vehicle. It is possible that the damage by n-PXL is different in nature and possibly more transient than that associated with c-PXL. The increased marrow suppression associated with c-PXL may also reflect the cremophor-influenced pharmacokinetics of the drug. Cremophor distribution is limited to the circulation where it forms micelles in vivo. This likely ends up delivering more drug to the bone marrow, which is part of the circulatory system.

4. Lesson Learned from Nanoparticle Formulation of Traditional Chemotherapy Drugs

The development of PLD and n-PXL, nanoparticle formulations of traditional chemotherapy drugs, demonstrates the potential of nanoparticles to improve cancer therapies. In the case of PLD, the altered pharmacokinetics resulting from the liposomal formulation dramatically affected the toxicity profile and the efficacy of the parent drug, although the improvement in efficacy was demonstrated only in the case of ARKS. Cancer cell killing is a complex phenomenon involving many factors including threshold concentration effects, growth rates, drug resistance mechanisms, features of the tumor microenvironment, the host immune response, and doubtless many other factors not understood at present. Thus it is not surprising that PLD did not show a significant increase in efficacy against most of the tumors tested, but its improved toxicity profile, particularly its reduced risk of cardiotoxicity, has earned it a well-established position amongst cancer chemotherapy drugs. N-PXL accomplished the desired design objective – the elimination of the problematic formulation of PXL with cremophor, a toxic and cumbersome vehicle for delivery of hydrophobic cancer drugs. The metastatic breast cancer trial leading to the drug's approval demonstrated a statistically significant improvement in response rate with n-PXL, suggesting that trapping of drug in the circulation by cremophor micelles and lower tumor tissue levels with c-PXL interfered with the killing effect of the parent drug. There was no significant improvement in overall survival, however, and with n-PXL costing 25 times more than c-PXL, it has enjoyed rising sales but has not been adopted as a standard replacement for c-PXL (20).

PLD and n-PXL are the first generation of nanoparticle-formulated cancer chemotherapy drugs. They do not exploit all the potential of nanoparticles to control the pharmacokinetics and pharmacodynamics, selectivity, and avoidance of drug resistance inherent in this technology (21–23). PLD relies on the enhanced permeability characteristic of the vasculature of many tumors to passively concentrate the drug (24). N-PXL provides more classical pharmacokinetics by avoiding the complications of the cremophor formulation currently in general use; although formulation with albumin may offer some degree of tumor selectivity, this has not been proven. Many potentially more targeted and selectively toxic nanoparticle formulations are undergoing development or preliminary testing in hopes that the full promise of this technology for cancer therapy will be realized.

References

1. Arcamone, F. (1981) *Doxorubicin: Anticancer Antibiotics*. Academic Press, New York.
2. Singal, P. K. and Iliskovic, N. (1998) Doxorubicin-induced cardiomyopathy. *N Engl J Med* **339**, 900–905.
3. Gabizon, A. A. (2001) Pegylated liposomal doxorubicin: metamorphosis of an old drug into a new form of chemotherapy. *Cancer Invest* **19**, 424–436.
4. Northfelt, D. W., Martin, F. J., Working, P., et al. (1996) Doxorubicin encapsulated in liposomes containing surface-bound polyethylene glycol: pharmacokinetics, tumor localization, and safety in patients with AIDS-related Kaposi's sarcoma. *J Clin Pharmacol* **36**, 55–63.
5. Symon, Z., Peyser, A., Tzemach, D., et al. (1999) Selective delivery of doxorubicin to patients with breast carcinoma metastases by stealth liposomes. *Cancer* **86**, 72–78.
6. O'Brien, M. E., Wigler, N., Inbar, M., et al. (2004) Reduced cardiotoxicity and comparable efficacy in a phase III trial of pegylated liposomal doxorubicin HCl (CAELYX/Doxil) versus conventional doxorubicin for first-line treatment of metastatic breast cancer. *Ann Oncol* **15**, 440–449.
7. von Moos, R., Thuerlimann, B. J., Aapro, M., et al. (2008) Pegylated liposomal doxorubicin-associated hand-foot syndrome: recommendations of an international panel of experts. *Eur J Cancer* **44**, 781–790.
8. Suffness, M. (1995) *Taxol: Science and Applications*. CRC Press, Boca Raton.
9. Rowinsky, E. K. and Donehower, R. C. (1995) Paclitaxel (taxol). *N Engl J Med* **332**, 1004–1014.
10. ten Tije, A. J., Verweij, J., Loos, W. J., and Sparreboom, A. (2003) Pharmacological effects of formulation vehicles: implications for cancer chemotherapy. *Clin Pharmacokinet* **42**, 665–685.
11. Webster, L., Linsenmeyer, M., Millward, M., Morton, C., Bishop, J., and Woodcock, D. (1993) Measurement of cremophor EL following taxol: plasma levels sufficient to reverse drug exclusion mediated by the multidrug-resistant phenotype. *J Natl Cancer Inst* **85**, 1685–1690.
12. Straubinger, R. M. (1995) Biopharmaceutics of paclitaxel (taxol): formulation, activity and pharmacokinetics. In Suffness M., eds. Taxol: science and applications. CRC Press, Boca Raton.
13. Hawkins, M. J., Soon-Shiong, P., and Desai, N. (2008) Protein nanoparticles as drug carriers in clinical medicine. *Adv Drug Deliv Rev* **60**, 876–885.
14. Ibrahim, N. K., Desai, N., Legha, S., et al. (2002) Phase I and pharmacokinetic study of ABI-007, a Cremophor-free, protein-stabilized, nanoparticle formulation of paclitaxel. *Clin Cancer Res* **8**, 1038–1044.
15. Sparreboom, A., Scripture, C. D., Trieu, V., et al. (2005) Comparative preclinical and clinical pharmacokinetics of a cremophor-free, nanoparticle albumin-bound paclitaxel (ABI-007) and paclitaxel formulated in Cremophor (Taxol). *Clin Cancer Res* **11**, 4136–4143.
16. Desai, N., Trieu, V., Yao, Z., et al. (2006) Increased antitumor activity, intratumor paclitaxel concentrations, and endothelial cell transport of cremophor-free, albumin-bound paclitaxel, ABI-007, compared with cremophor-based paclitaxel. *Clin Cancer Res* **12**, 1317–1324.
17. Gardner, E. R., Dahut, W. L., Scripture, C. D., et al. (2008) Randomized crossover pharmacokinetic study of solvent-based paclitaxel and nab-paclitaxel. *Clin Cancer Res* **14**, 4200–4205.
18. Winer, E. P., Berry, D. A., Woolf, S., et al. (2004) Failure of higher-dose paclitaxel to improve outcome in patients with metastatic breast cancer: cancer and leukemia group B trial 9342. *J Clin Oncol* **22**, 2061–2068.
19. Gradishar, W. J., Tjulandin, S., Davidson, N., et al. (2005) Phase III trial of nanoparticle albumin-bound paclitaxel compared with polyethylated castor oil-based paclitaxel in women with breast cancer. *J Clin Oncol* **23**, 7794–7803.

20. Hope, at $4,200 a Dose – New York Times. 2008. http://www.nytimes.com/2006/10/01/business/yourmoney/01drug.html?pagewanted=1
21. Heath, J. R. and Davis, M. E. (2008) Nanotechnology and cancer. *Annu Rev Med* **59**, 251–265.
22. Peer, D., Karp, J. M., Hong, S., Farokhzad, O. C., Margalit, R., and Langer, R. (2007) Nanocarriers as an emerging platform for cancer therapy. *Nat Nanotechnol* **2**, 751–760.
23. Lammers, T., Hennink, W. E., and Storm, G. (2008) Tumour-targeted nanomedicines: principles and practice. *Br J Cancer* **99**, 392–397.
24. Maeda, H., Wu, J., Sawa, T., Matsumura, Y., and Hori, K. (2000) Tumor vascular permeability and the EPR effect in macromolecular therapeutics: a review. *J Control Release* **65**, 271–284.

SUBJECT INDEX

A

Active targeting 3, 14, 76–77, 132, 376, 379
Adsorbed species 2, 55, 58
Aerosol 49, 69, 153, 267–279
Agglomeration 2, 44, 49–50, 55, 184, 191
Albumin-bound paclitaxel 388
Angiotensin II 26–28
Annexin-A5 .... 331, 334
Antibody/Antibodies 3, 14–18, 70, 72, 77, 84, 92–93, 108, 113, 115–116, 136–140, 156–158, 160, 166, 171, 182, 184–191, 196, 198–200, 202–207, 236, 282, 295–307, 311, 319–320, 349–352, 354, 362, 365–366, 368, 370
Antibody conjugation...113, 115–116, 182, 186–189, 199, 205, 349
Apoptosis 13, 16, 19–20, 325–338, 360, 363, 366, 370, 378
Atomic arrangement 52–54
Atomic composition 57

B

Bevacizumab 17–18
Bioconjugation 70, 72, 93, 122, 152, 156–158, 236, 311
Biodistribution 2, 4, 14, 21, 26, 35, 128, 132, 172–173, 261
Bradykinin 26–29
Bulk properties 57–62

C

CA19-9 362
Cancer
   characterization 39–62
   description 1–34
   imaging/therapy
      fluorescent silica nanoparticles for 151–160
      gold nanocages for 83–98
      gold nanoparticles for 177–191
      gold nanorods for..... 119–128, 343–356, 375–382
      LHRH-targeted nanoparticles for 281–293
      nanoparticle formulations................. 385–391
      nanoshells for photothermal therapy 101–117
      targeting and detection 235–247
Carbon nanotubes 5–6, 40, 320, 322, 363, 370
Cardiovascular disease 136, 327, 330, 334–336, 338, 386–387
Catalysis 83, 155, 178
Cell surface antigen 14
Cell surface receptors 3, 18–19, 21, 378

Cetuximab 16, 368, 370
Chemical properties............................57–62
Chemotherapy 5, 11–12, 16, 18, 25, 250, 268, 281, 360, 363, 385–391
Chitosan 133–134, 224, 230–231
Chlorotoxin .... , 370
c-Kit .... , 17
Colloidal gold 119, 182, 363, 375–382
Confocal microscopy 244–245, 260, 282, 291
Contrast agent 4–5, 67–79, 84, 96, 113, 119–120, 136, 142, 311, 317–320, 322, 328–330, 332–338, 350
Copolymers 27, 132–134, 163–164, 167, 169, 223, 231, 250
Critical micelle concentration 132, 135, 137, 139–142
Crystallinity................................... 57, 61
c-Src 20
CYT-6091 379–382
Cytotoxicity assay 144–145, 172

D

Darkfield microscopy 178, 181, 190
Delay-and-sum beam forming algorithm 312
Dendrimer 2, 5, 51, 56, 134, 163, 223–230, 232, 250, 263, 282–289, 291–293, 329
Dimerization 14–15, 17, 206
Dispersion 2, 43, 49–50, 70, 72, 76, 78, 91, 122–123, 125–126, 128, 144, 182, 186–187, 273–274
DNA 12–13, 84, 93, 113, 134, 158, 160, 165, 171, 197–198, 200–201, 204, 206, 238–240, 246, 270–271, 273–274, 278, 285, 326, 361, 370, 386
DNA microarray......... 13, 197–198, 200–201, 206–208
Doxorubicin 16, 31, 32–34, 134, 165, 168, 170, 211–218, 296, 385–391
Drug delivery 4–5, 14, 83, 163–174, 223, 251, 281, 320, 375–377, 388
Dynamic light scattering 42, 45–46, 140, 169, 181–182, 186, 189, 217, 305

E

Electromagnet 102, 268–269, 271–273, 278, 319, 328, 343, 365, 367–368
Encapsulation............... 168, 211, 213–214, 216–218
Endosomal 171, 251
Endothelium 3, 389
Enhanced permeability and retention (EPR)....14, 25–36, 76, 84, 132, 136, 250, 318, 354
Epidermal growth factor (EGF) 14
Epidermal growth factor receptor (EGFR) 15–17, 350, 368–369

S.R. Grobmyer, B.M. Moudgil (eds.), *Cancer Nanotechnology*, Methods in Molecular Biology 624,
DOI 10.1007/978-1-60761-609-2, © Springer Science+Business Media, LLC 2010

F

F-19 .... 187–188, 190
Fibroblast activation protein (FAP) 187, 301
Fibroblast growth factor (FGF) 14
Fibronectin 57
Finite-element based algorithm 312–315
Flavopiridol 16
Flow cytometry 84, 95, 160, 236, 240, 260, 301,
   305–306, 331–332, 334, 366
Fluorescent/Fluorescence 5, 35, 59–60, 68, 70–72,
   74–75, 77, 84, 87, 93–95, 121, 141–142,
   151–160, 171, 173–174, 178–179, 198–199,
   200, 204–205, 216–217, 236, 238–239, 244,
   246–247, 260, 282, 284, 292, 300–301,
   303–304, 306–307, 329–330, 332–335, 337,
   352, 362, 365–366
Fluorescent silica nanoparticles 151–160, 236
Focal adhesion kinase (FAK) 19–20
Focal adhesion kinase inhibitor 20
Folate receptor 3, 160, 249–263

G

Gelatin 224, 231–232
Gemcitacine 363
Gene expression profiling 197, 200–201
Gold
   nanoparticle 6, 124, 177–191, 311, 317–318, 320,
      343–345, 347, 351, 362–370, 376–377,
      379–382
   speckled silica nanoparticles 69–70, 75

H

Heat shock proteins (HSPs) 360
HER2 .... 15–16, 85, 92, 108–110, 113
High pressure extrusion method 217
Hypertension 26–27, 35

I

Immunocytochemistry 198–200, 204–206
Immunoliposomes 218, 295–307
Immunomicelles 136–140, 144–145
Insulin like growth factor (IGF) 14, 18–20
Insulin like growth factor receptor (IGFR) 20
Iron oxide 241, 268, 270–271, 318, 322,
   329–332, 338, 362–363
Isoelectric point 55–56

L

Laser 4, 44–46, 57, 60, 87, 90, 92, 94–95,
   106–110, 112–113, 120–121, 159, 165,
   181–182, 244, 309–310, 316, 347, 352–354,
   360, 363
Lipid 2, 18, 135–140, 212, 214–215, 218, 223,
   232, 257, 262–263, 295–296, 300–301,
   303–307, 327–328, 333–334, 336, 361,
   367, 386
Liposomes 5, 136, 211–218, 223–224, 232, 250,
   257, 260, 263, 295–296, 301, 303–307,
   329–330, 333–334, 336, 376, 386
Luciferasae 271, 276–277, 279

Lung cancer 160, 267–268, 292, 388
Luteinizing hormone-releasing hormone
   (LHRH) 281–293

M

Magnetic aerosol targeting 267–279
Magnetic nanoparticle (MNP) ... 236, 238–239, 241–245,
   337–338
Magnetic resonance imaging (MRI) 4–5, 58, 68,
   70–73, 136, 142–143, 165, 169, 323, 325–338,
   362
Magnetic resonance thermal imaging (MRTI) 107
Matrix metalloproteinases 26, 28
Micelles 31–35, 68, 70, 72, 75, 131–146, 226, 250,
   256, 263, 296, 301, 304–305, 329–330, 334,
   349, 390
Microfluidics 165, 168–169
Mie theory 102, 343
Molecular targeted therapy 11–21
Monoclonal 15–18, 113, 136, 158, 166, 171,
   186–187, 190, 196, 202, 299, 352, 370
Mouse 5–6, 16, 20, 27, 30–32, 72–73, 85,
   106–107, 110, 113, 120, 136–138, 144, 164,
   166, 171–174, 190, 199, 252, 261–263, 271,
   273–277, 292, 320, 335–338, 354, 380, 389

N

Nanocages 5, 83–98
Nanomagnetosols 267–279
Nanoparticles 2–6, 14, 20–21, 39–62, 69–72, 75–76,
   101–102, 114–115, 119, 121, 124–125, 127,
   136, 151–160, 163–174, 177–191, 209,
   223–224, 230–231, 235–247, 249–263,
   267–279, 281–293, 295–307, 309–323,
   328–332, 334–338, 343–350, 359–371,
   375–382, 385–391
Nanorod 6, 119–129, 311, 318, 320, 343–356
Nanoshells 6, 101–117, 311, 318–320, 355, 363–364
Nanotechnology 1–3, 5–7, 11–21, 39–63, 67,
   325–338, 362, 375
Nanotoxicology 2–3, 41
National Institute of Standards and Technology
   (NIST) 42–43
Near infrared (NIR) 6, 68, 75, 84, 87, 105–108,
   110, 112, 119–121, 127–128, 179, 282,
   310–311, 319–320, 335, 345, 347, 352,
   354–355, 363
Nerve growth factor (NGF) 14
Nitric oxide 26, 28

O

Oncogenes 12, 14, 17
Opsonization 51–52, 57
Optical coherence tomography (OCT) 109–111,
   119–120
Optical imaging (OI) 68, 102, 109, 120, 182, 190–191,
   310–311

P

p53 .... 13, 19
Paclitaxel 133–134, 136–137, 139–142, 144, 164,
   167, 172, 283, 286, 289–291, 385–391

PAMAM dendrimers 226–227, 232, 285–289
Pancreatic cancer 19, 187, 190, 195–209
Particle size distribution................41, 43–45, 50, 70
Passive targeting 3, 14, 132, 376
PEGylation 185–186, 221–223, 226–228, 230
Peptide ligands...............................196, 209
Peptides 3, 17, 70, 72, 77, 84, 137, 156–157, 160, 196–197, 202, 209, 224, 236, 254–255, 282–283, 286–287, 292, 322, 331, 362, 368, 370
Pharmacodynamics 385, 390
Phase I clinical trial............................381–382
Phospholipid phosphatidylserine 326–327
Photoacoustic tomography (PAT) 4–5, 68–70, 75–77, 119–121, 309–323
Photodynamic therapy (PDT) 28–30, 35
Photothermal therapy 6, 77, 83–84, 92–95, 105–113, 343–356
Plasmon resonance 7, 84, 104–105, 119–120, 127–128, 180–181, 311, 334, 343–345, 352, 363, 365, 368
Platelet derived growth factor 14, 17
PLGA.....................163–165, 167–171, 173, 224, 231, 233
Polyethylene glycol (PEG) 3, 50, 76, 84, 92, 110, 115–116, 128, 131–146, 164–165, 167–171, 182, 184–186, 212, 221–223, 227–232, 250, 256, 295–296, 298–299, 301, 303–304, 332, 334, 376, 380, 386, 388
Polymer...............3, 35, 132–135, 141, 155, 164–165, 167–169, 173, 184, 221, 223, 230–231, 279, 345, 349, 380
Polymeric micelles........................131–146, 163, 250, 263
Polymeric nanoparticles...........51, 163–174, 223–224, 362, 388
Porosity 51
Positron emission tomography (PET) 196, 362
PPI dendrimer 227–230
Prodrugs 281
Prostaglandins 26
Prostate specific membrane antigen.............164–165
Pteroic acid synthesis 251–252

Q

Qdots.....................................70, 72–74, 77
qRT-PCR................................198, 200, 204
Quantum dots 70, 72–73, 75, 79, 178, 184, 263, 330, 334, 338, 362
Quaternization 285

R

Radiofrequency
 ablation 4, 6, 361
 field 6, 365
Radiotherapy..................................6, 327
Raman spectroscopy.................................58
Reticuloendothelial system 14, 250, 356, 376
RuBpy 69, 71–73, 152, 155–158, 237, 242–243, 247

S

Seed growth 115
SELEX......................................236–239
Sentinel nodes 84
Shape 2–3, 41, 43–46, 48–49, 69, 97, 122, 127, 135, 181, 183, 186, 236, 239, 291, 311–312, 343–344, 368
Shell formation 115
Silica 5, 61, 69–76, 78, 85, 105, 113–115, 151–160, 236–237, 241–242, 246–247, 262, 269, 276, 319, 363
 nanoparticle 69–71, 75–76, 114, 151–160, 236
Single-chain Fv fragments.....................296, 300
Size............2–3, 14, 26–27, 31, 35, 40–50, 56–57, 61, 69–71, 76, 102, 105–106, 108, 110, 112, 114, 116, 122, 127, 131–132, 135–137, 139–142, 152–159, 165, 167, 169, 178–179, 181–184, 186, 188–189, 209, 211, 213–217, 236, 247, 257, 269–270, 291–292, 305, 318–319, 329, 331–332, 334, 336–337, 343, 347–348, 376, 379, 386
 distribution analysis 140, 215
Size exclusion chromatography (SEC) .. 47, 182, 184, 186, 188–189, 291
STI571 17
Stober method...........................105, 114, 157
Structure....................2, 41, 52–54, 58–59, 61–62, 132, 135, 164, 190, 196, 200, 202, 226, 285, 320, 329
Superparamagnetic iron oxide nanoparticles 136, 268, 270, 271, 322
Surface
 area...................40, 44–45, 48–49, 51, 56, 181, 236, 375
 charge 2, 55, 56, 155, 184
 composition 51–54, 58
 energy 45, 52, 55
 modification 70, 72, 76–77, 85, 92, 156, 158, 182, 184, 222, 362
 plasmon resonance 7, 84, 119, 334, 343–345, 352, 368
 properties 21, 40–41, 49, 51–52, 55, 155, 183
 reactivity 41, 56
Surfactant..........43, 69, 71–72, 78–79, 122–123, 132, 136, 139, 153, 156–157, 160, 183–184, 224

T

Taxane 16
Theranostics...6
Thermal tumor ablation 360
Tissue microarray.............................198, 200
Total extinction coefficient...........................179
Toxicity 2, 4–6, 17, 26, 35, 40–41, 43, 48, 61, 74, 132, 200, 207, 222, 261–262, 338, 363, 375, 377–382, 387, 389–390
Transferrin receptors..................................3
Transforming growth factor alpha (TGF-alpha) 16
Transforming growth factor β (TGFβ).............18–19
Transmembrane pH gradient...............211, 217–218
Transmission electron microscopy.........47, 54, 61, 177, 181, 189, 213–215, 217, 365–366
Trastuzumab.......................................16
Tumor necrosis factor (TNF) 326, 363, 377–382

Tumor stroma 187, 191
Tyrosine kinase inhibitor 15–16, 18

U

Ultrasound 4, 120, 195, 309–310, 316, 320, 322, 361

V

Vascular endothelial growth factor 16–17, 26, 376
Vasculature 3, 26, 34–35, 76, 106–107, 132, 136, 196, 320, 336, 368, 370, 376, 378–379, 381, 390

W

Water-in-oil microemulsions 68, 69
Wettability 52, 55

X

Xenograft 20, 164, 262, 282, 292, 354, 355, 380

Z

Zeta potential 46, 55–56, 72, 155, 169, 380